The Physician as a Rebellious Intellectual

Beihefte zur

MEDIAEVISTIK

Monographien, Editonen, Sammelbände

Herausgegeben von Peter Dinzelbacher

Band 18

PETER LANG
EDITION

N. Peter Joosse

The Physician as a Rebellious Intellectual

The Book of the Two Pieces of Advice or *Kitāb al-Naṣīḥatayn* by ᶜAbd al-Laṭīf ibn Yūsuf al-Baghdādī (1162–1231)

Introduction, Edition and Translation of the Medical Section

PETER LANG
EDITION

Bibliographic Information published by the Deutsche Nationalbibliothek
The Deutsche Nationalbibliothek lists this publication in the Deutsche Nationalbibliografie; detailed bibliographic data is available in the internet at http://dnb.d-nb.de.

Library of Congress Cataloging-in-Publication Data

Joosse, N. Peter, author, translator.
The physician as a rebellious intellectual : The book of the two pieces of advice, or, Kitab al-Nasihatayn by 'Abd al-Latif ibn Yusuf al-Baghdadi (1162-1231) : introduction, edition, and translation of the medical section / N. Peter Joosse.
pages cm. -- (Beihefte zur Mediaevistik ; Band 18)
Includes bibliographical references and index.
ISBN 978-3-631-64285-6
1. 'Abd al-Latif al-Baghdadi, Muwaffaq al-Din, 1162-1231. Kitab al Nasihatayn. 2. Medicine, Arab--Philosophy. 3. Physicians' writings, Arabic--Criticism and interpretation. I. 'Abd al-Latif al-Baghdadi, Muwaffaq al-Din, 1162-1231, author. II. 'Abd al-Latif al-Baghdadi, Muwaffaq al-Din, 1162-1231. Kitab al Nasihatayn. Selections. III. 'Abd al-Latif al-Baghdadi, Muwaffaq al-Din, 1162-1231. Kitab al Nasihatayn. Selections. English. IV. Title. V. Series: Beihefte zur Mediaevistik ; Bd. 18.
R128.3.J66 2013
610.1--dc23

2013039166

Cover image:
A portrait of ᶜAbd al-Laṭīf al-Baghdādī lecturing on medicinal plants to a group of students seated in a so-called Study Circle at the Umayyad Mosque of Damascus, Syria. The original of this drawing is found in The Museum of Arab Medicine and Sciences, Damascus, Syria (date of production and artist: unknown)

ISSN 1617-657X
ISBN 978-3-631-64285-6 (Print)
E-ISBN 978-3-653-03127-0 (E-Book)
DOI 10.3726/978-3-653-03127-0

Peter Lang Edition is an Imprint of Peter Lang GmbH.

Peter Lang – Frankfurt am Main · Bern · Bruxelles · New York · Oxford · Warszawa · Wien

www.peterlang.com

Table of Contents

The Physician as a Rebellious Intellectual: The *Book of the Two Pieces of Advice* or *Kitāb al-Naṣīḥatayn* by ʻAbd al-Laṭīf ibn Yūsuf al-Baghdādī (1162-1231): Introduction, Edition & Translation of the Medical Section 7

History of Research 7

Dating the Manuscript & Principle of Edition 9

Brief Survey of the Contents 10

ʻAbd al-Laṭīf's Life and Medical Work 11

The *Kitāb al-Naṣīḥatayn*: Topoi as Sources? 12

The Physician and the Ruler 17

ʻAbd al-Laṭīf al-Baghdādī and his Relation to Alchemy 29

The *Book of the Two Pieces of Advice* or *Kitāb al-Naṣīḥatayn* by ʻAbd al-Laṭīf ibnYūsuf al-Baghdādī (1162-1231): Annotated Translation of the Medical Section - Ms. Bursa (Turkey): Hüseyin Çelebi 823 (fol. 62r-78r)......................... 63

The *Book of the Two Pieces of Advice* or *Kitāb al-Naṣīḥatayn* by ʻAbd al-Laṭīf ibn Yūsuf al-Baghdādī (1162-1231): Arabic Edition of the Medical Section on the basis of the unique Ms. Bursa (Turkey): Hüseyin Çelebi 823 (fol. 62r-78r) 95

Bibliography 113

1. ʻAbd al-Laṭīf al-Baghdādī: manuscripts consulted 113
2. ʻAbd al-Laṭīf al-Baghdādī: autobiographical and biographical information 114
3. ʻAbd al-Laṭīf al-Baghdādī and his milieu: editions, studies & translations 117
4. Primary sources 126
5. Secondary sources 131

Index of Terms Relating to the English Translation of the Medical Section of the *Kitāb al-Naṣīḥatayn* 163

Index of Authors and Works Cited in the Medical Section of the *Kitāb al-Naṣīḥatayn* 167

Appendix: The Arabic Originals of the Medical Section of the *Kitāb al-Naṣīḥatayn* - Ms. Bursa (Turkey): Hüseyin Çelebi 823 (fol. 62r-78r) 169

The Physician as a Rebellious Intellectual: The *Book of the Two Pieces of Advice* or *Kitāb al-Naṣīḥatayn* by ʻAbd al-Laṭīf ibn Yūsuf al-Baghdādī (1162-1231)[1] : Introduction, Edition & Translation of the Medical Section

History of Research

In 1962 Samuel Miklos Stern presented the scholarly community with the first ever description of the *Book of the Two Pieces of Advice* or *Kitāb al-Naṣīḥatayn* by the well-known grammarian, lexicographer, philosopher, and physician ʻAbd al-Laṭīf ibn Yūsuf al-Baghdādī.[2] A couple of years later, the German scholar Albert Dietrich gave a very short description of the *Kitāb al-Naṣīḥatayn* without referring thereby to Stern's prior publication.[3] Eight years later, in the year 1972, the physicians and medical historians Paul Ghalioungui and Said Abdou presented us with a brief

---

1 This monograph, including the edition and translation, was made possible by the Vereniging Nederlands Tijdschrift voor Geneeskunde (NTvG), the leading Dutch medical journal: it provided the financial support for the research project "The physician as a rebellious intellectual: ʻAbd al-Laṭīf al-Baghdādī (1162-1231) and the Arabic medicine of his time", which the present author carried out as a SRF at the Faculty of Arts of Leiden University, The Netherlands. The author wishes to express his gratitude to the above institutions for their kind assistance. Thanks also goes out to emeritus Prof. dr. Remke Kruk for initiating and realizing the aforementioned project. The author would also like to thank the following persons for their contributions to the translation of the medical section of the *Kitāb al-Naṣīḥatayn*: Hans Daiber (Düsseldorf); Rob Hilders (Schellinkhout); Remke Kruk (Leiden); Peter E. Pormann (Manchester); and Wim Raven (Marburg). Thanks are also due to my wife Farida Bhayat (Amsterdam) for preparing the CRC of this manuscript. The monograph is dedicated to my grandfather, Nanne Pieter Joosse (1888-1980), who was never given a proper chance to learn, but would have made a terrific learner.

2 Samuel Miklos Stern, 'A Collection of Treatises by ʻAbd al-Laṭīf al-Baghdādī', in: *Islamic Studies*, (Karachi), vol. 1 (1962), 53-70, at 59-66 [Reprint in: Samuel Miklos Stern, *Medieval Arabic and Hebrew Thought* (London 1983): Variorum Reprints CS 183 under No. XVIII].

3 Albert Dietrich, *Die arabische Version einer unbekannten Schrift des Alexander von Aphrodisias über die Differentia specifica* (Nachrichten der Akademie der Wissenschaften in Göttingen: I. Philologisch-historische Klasse, Jahrgang 1964; Nr. 2, Göttingen) (Göttingen 1964), 88-148, at 105.

description of the *Kitāb al-Naṣīḥatayn* in the Arabic language.[4] Although the initial section of the book must be regarded as one of the forgotten masterpieces of Arabic-Islamic medicine, it took 35 years, until 2007, before the next publication on the subject announced itself in the form of the present author's English translation of a lengthy passage dealing with the untimely death of the prince al-Malik al-Ẓāhir Ghāzī ibn Yūsuf of Aleppo,[5] which in the same year was followed by his elaborate description of the *Kitāb al-Naṣīḥatayn* in the Dutch language.[6] In the year 2008, the present author and Peter E. Pormann co-authored a brief article on the so-called "mathematical fragment".[7] This publication was soon followed by another article, likewise co-authored by Joosse and Pormann, which challenges the idea that Islamic medicine declined after the twelfth century A.D. Moreover, the article also sheds important new light on questions regarding the social history of medicine, and discusses a number of quotations from the *Book of the Two Pieces of Advice*.[8] Dimitri Gutas recently has published a study on the philosophical contents of the treatise,[9] and is in the course of preparing an edition and translation of the autobiography of ʻAbd al-Laṭīf as present in the philosophical section of the *Kitāb al-Naṣīḥatayn* in which he *inter alia* shall comment on the linguistic peculiarities of

---

4 Paul Ghalioungui and Said Abdou, *Maqālatān fī l-Ḥawāss wa-Masā'il Ṭabi'ya/Risāla li l-Iskandar fī l-Faṣl/Risāla fī l-maraḍ al-Musammā Diābīṭis by Abd Al-Latif Al-Baghdadi*, [= The Arab Heritage series: Wizārat al-Iʻlām/Ministry of Information No. 18] (Kuwait 1392 A.H./1972 A.D.), at 29-32.

5 N. Peter Joosse, "Pride and Prejudice, Praise and Blame'. ʻAbd al-Laṭīf al-Baghdādī's Views on Good and Bad Medical Practitioners', in: Arnoud Vrolijk and Jan P. Hogendijk (editors*): O ye Gentlemen: Arabic Studies on Science and Literary Culture in Honour of Remke Kruk* (Leiden/Boston 2007), 129-141. [= Hans Daiber (general editor): Islamic Philosophy, Theology and Science. Texts and Studies, Volume LXXIV]. Stern announced already in 1962 that he would publish this account in full on another occasion. However, he never fulfilled his promise; cf. Stern, *A Collection of Treatises*, at 61.

6 N. Peter Joosse, "De Geest is uit de Fles'. De middeleeuwse Arabische arts ʻAbd al-Laṭīf ibn Yūsuf al-Baghdādī: zijn medische werk en zijn bizarre affiliatie met het twintigste-eeuwse spiritisme'; [English] title: "The spirit has left the bottle': the medieval Arabic physician ʻAbd al-Laṭīf ibn Yūsuf al-Baghdādī: his medical work and his bizarre affiliation with twentieth-century spiritualism', in: *Gewina* 30: 4 (2007), 211-29, at 216-221.

7 N. Peter Joosse and Peter E. Pormann, 'Archery, mathematics, and conceptualising inaccuracies in medicine in 13th century Iraq and Syria'. Available from: www.jameslindlibrary.org eds. Sir Iain Chalmers and Jan P. Vandenbroucke. [Republished as: 'Archery, mathematics, and conceptualizing inaccuracies in medicine in 13th century Iraq and Syria', in: *Journal of the Royal Society of Medicine* 101 (2008), 425-27].

8 N. Peter Joosse and Peter E. Pormann, 'Decline and Decadence in Iraq and Syria after the Age of Avicenna? ʻAbd al-Laṭīf al-Baghdādī (1162-1231) between Myth and History', in: *BHM* 84 (2010), 1-29.

9 Dimitri Gutas, 'Philosophy in the Twelfth Century: one View from Baghdad, or the Repudiation of al-Ghazālī', in*: In the Age of Averroes: Arabic Philosophy in the Sixth/Twelfth Century*, ed. Peter Adamson (London/Turin 2011), 9-26.

the treatise and on the philological details concerning the readings of the Bursa MS. Cecilia Martini Bonadeo's recent study (2013) on 'Abd al-Laṭīf's philosophical thought contains amongst others a partial English translation of the philosophical section of the *Kitāb al-Naṣīḥatayn* as well as an extensive commentary on it.

Dating the Manuscript & Principle of Edition

The medical section of the *Kitāb al-Naṣīḥatayn* has been preserved only in the unique manuscript: Bursa (Turkey), Hüseyin Çelebi 823, fol. 62r-78r. This MS is a so-called *majmū'a*, a collection of texts, which contains nine more treatises on a variety of subjects by 'Abd al-Laṭīf and another one by the Greek philosopher Alexander of Aphrodisias on the *differentia specifica*. It is stated in the colophon of the manuscript that it was copied in the Anatolian city of Erzinjān, in the country of the Rūm Saljūqs,[10] in the year 622 A.H./1225 A.D. The title page refers to the fact that text no. 2: *Qaul li-'Abd al-Laṭīf b. Yūsuf 'alā ḥāl Ibn Khaṭīb ar-Raiyī fī tafsīr sūrat al-ikhlāṣ* was written in Aleppo in the year 613 A.H./1216 A.D. The *Kitāb al-Naṣīḥatayn*, or Bursa no. 5, must have been written in Aleppo after the death of the prince al-Malik al-Ẓāhir Ghāzī ibn Yūsuf that is, after the month of October 1216 A.D.

The medical section of the *Kitāb al-Naṣīḥatayn* as presented by the single manuscript Bursa 823 is entirely intact. It is completely undamaged and very well legible. Its text was, moreover, written by an exceptionally careful scribe. The editor only had to make a single major correction to it (cf. fol. 77r in the ed. and trl.). The original Arabic manuscript of the medical section of the treatise has been attached as an appendix. It mainly serves as a control mechanism to my edition of the Arabic text (cf. pages 95-112).

The principle of edition used for the medical section of the *Kitāb al-Naṣīḥatayn* is as follows: The manuscript's reading of *hamza, madda* has been adapted to Classical Arabic [CA] standards. The manuscript's reading of *shadda* is omitted, except for isolated cases. The diacritical dots, where lacking, are supplied. The dots of *tā' marbūṭa*, where lacking, are likewise supplied. The vocalization of the text is generally omitted, but is provided in those instances where this is deemed necessary in illustration of a specific form. The use of deviating forms of verbs, irregular plurals of nouns and full writing of long vowels in words which according to CA require short vowels, is not maintained.

---

10 The best study available on the Saljūqs of Rūm still is: Claude Cahen, *The Formation of Turkey: The Seljukid Sultanate of Rum: Eleventh to Fourteenth Century* (Harlow, Essex 2001); cf. also the recent study by Songül Mecit, *The Rum Seljuqs: Evolution of a Dynasty* (Abingdon [Ox]/New York 2014). Unfortunately, I have not been able to check this source.

Brief Survey of the Contents

ʿAbd al-Laṭīf al-Baghdādī composed his *Kitāb al-Naṣīḥatayn* as a diatribe directed against false knowledge, which according to the author is worse than ignorance. As the title suggests, it is divided into "two pieces of advice", that is, "advice" for would-be physicians and would-be philosophers, respectively.[11] Both incur ʿAbd al-Laṭīf's scathing criticism and find themselves lambasted in no uncertain terms. The first part, rebuking the doctors of his day, contains four main themes:

1. medical epistemology;
2. medical deontology: the discussion of the methods and practices of charlatans and quacks, called "spongers (*mustarziqa*)" by ʿAbd al-Laṭīf;
3. the idea that book-learning is not sufficient for practising medicine; and
4. the danger of prescribing and using purgatives without having the necessary skills and the full knowledge of the facts.

ʿAbd al-Laṭīf laments the pitiful state of medicine. He does not tire to extol the virtues of the ancient Greek doctors such as Hippocrates, Dioscorides, and Galen of Pergamon. Their skills and know-how form a stark contrast to the inability of his contemporaries. The medical section of the work thus is intended to advise and recommend to physicians and students of medicine to abandon the medicine of those who do not fully master the medical art and are moreover frequently motivated by money more than the welfare of their patients. ʿAbd al-Laṭīf also criticises the medical education of his day: according to him students rely too much on a restricted number of textbooks such as the *Canon* by Ibn Sīnā (Avicenna, d. 1037 A.D.) or imperfect abridgments. Students should therefore master the writings of the ancient Greek doctors in order to gain a comprehensive understanding of medicine.[12]

ʿAbd al-Laṭīf's *Kitāb al-Naṣīḥatayn* without any doubt belongs to the genre of advice-literature and therefore may well represent a so-called 'multiple mirror': a mirror for physicians, a mirror for philosophers and a mirror for princes [*lege*: rulers]. The latter aspect becomes clear from the fact that the treatise strives to 'give sincere advice and to (also) bring guidance…to kings of faraway regions, governors and princes, and furthermore to everyone who wishes the best for himself, and desires happiness. To all these people it [this treatise] brings love, solidarity, rejection of blind authority and fanaticism, by way of using insight, contemplation and consideration' (fol. 62v, lines 2-7).

---

11 For the very common parallel between philosophy as medicine of the soul and medicine as medicine of the body, see: N. Peter Joosse, "ʿAbd al-Laṭīf al-Baghdādī as a Philosopher and a Physician: Myth or Reality, Topos or Truth?', in: *In the Age of Averroes: Arabic Philosophy in the Sixth/Twelfth Century*, ed. Peter Adamson (London/Turin, 2011), 27-43.

12 See: Joosse and Pormann, *Decline and Decadence*, 6-8 and 21-23.

ʻAbd al-Laṭīf's Life and Medical Work

The polymath ʻAbd al-Laṭīf ibn Yūsuf al-Baghdādī (1162-1231 A.D.) was largely active in Iraq, Syria, and Egypt. He was born in Baghdād in the aftermath of the Second Crusade (1147-49 A.D.) and lived through the Third, Fourth and Fifth Crusade. He grew up in an upper class Shāfiʻī family that possessed strong links with the *Niẓāmīya* College [*madrasa*] in his hometown. He continued to move in fashionable and influential circles all his life and maintained a close relationship with the Ayyūbid rulers of his time (for instance with Ṣalāḥ al-Dīn and his sons) whose patronage he enjoyed and by whom he was supplied with ample means of sustenance and employment in high positions. The generous patronage that he enjoyed allowed him to devote his life to research and study, without having to worry about the material aspects of his private and professional existence.

He passed away in Baghdād on Sunday 12 *Muḥarram* 629 A.H. [9 November 1231 A.D.], where he intended to present a collection of his works to the Abbasid Caliph al-Mustanṣir b. al-Zāhir (1226-42 A.D.). He became sixty-nine years old, and was buried next to his father Yūsuf in the *Wardīyah* cemetery in his beloved hometown.

Some of ʻAbd al-Laṭīf's more famous students included the biographer and chronicler Ibn Khallikān (d. 1282 A.D.); the historian and statesman Ibn al-ʻAdīm (d. 1262 A.D.); the botanist Ibn al-Sūrī (d. 1242 A.D.); the judge al-Tīfāshī (d. 1253 A.D.), noted for his works on magic, precious stones, sexual hygiene and eroticism; and the *ḥadīth* scholar al-Birzālī (d. 1239 A.D.).[13] One of his lesser known pupils was the medical student al-Marāġī.[14]

The latter is the author of a short manual (*tadhkira*) in twelve chapters on the basics of medicine.[15]

ʻAbd al-Laṭīf produced a number of remarkable works not only on medicine, but also on alchemy, philosophy and grammar. His works portray him as an independent spirit and an innovative mind. Unfortunately, most of ʻAbd al-Laṭīf's medical oeuvre is lost today. We are however fortunate to have a number of interesting and important books and treatises by him. Apart from the passages on

---

13 Cf. also Joosse and Pormann, *Decline and Decadence*, 5-6.

14 N. Peter Joosse and Peter E. Pormann, ''Abd al-Laṭīf al-Baġdādī's *Commentary on Hippocrates' 'Prognostic'*: A Preliminary Exploration', in: *>Epidemics< in Context: Greek Commentaries on Hippocrates in the Arabic Tradition*, ed. Peter E. Pormann (Berlin/Boston 2012) [= Scientia Graeco-Arabica Band 8], 251-283 at 254-55 and 266-67; Albert Dietrich, *Medicinalia Arabica. Studien über arabische medizinische Handschriften in türkischen und syrischen Bibliotheken* (Göttingen 1966), 217-236.

15 Dietrich, *Medicinalia Arabica*, at 224-28. This medical manual is preserved in the *majmūʻa* MS Manisa: *Kitapsaray* 1781/6, fol. 130b-153b. It was read, collated and approved by ʻAbd al-Laṭīf ibn Yūsuf al-Baghdādī in the Anatolian city of Erzinjān in the month of *Rajab* of the year 617 H.

medicine in his book on Egypt, the *Kitāb al-Ifāda wa-l-iʻtibār fī-l-umūr al-mushāhada wa-l-ḥawādith al-muʻāyana bi-arḍ Miṣr* or *Mukhtaṣar akhbār miṣr*[16] and the large medical section of his *K. al-Naṣīḥatayn* which among others contributes greatly to our understanding of the social history of medicine in the geographical areas of Islam, they are the following: a massive book "On the Principles of Simple Medical Substances and their Natural Qualities" (*Fī Uṣūl mufradāt al-ṭibb wa-kaifīyāt ṭabā'iʻhā*), as well as a shorter treatise entitled "Medical Aphorisms Extracted by ʻAbd al-Laṭīf" (*Fuṣūl ṭibbīya intazaʻahā ʻAbd al-Laṭīf*); a didactic treatise entitled "Questions on Natural History" (*al-Masā'il al-ṭabīʻīya*), dealing with problems of natural history in the large sense (that is, including certain aspects of medicine); a commentary on Ḥunayn Ibn Isḥāq's "Medical Questions" (*al-Masā'il al-ṭibbīya*); a medium-length treatise "On the Disease Called Diabetes" (*Fī l-maraḍ alladhī yusammā diyābīṭā*); a critique on Fakhr al-Dīn al-Rāzī's commentary on the first section of Avicenna's "Canon of Medicine" discussing generalities (*Kullīyāt*); two commentaries on works by Hippocrates, namely the "Book on Aphorisms" (*Kitāb al-Fuṣūl*), and the "Book on Prognostic" (*Kitāb Taqdimat al-maʻrifa*); and a "Book on the Senses" (*Maqāla fī al-Ḥawāss*) investigating sense-perception, which seems to have a rather limited medical significance.[17]

The *Kitāb al-Naṣīḥatayn*: Topoi as Sources?

Within the history of medicine, be it in Chinese, Indian, ancient Greek and Roman, Byzantine, or Medieval and Renaissance European medicine, we find without a single exception communications about arguing and competing physicians, who cannot stand each other and do not give each other the time of day. Arabic medicine is no exception to that rule and does not provide us with a different picture. Within

---

16 This work contains ʻAbd al-Laṭīf's famous criticism of Galen with respect to certain anatomical data. ʻAbd al-Laṭīf's discoveries were, however, not widely accepted. Only future research will provide us with the answer as to whether later Arabic physicians reacted to ʻAbd al-Laṭīf's ideas and how Arabic-Islamic medicine developed in the so-called post-classical age (i.e. after 1200 A.D. and onwards). Similarly, it is not at all known whether ʻAbd al-Laṭīf's ideas and works ever transferred to the Latin West during the Middle Ages and the Renaissance. It will be interesting to find out whether ʻAbd al-Laṭīf, directly or indirectly, influenced for example Renaissance authors such as the physician and botanist Prospero Alpini/Prosper Alpinus (Marostica/Venice 1553 A.D. - Padua 1617 A.D.) whose works cover similar topics, cf. his *De medicina aegyptiorum, De plantis aegypti liber, De rhapontico, and Rerum aegyptiarum libri quattuor.* Like ʻAbd al-Laṭīf, Alpini also composed a large work on the Hippocratic *Prognostic: De praesagienda vita et morte aegrotantium libri septum* [English translation: The presages of life and death in diseases. In seven books…Translated from the last Leyden edition, revised and published by Gaubius, at the request of Dr. Boerhaave. By R. James (London 1746)].

17 Cf. also Joosse and Pormann, *Decline and Decadence*, 6-8.

the Arabic setting we can also read about medical controversies, rivalry, and professional jealousy. Likewise we might come across physicians who pester the life out of each other, bombard each other with scathing criticism, and look upon each other with feelings of envy and enmity such as often prevail between men who are prominent in the same profession. On the one side, we will encounter physicians who sing each others praises. On the other side, we will meet those who pour scorn on each other, slander each other, and accuse each other of being a charlatan, a quack, a mountebank or a sponger with the sole purpose of making the other look bad in the eyes of his colleagues. The other becomes then a perfect doctor, or a fraud, a trickster or a charlatan, but merely in a subjective way, namely only in the eye of the beholder.[18]

The thirteenth century Syriac author Bar Hebraeus, who was besides a high-placed cleric and many other things a well-trained physician himself, advised his readers that:

Learned men behave deceitfully towards each other. They are frequently very wicked and act stingy with regard to their respective science, or with respect to that which they have confirmed through their science, for they are afraid that other persons who come into possession of science will become more skilled in it than them, or because they want to be singularly esteemed in their time, or the one man of their time, or because they fear that their role in science will be reduced if it has to be shared with many people, or merely because of jealousy.[19]

The theme of the physician who compels recognition against the incompetent and the inept, and who succeeds when all the other doctors have failed, is a literary *topos* which was popular and much savoured.[20]

The topic of the praise of the good physician and the blame of the bad physician is another traditional theme.[21]

---

18 During my late teens I sojourned in Bombay (India) with my parents. On Bombay's streets, I often witnessed practitioners of one of the most curious forms of charlatanism: the *karaklaxmi* – people (mostly a pair: a male adult and a child) who transfer light ailments, like for instance headaches, ear-aches, and muscle pains, by looking deeply into the eyes of their patients and absorbing their pain through the cracking of a whip.

19 N. Peter Joosse, *A Syriac Encyclopaedia of Aristotelian Philosophy*. Barhebraeus (13th c.), *Butyrum sapientiae*, Books of Ethics, Economy and Politics. A Critical Edition, with Introduction, Translation, Commentary and Glossaries (Leiden/Boston 2004), 167-69 [= Hans Daiber and Remke Kruk (editors): Aristoteles Semitico-Latinus Volume 16].

20 Françoise Micheau, 'Great Figures in Arabic Medicine According to Ibn al-Qifṭī', in: Sheila Campbell, Bert Hall and David Klausner (editors): *Health, Disease and Healing in Medieval Culture* [Center for Mediaeval Studies, University of Toronto] (Basingstoke and London 1992), 169-185, at 172.

21 That this is also a universal theme can be extrapolated from Indian medicine. The earliest surviving Sanskrit medical manual by Caraka (first or first half of the second century A.D.), already mentions 'that fashionably dressed *vaidyas* (doctors of the traditional type) would walk the streets in the hope of finding patients. Immediately on hearing that someone is ill, they swoop down on him from all quarters and in his hearing speak loudly of their medical attainments. If a certain doctor is already in attendance (...) they make

Franz Rosenthal made mention of the fact that its roots lie in Classical Antiquity, in those centuries of late Hellenistic civilization preceding the coming of Islam.[22]

Peter E. Pormann has remarked that Arabic medical writers often referred to a glorious Greek past, which was not infrequently more imagined than real, when forming their own medical traditions and institutions.[23]

J. Christoph Bürgel and Ursula Weisser bring to mind that the theme of the complaint about the times could also well be a sheer echo of a topic already extant in the writings of Galen and even in those of Hippocrates.[24]

It was habitual for writers on medical deontology, which is the area of medical writing in which doctors discuss quackery, to start out with bitter complaints about the circumstances that existed in their day and age. They complained that medicine was in a state of decay. Ancient medicine, especially the work of Galen and Hippocrates, is the idealized picture for aspiring doctors. The decline of medicine is continual and progressing. The physician's morale has fallen low. The medicaments of the ancients have become forgotten or have been tampered with. The authorities do not exert pressure on the druggists and turn a blind eye towards them. The medical handbooks of important doctors from the magnificent past have been given way to the poor and weak compendia of simple and uneducated souls. The doctors do not attach great value anymore to solid education or to solid instruction. Many of the doctors joined the medical profession only to become loaded with money. The wrongdoers are the rulers who do not care about the decline of the medical profession, but also the patients themselves. People, who would immediately consult a veterinary for their donkey when it is sick, refuse to visit a doctor when they feel in poor health themselves or trust the first swindler which they come across. The authors of these and similar texts feel, because of all these abuses and wrongs, an obligation to elevate medicine and raise it to its former lustre.

For this reason they have to defend medicine against sceptics and despisers and convince the indifferent to pay more attention to medicine than to other matters.

---

mention of his failings', cf. Arthur Llewellyn Basham, 'The Practice of Medicine in Ancient and Medieval India', in: Charles Leslie (editor): *Asian Medical Systems: A Comparative Study* (Berkeley/Los Angeles/London 1976), 18-43, at 30. The texts of Caraka were known to the ninth-century Arab physician 'Alī b. Sahl Rabban aṭ-Ṭabarī who refers to them in his *Firdaus al-ḥikma fī ṭ-ṭibb*; cf. also Fuat Sezgin (ed.): *GAS = Geschichte des arabischen Schrifttums*, vols. 1-9: (Leiden 1967-84); Indices: (Frankfurt am Main 1995); vols. 10-12: (Frankfurt am Main 2000), vol. 3, at 198.

22 Franz Rosenthal, 'The Physician in Medieval Muslim Society' – The Fielding H. Garrison Lecture, in: *BHM* 52 (1978), 475-491, at 485-86.

23 Peter E. Pormann, 'The Physician and the Other: Images of the Charlatan in Medieval Islam', in: *BHM* 79 (2005), 189-227, at 195-199.

24 J. Christoph Bürgel, 'Secular and Religious Features of Medieval Arabic Medicine', in: Charles Leslie (editor): *Asian Medical Systems: A Comparative Study* (Berkeley/Los Angeles/London 1976), 44-62, at 50; Ursula Weisser, 'Unter den Künsten die nützlichste: Aspekte des ärztlichen Berufs im arabisch-islamischen Mittelalter', in: *Medizinhistorisches Journal* 26 (1991), 3-25, at 7; cf. also Rosenthal, *The Physician*, 484.

Moreover, they have to stimulate the sensible and skilful youngsters to learn and study the noble art of medicine. Frequently combined with the previous themes, is the *topos* of the incompetent and often elderly doctor who suggests a different treatment to his colleagues. The treatment of the one doctor is then pursued in spite of the fact that all the other doctors were in agreement about the procedure to follow, as a result of which everything is going haywire and the patient runs a great risk of dying in the process or actually passing away. A faint and rather unusual echo of this theme (combining a theological and a medical issue) glimmers through in medieval English medicine:

In the summer of the year 1205, Hubert Walter, archbishop of Canterbury, suddenly fell ill with a deadly fever and carbuncle (anthrax) while travelling to Boxley in Kent. The carbuncle erupted around his waist, at the third-from-last vertebra of his back, with the inflammation extending around so as to threaten his private parts. In his illness, Hubert was attended by Master Gilbert Eagle (also called Gilbertus Anglicus), a prominent physician who was the author of a massive medical and surgical text, the Compendium medicine, one of the first works to take advantage of new Latin translations of Arabic medical and philosophical texts. Gilbert, worried that his patron's fever would rise, advised him to confess his sins. On doing so, the fire of the archbishop's remorse and charity rose up and caused the moisture in his brain to dissolve, bringing forth from him a torrent of tears and great relief. After this, he was able to eat and drink a bit. Gilbert then advised him to make out his will, which he did in good order. At dawn the next day, Gilbert secretly observed the ill man and advised Hubert to receive last rites. Another physician, Henry le Afaitie, disagreed and advised him to wait. Then, the poisonous matter that was causing the fever went to the archbishop's brain and he became delirious. He had to be brought back to himself with "physical remedies" and shortly thereafter followed Gilbert's advice. After last rites, Hubert was much relieved, and joined others in praying and rejoicing...[25]

The unusual aspect of this account is of course the fact that the doctor in attendance Master Gilbert Eagle did not prescribe any medicaments. He did not administer drugs, view the patient's urine or take his pulse. Just by observing the patient closely, he could tell that there was no hope that the archbishop would recover and that death was around the bend. The other remarkable feature is that the second doctor Henry le Afaitie did not offer an alternative remedy, but just advised to wait a little bit longer with the last sacraments. He thus suggested a different 'treatment', but this 'diagnosis' exacerbated the illness. Only when Master Gilbert Eagle's suggestion was pursued to let the archbishop receive the last sacraments, the latter slightly felt better. Then the fever came back and soon the archbishop embarked on his last journey. Confession and not potions and drugs brought the archbishop relief. Master Gilbert Eagle used his learned judgment to recognize that death was unavoidable in this particular case.[26]

The archbishop's death was not caused by the carelessness of the attending physicians. The reverse is true: due to untold suffering the patient and the doctors welcomed death's release.

---

[25] Faye Getz, *Medicine in the English Middle Ages* (Princeton 1998), 3-4.

[26] Getz, *Medicine in the English Middle Ages*, 4.

Occasionally, the incompetent doctor is depicted in Arabic literature as an old man in years (often originating from North Africa, a *maghribī*) with the knowledge and the mind of a child.[27] The aforementioned *topoi* are all widely and vividly present in the writings of ʻAbd al-Laṭīf al-Baghdādī, in particular in his *Book of the Two Pieces of Advice to the Public at large*, but for instance also in the "Treatise to Ṣalāḥ ad-Dīn on the Revival of the Art of Medicine" (*al-Maqāla aṣ-ṣalāḥīya fī iḥyā' aṣ-ṣināʻa aṭ-ṭibbīya*) by the Jewish physician Abū l-Makārim Hibat Allāh ibn Jumayʻ (d. 1198 A.D.), a tractate of which the framework may well have served as one of the models for ʻAbd al-Laṭīf's *Kitāb al-Naṣīḥatayn.*[28]

In the *Kitāb al-Naṣīḥatayn*, ʻAbd al-Laṭīf al-Baghdādī quotes lavishly from the works of the ancient Greek authors Hippocrates, Dioscorides and Galen, and specifically from the latter's *K. fī Imtiḥān aṭ-ṭabīb* (*Book on the Examination of the Physician*) which in hindsight is nothing else than the *K. fī Miḥnat afḍal al-aṭibbā'.*[29] We have also found two quotations of Plato[30] and two references to the *ḥadīth qudsī*. Except for a single reference to the physician Abū Bakr ar-Rāzī (d. c. 925 A.D.), no other Arab author has been quoted. In an isolated case, the author refers to a book that he has composed himself. Nevertheless, ʻAbd al-Laṭīf highly praises a few Arabic medical handbooks, namely those of Ibn Serapion, that is Ibn Sarābiyūn (fl. c. 870s), and Abū Sahl al-Masīḥī (d. 1010 A.D.). He moreover extols the Arab physician Abū Jaʻfar Aḥmad ibn Muḥammad ibn abī l-Ashʻath (d. circa 970 A.D.).

---

27 This is a *topos* of which we can also encounter echoes in Medieval and Renaissance texts, for instance in Julius Caesar Scaliger's scathing criticism of the famous Italian physician Gerolamo Cardano (Pavia 1501-Rome 1576) here presented through his contemporary, the historian Jacques de Thou (Jac. Augustus Thuani): 'Julius Caesar Scaliger, who (…) in all fields exactly pinpointed Cardano's instability, and believed that this (old) man knew more than anyone in certain expertises, but in others he knew less than a small child', cf. Gerolamo Cardano, *Mijn leven* [*De propria vita*] (Amsterdam 2000), at 61.

28 Ibn Jumayʻ (or sometimes: Ibn Jamīʻ), *Al-Maqāla al-ṣalāḥīya fī iḥyā' al-ṣināʻa al-ṭibbīya: Treatise to Ṣalāḥ ad-Dīn on the Revival of the Art of Medicine*. Edited and translated by Hartmut Fähndrich (Wiesbaden 1983). [= Abhandlungen für die Kunde des Morgenlandes XLVI, 3]; Max Meyerhof, 'Sultan Saladin's Physician on the Transmission of Greek Medicine to the Arabs', *BHM* 18 (1945), 169-178. [Reprint in: Penelope Johnstone (editor): Max Meyerhof, *Studies in Medieval Arabic Medicine: Theory and Practice* (Variorum Reprints) (London 1984) under No. III].

29 Galen, *On How to Recognise the Best Physician (De optimo medico cognoscendo)*, Albert Z. Iskandar (editor) [Corpus Medicorum Graecorum, Supplementum orientale 4] (Berlin 1988). The present author will endeavour to allude to the identification of the different quotations in another study.

30 The "quotations" from Plato at first view seem spurious, but may come from a collection of sayings attributed to Plato.

We encounter a completely different situation in text no. 11 of the Bursa MS: *(Fī) l-maraḍ al-musammā diyābīṭā*, or "On the disease called Diabetes".[31] There all the sources have been summed up in the text.

The German editor Hans-Jürgen Thies, moreover, did a marvelous job in matching the sources to their exact references. The diabetes-text reveals the following sources: Qahlamān, Theodokos (Tīyadhūq), Ahrun, Oribasius of Pergamon, Philagrios, Galen, Hippocrates, Dioscorides, Rufus of Ephesus, Jibrīl ibn Bukhtīshū', Jurjīs ibn Jibrīl ibn Bukhtīshū', Ibn Sarābiyūn, Thābit ibn Qurrah, 'Alī al-Majūsī, Yūḥannā ibn Māsawayh, Abū Bakr ar-Rāzī, Ibn Samajūn, Ibn Idrīs aṣ-Ṣiqillī al-Māzarī and Ibn Sīnā. Thies was not able to identify two of the sources, namely the *ṣāḥib kitāb al-bustān* (i.e. the author of the book called "The Garden"), and Aḥmad al-Fārisī i.e. Ahmed the Persian. The former description might either fit Ẓahīr al-Dīn al-Bayhaqī (d. 1169 A.D.) or Ilyās ibn al-Muṭrān (d. 1191 A.D.).[32] The latter description may refer to the aforementioned Ibn abī l-Ash'ath whose first name was Aḥmad, and who originated from Persia.[33] Rainer Degen added hereto that the sections on the quince from Galen's *De alimentorum facultatibus*, Hippocrates' *De victu*, Dioscorides' *De materia medica* and Rufus of Ephesus' *De victu* were not directly taken from the original Greek versions, but from one and the same Arabic source, viz. the *Book on Foods* or *K. al-Aghdhiya* by Ḥunayn ibn Isḥāq (d. c. 873 or 877 A.D.).[34]

The Physician and the Ruler

In this paragraph, we shall discuss 'Abd al-Laṭīf al-Baghdādī's relation to the highly esteemed Jewish doctor Abū l-Ḥajjāj Yūsuf ibn Yaḥyā ibn Isḥāq al-Sabtī al-Maghribī (d. 1226 A.D.), the favourite pupil of the famous Jewish philosopher and physician Moses Maimonides (d. 1204 A.D.) and the intimate friend of the chronicler and vizier Ibn al-Qifṭī (d. 1248 A.D.),[35] and their relationship to the

---

31 Hans-Jürgen Thies, *Der Diabetestraktat 'Abd al-Laṭīf al-Baġdādī's. Untersuchungen zur Geschichte des Krankheitsbildes in der arabischen Medizin* (Bonn 1971) [= Bonner Orientalistische Studien, Neue Serie, hsgb. von Otto Spies, Bd. 21].

32 However, the wording of 'Abd al-Laṭīf's text is not in agreement with the passage on diabetes as found in my manuscript of Ibn al-Muṭrān's *Bustān al-aṭibbā' wa-rawḍat al-alibbā'*, i.e. the facsimile edition of the manuscript held at Malik National Library and Museum (Teheran) with an introduction by Dr. Mahdi Muhaghghigh (Tehran 1989) [= Encyclopaedia Islamica Foundation: Center for the Publication of Manuscripts No. 5], at 320-22.

33 Remke Kruk, 'Ibn abī l-Ash'ath's *Kitāb al-Ḥayawān*: a Scientific Approach to Anthropology, Dietetics and Zoological Systematics', in: *ZGAIW*, 14 (2001), 119-168, at 119.

34 Rainer Degen, 'Zum Diabetestraktat des 'Abd al-Laṭīf al-Baġdādī', in: *Annali Istituto Universitario Orientale di Napoli* 37 (1977) [N.S. 27], 455-462, at 455.

35 Salomon Munk, 'Notice sur Joseph ben-Iehouda ou Aboul'hadjādj Yousouf ben-Ya'hya al-Sabti al-Maghrebi, disciple de Maïmonide,' in: *JA* Série 3; Tome XIV (1842), 5-70; cf.

prince al-Malik al-Ẓāhir of Aleppo and other members of the Ayyūbid royalty and the royal administration.

Abū l-Ḥajjāj is better known by the name Ibn Sham'ūn, and is very often called by his Hebrew name: Rabbi Joseph ben Judah.[36] Ibn al-Qifṭī dedicated an entry to his good friend in his biographical dictionary the *Ta'rīkh al-ḥukamā'* of which the outlines match 'Abd al-Laṭīf al-Baghdādī's statement. Joseph ben Judah and Ibn al-Qifṭī apparently met each other at social gatherings [*majālis*] at the house of the emir Fāris al-Dīn Maymūn al-Qaṣrī in Aleppo. They were not just good friends, but real 'chums' as the following anecdotes may show: In the first anecdote, Joseph tells Ibn al-Qifṭī in confidence that after having had two girls, he would now prefer to have a boy. Thereupon, Ibn al-Qifṭī gives him 'a recipe', a technique which Joseph has to employ during sexual intercourse. In the following years indeed three sons were born to him. In the second anecdote, the two men promise each other that the one who passes away first should inform the other about the hereafter. Joseph is the first to die and shortly after his death he appears to his friend Ibn al-Qifṭī in a dream. He is completely dressed in white and speaks the enigmatic words: 'the universal has joined the universal and the particular stayed behind in the particular'. This indicates to Ibn al-Qifṭī that the soul has returned to the universal, while the body has rested in the grave.[37]

In his work entitled "The information of the narrators on renowned grammarians" (*Inbāh al-ruwāt 'alā anbāh al-nuḥāt*) Ibn al-Qifṭī attacked 'Abd al-Laṭīf al-Baghdādī in a most vicious manner. The ground for this attack was that Ibn al-Qifṭī wanted to take revenge for 'Abd al-Laṭīf al-Baghdādī's accusation that Joseph intentionally killed his royal patient, the prince al-Malik al-Ẓāhir. Ibn al-Qifṭī of course intended to protect his best friend's honour, but what was 'Abd al-Laṭīf al-Baghdādī's motive for blaming Joseph? Was it frustration, professional jealousy or hate against a Jew, who had once apostatized and lived as a Muslim, but practiced the Jewish faith in secret?

Stern and Eddé seem to hold the view that it was an act of racism or xenophobia.

Other scholars illustrated that the early Ayyūbid period rather saw an intellectual revival which paved the way for unconstrained contacts between the members of

---

for instance also Jamāl al-Dīn ibn al-Qifṭī, *Ta'rīkh al-ḥukamā'*, ed. Julius Lippert (Leipzig 1903), 392-94; Barhebraeus (Ibn al-'Ibrī), *Ta'rīkh mukhtaṣar al-duwal*, ed. A. Ṣālḥānī (Beirut 1890), 242.

36 Max Meyerhof has identified Joseph ben Judah with Joseph ibn 'Aqnin, a Jewish author living in Morocco in the 12th century. This identification is incorrect since Ibn 'Aqnin is said never to have left his homeland, cf. Max Meyerhof, 'Mediaeval Jewish Physicians in the Near East, from Arabic Sources', in: *Isis* XXVIII (1938), 432-460, especially 451-52. [Reprinted in: Penelope Johnstone (editor): Max Meyerhof, *Studies in Medieval Arabic Medicine: Theory and Practice* (Variorum Reprints) (London 1984), under No. VII].

37 Anne-Marie Eddé, *La principauté Ayyoubide d'Alep (597/1183 – 658/1260)* [= Freiburger Islamstudien; Bd. 21] (Stuttgart 1999), 476.

different religions,[38] but laid stress on the ephemeral character of these contacts which almost never led to close personal relationships.

Goitein asserted 'that the general trend was towards segregation, discrimination, and, finally outright persecution…The thirteenth century witnessed the definite turn for the worse. With the fourteenth, the night of the Middle Ages had become total'.[39] But was this actually the case?

Mark R. Cohen pointed out that Christians were more persecuted by Muslims than were Jews and that the persecution of Jews by Muslims was 'less frequent and less brutal than anti-Jewish persecution in Christendom'.[40] Cohen emphasizes the fact that Jewish doctors 'were found in Arab society in numbers disproportionate to the Jewish presence in the population at large'.[41] Muslim admiration for Jewish physicians is plentiful in Arabic biographical dictionaries and Muslim and Jewish physicians worked together in good harmony at the city hospitals. Moreover, Jewish physicians were consulted by private patients who were Muslims, both dignitaries at court and common people. According to Cohen, these meetings 'provided considerable opportunity for Jewish-Muslim sociability which seems not to have been accompanied by suspicion of the inimical intentions of Jewish doctors that had its root in late antique Christianity…'.[42]

The intimate relationship between Joseph ben Judah and Ibn al-Qifṭī is another good example of the sound interrelations between Jews and Muslims. Social bonding and deep friendships between members of both these religions were clearly not always ephemeral, but also frequently lasting and intense.

With regard to 'Abd al-Laṭīf al-Baghdādī's motive for blaming Joseph, I rather would start from the idea that there is some truth in the old saying that there is no smoke without fire, and consequently I would like to raise some slight reservations about the flawlessness of Joseph's character.

---

38 The Syrian (Syriac) Orthodox prelate and scholar Barhebraeus (1225/6-1286 A.D.) lived through this period in the history of the Near East which, from a Syrian (Syriac) point of view, is sometimes called 'The Syrian (Syriac) Renaissance' (± 1026-1318 A.D.), the main characteristics of which have been described as openness towards fellow Christians as well as receptivity to the world of Islam; cf. Herman Teule, 'Gregory Barhebraeus and his Time: The Syrian Renaissance', in: *Journal of the Canadian Society for Syriac Studies* 3 (2003), 21-43, at 37; cf. also N. Peter Joosse, 'Expounding on a Theme: Structure and Sources of Bar Hebraeus' 'Practical Philosophy' in *The Cream of Wisdom*', in: Herman Teule, Carmen Fotescu Tauwinkl with Bas ter Haar Romeny, and Jan van Ginkel (editors): *The Syriac Renaissance* (Louvain 2010), 135-50.

39 Shlomo Dov Goitein, 'The Moses Maimonides – Ibn Ṣanā' al-Mulk Circle (A Deathbed Declaration from March 1182)', in: Moshe Sharon (editor): *Studies in Islamic History and Civilization in Honour of Professor David Ayalon* (Jerusalem/Leiden 1986), 399-405, at 404.

40 Mark R. Cohen, *Under Crescent & Cross: the Jews in the Middle Ages* (Princeton 1994), 163; cf. also Pormann, *The Physician and the Other*, 212-13, at note 60.

41 Cf. Cohen, *Under Crescent & Cross*, 134.

42 Cohen, *Under Crescent & Cross*, 134-35.

In a letter addressed to Joseph, Maimonides had to restrain his student and warned him against insulting Samuel ben Eli, the principal of the rabbinic academy in Baghdād, a man who, despite all his limitations, was much older, held a dignified post, and was respected by society.[43]

In another letter, Maimonides responds to Joseph's dark complaint that he had been the subject of false tales spread by his enemies [*sic*!]. Thereupon, his master advised him to learn to control his temper and to forgive his foes.[44] Joseph was apparently not 'very forgiving' for on another occasion his master had to reprimand him again.

The most interesting, but unfortunately somewhat murky statement comes from the *Taḥkemoni* by the poet and translator Judah al-Ḥarizi, who visited Aram Zova (Aleppo) in the beginning of the year 1217 A.D. not so long after the death of prince al-Malik al-Ẓāhir. He found Joseph (the Westerner i.e. *al-maghribī*) at the peak of his glory, but the physician was in a state of distress because one of his disciples[45] had shown ingratitude towards him in a rather nasty and hateful manner.[46] In the new translation of the *Taḥkemoni* by David Simha Segal it has been expressed as follows:

Now one of his students, an ingrate and overreacher, rebelled against his teacher with forehead of brass and heart of wood, returning evil for good, forgetting how Joseph had drawn him out, sought him, whence he had brought him, and how much he had taught him; for he had raised him from a heap of dung to set him among thinkers, seers, and giants, only to merit such defiance.[47]

Could ʻAbd al-Laṭīf have been the disciple in question? Or was this disciple a certain doctor Elazar who has also been spoken of in the *Taḥkemoni*?[48] Judah al-Ḥarizi utilises the following words:

Now, having succinctly set forth this bastard's shame, this dastard's claim to fame, I add how, long years ago, he swelled with pride and sallied forth, a snorting ram pushing south and

---

[43] Herbert Alan Davidson, *Moses Maimonides. The Man and His Works* (Oxford 2005), 520; cf. Moses ben Maimon, *Epistulae*, ed. D.H. Baneth (Jerusalem 1946), 61-62.

[44] Davidson, *Moses Maimonides*, 547-48; cf. Moses ben Maimon, *Epistulae*, 49-50.

[45] Could it be that the term 'disciple' or 'student' has been misunderstood or interpreted wrongly, and that instead thereof the word 'colleague' is meant? Both men fell under the patronage of prince al-Malik al-Ẓāhir Ghāzī and can thus be seen as colleagues of each other.

[46] Munk, *Notice*, 54; cf. Judah al-Ḥarizi, *Sefer Taḥkemoni*, ed. Y. Toporovsky, (Tel Aviv 1952); Davidson, *Moses Maimonides*, 265, 427. Judah al-Ḥarizi has also mentioned another Jewish physician who was present at the court of al-Malik al-Ẓāhir Ghāzī: a man called Master Elazar, the king's physician; cf. Eddé, *La principauté Ayyoubide*, 467; cf. also Judah al-Ḥarizi, *The Book of Taḥkemoni*. Jewish Tales from Medieval Spain translated, explicated, and annotated by David Simha Segal (Oxford/Portland, Oregon 2001), 350.

[47] Judah al-Ḥarizi, *The Book of Taḥkemoni*, 348.

[48] This Dr Elazar should not be confused with Master Elazar, the king's physician. Apparently both these men lived in Aleppo at the time of Judah al-Ḥarizi's visit to the city. The use of *Decknamen* or pseudonyms should not be excluded here.

north; and lo, a lion sprang up from the west, wondrous in size, and bitter smote the ram, broke his two horns and put out his eyes; he was the great doctor, Master Joseph the Westerner, who forced the fool to see his own tumidity, then showed the world his singular stupidity.[49]

At present, little or nothing is known about the pupil-tutor relationship of ʻAbd al-Laṭīf and Joseph ben Judah. The newly translated medical section of the *Kitāb al-Naṣīḥatayn*, which is presented here for the very first time, has unfortunately not changed this particular state of affairs. ʻAbd al-Laṭīf nowhere clearly indicates that he had once been a pupil of the Jewish doctor, although he gives the following statement at the end of the medical section of the *K. al-Naṣīḥatayn*:

I have witnessed some of the physicians of Cairo and Baghdād and of (certain) places which lie in between these cities, and I took a close look at some of the matters which I (still) remember to have taught them and which they (may have) taught me, but I can (truthfully) state that I have never experienced a doctor who was any worse than this damned North African [*maghribī*] devil who (nowadays) resides in Aleppo.

The two (auto)biographical texts and the few scattered fragments which we still possess do not reveal any encounter of ʻAbd al-Laṭīf and Joseph ben Judah before the year 1216 A.D., which raises the question where they possibly could have met each other before that particular date. For this purpose it is essential to take a somewhat closer look at Joseph ben Judah's life history. Joseph was born in Ceuta, North Africa in a time in which Ceuta was under control of the much feared Almohad movement. He had to flee his homeland because of the brutal persecutions of the Jews and Christians under these bold religious fanatics. The *dhimmī* status – the legal status of toleration– which these groups had traditionally enjoyed under Muslim law had been lifted and the Jewish and Christian populations of North Africa were offered the choice between converting to Islam and death.[50] Joseph made an alternative choice and escaped to Egypt. He arrived in Alexandria. From there he sent letters and literary compositions to Maimonides in order to introduce himself. Thereupon, he set out for Cairo and ultimately joined Maimonides at the latter's residence in Fusṭāṭ. As a student of Maimonides, Joseph chiefly studied mathematics and logic. Maimonides may have allowed him a foretaste of scriptural and haggadic texts, but resisted his desire to go ahead with scientific and philosophic studies.[51] In the mid- or rather late 1180s Joseph ben Judah left Egypt for Syria. According to the sources he arrived in Aleppo around the year 1187 A.D. He stayed there for some years and married. After that he decided to go on a long business trip to Iraq which he must have reached around 1191-92 A.D. By the early 1190s he is supposed to have been fully trained in medical theory, and in a letter of Maimonides written around this period (most probably from October 1190 A.D.) Joseph is advised to support himself by teaching medical texts.[52] In this letter, Maimonides also suggests to Joseph to abandon the idea to open a school for Jewish

49 Judah al-Ḥarizi, *The Book of Taḥkemoni*, 349.
50 Davidson, *Moses Maimonides*, 15.
51 Davidson, *Moses Maimonides*, 330-32.
52 Davidson, *Moses Maimonides*, 472-75, especially 473.

religious studies in Baghdād. One of the reasons he gives is that Joseph would be too busy with the school to be able to continue his trading activities. Therefore, he advises Joseph to apply himself instead to religious and medical studies, and to continue his trading activities in order to keep himself financially and spiritually independent.[53]

Joseph seemed to have lived on and off in Baghdād.[54] It has been alleged that he continued to undertake business trips, perhaps even as far as India. When he returned permanently to Aleppo, he was already fairly advanced in years. He became the physician of one of the most powerful and influential men within the Ayyūbid hierarchy, the emir Fāris al-Dīn Maymūn al-Qaṣrī,[55] lord of Sidon and Nablus, and formed part of a team of medical practitioners present at the court of prince al-Malik al-Ẓāhir Ghāzī ibn Yūsuf.

'Abd al-Laṭīf lived in Baghdād from his birth in 1162 to 1189 A.D. After February 1189 A.D., 'Abd al-Laṭīf, aged 27, left Baghdād only to return at the end of October 1231 A.D. after an absence of forty years.[56] Around 1182 A.D. he started to study medicine under (Raḍī al-Dawla Abū Naṣr) Ibn Hibat Allāh b. Ṣā'id, the son of the famous physician Amīn al-Daula ibn at-Tilmīdh. 'Abd al-Laṭīf did not reside in Baghdād during the years 1191-92 A.D. and cannot have met Joseph ben Judah there. We must, however, accept the fact that Joseph ben Judah was besides a doctor also a trader, as a result of which it is not unreasonable to conclude that he must have journeyed from east to west and from north to south. There was ample opportunity for them to have met during this time, although concrete evidence of their actual meeting is non-existent.

The first statement of the two men actually working together is dated Saturday the 10th September of the year 1216 A.D. On that day a team of physicians was called together at the Citadel, the Ayyūbid palace, of Aleppo to treat prince al-Malik al-Ẓāhir Ghāzī ibn Yūsuf who had suddenly become feverish, abandoned the

---

53 Elinor Lieber, 'Galen: Physician as Philosopher, Maimonides: Philosopher as Physician', *BHM* 53 (1979), 268-285, esp. 279-80.

54 Davidson, *Moses Maimonides*, 520.

55 Joseph ben Judah was in Aleppo the private physician of the emir Ṣalāḥīya Fāris al-Dīn Maymūn al-Qaṣrī (d. 1214). In Damascus this emir was, however, attended by Ibn al-Muṭrān, and later by the Melkite physician Ibn Siqlāb, cf. Etan Kohlberg and B.Z. Kedar, 'A Melkite Physician in Frankish Jerusalem and Ayyubid Damascus: Muwaffaq al-Dīn Ya'qūb b. Siqlāb', *Asian and African Studies* 22 (1988), 113-126, esp. 118; cf. also Johannes Pahlitzsch: 'Ärzte ohne Grenzen. Melkitische, jüdische und samaritanische Ärzte in Ägypten und Syrien zur Zeit der Kreuzzüge', in: Florian Steger and Kay Peter Jankrift (editors): *Gesundheit-Krankheit. Kulturtransfer medizinischen Wissens von der Spätantike bis in die Frühe Neuzeit* (Köln/Weimar/Wien 2004), 101-119 [= Beihefte zum Archiv für Kulturgeschichte; Heft 55].

56 For a detailed chronology and an itinerary of 'Abd al-Laṭīf's life, see: Shawkat M. Toorawa, 'Travel in the medieval Islamic world: the importance of patronage, as illustrated by 'Abd al-Latif al-Baghdadi (d. 629/1231) (and other littérateurs)', in: Rosamund Allen (editor): *Eastward Bound. Travel and travellers*, 1050-1550 (Manchester and New York 2004), 53-70, esp. 63-65.

drinking of fluids, decreased the intake of food and suffered from major sleeplessness. Both men held important post at or around the court of the prince, which they without a single doubt owed to their friendship and acquaintance with people in high positions. 'Abd al-Laṭīf enjoyed the patronage of Ṣalāḥ al-Dīn and his sons and was very well paid by them. He knew the Sultan's military judge Bahā' al-Dīn ibn Shaddād quite well and was on good terms with al-Qādī al-Fāḍil, Ṣalāḥ ad-Dīn's chief counsellor and the director of his chancellery, and 'Imād al-Dīn al-Kātib al-Iṣfahānī, Ṣalāḥ al-Dīn's famous scribe and personal secretary. Joseph ben Judah was on the other hand very well-acquainted with the emir Fāris al-Dīn Maymūn al-Qaṣrī and the vizier Jamāl al-Dīn ibn al-Qifṭī, who once was the private treasurer of the prince al-Malik al-Ẓāhir Ghāzī ibn Yūsuf and later became the head of the office of finances of the entire Ayyūbid principality. He was moreover on familiar terms with Tāj al-Dīn Zayd ibn al-Ḥasan Abū l-Yumn al-Kindī, a Hanafitic grammarian and prominent reciter of the Koran, who for his part was again befriended with the emir 'Izz al-Dīn Yūsuf ibn Ayyūb, a nephew to Ṣalāḥ al-Dīn.[57] Although the two men may only have met each other for the very first time at the court in Aleppo, there are sound reasons for assuming that Joseph ben Judah was informed about the existence of 'Abd al-Laṭīf at a much earlier date, namely through correspondence with his master Maimonides who met 'Abd al-Laṭīf in Cairo in the year 1191 A.D. 'Abd al-Laṭīf did not like the great Jewish philosopher and physician very much. He reports: 'When Maimonides came to see me, I found him to be tremendously learned, but overcome with the love of leadership and of service to worldly lords'.[58]

Herbert Davidson mentions in his work on the life and works of Maimonides that 'Abd al-Laṭīf was 'a prickly individual, and his impressions of others should always be taken with a grain of salt'.[59] In the last section of his book, Davidson returns to this subject by stating that ''Abd al-Laṭīf did not possess the sweetest of personalities and he does not hide his antipathy to Maimonides, which Maimonides may well have reciprocated on the occasion. What he says may, therefore, be taken with a grain of salt'.

However, Davidson admits that humility was not the quality that stood out when Maimonides spoke about his literary achievements. And thus, 'Abd al-Laṭīf's impression 'may therefore contain a grain or two of truth'.[60] Throughout his entire life Joseph ben Judah remained a dedicated, often fanatical, defender of his master Maimonides's values and views, who by no means would let anyone tarnish his master's legacy. The disagreeable incident between his master and 'Abd al-Laṭīf may have given Joseph ben Judah a negative portrait of the Iraqi scholar, as a result

---

57 Cf. Toorawa, *A Portrait of 'Abd al-Laṭīf al-Baghdādī's Education and Instruction*, 102.

58 Toorawa, 'The Autobiography of 'Abd al-Laṭīf al-Baghdādī (1162-1231): Selections from the Autograph Notes of 'Abd al-Laṭīf al-Baghdādī', in: Dwight Fletcher Reynolds (editor); coauthored by Kristen Brustad [et al.], *Interpreting the self: autobiography in the Arabic literary tradition* (Berkeley-Los Angeles-London 2001), 161.

59 Davidson, *Moses Maimonides*, 70.

60 Davidson, *Moses Maimonides*, 549-50.

of which a normal relation between the two men remained an illusion and could never take off.

Ullmann has suggested that ʻAbd al-Laṭīf must have lived in Aleppo from 1216 to 1220 A.D.[61] Toorawa rather opted for a date somewhere after February 1212 A.D., or March 1212 A.D.[62] I wholly agree with the dating proposed by Toorawa, but like to specify the date even further due to some facts that have arisen out of the historical context. It is clear from ʻAbd al-Laṭīf's autobiography that he was often in the fortunate position to observe the making of history from nearby, for on many important occasions he turned up at the right place and at the right time. This of course was only possible for ʻAbd al-Laṭīf because he received the patronage of highly placed persons.[63] He was for instance in Damascus on the day that Sultan Ṣalāḥ al-Dīn died and similarly he was in Aleppo when Sultan al-Malik al-Ẓāhir passed away. He moreover visited Egypt at the time of the plague and witnessed the famine and its accompanying horrors. From 1204 until 1212 A.D. ʻAbd al-Laṭīf remained in Damascus where he taught law at the *Madrasa al-ʻAzīzīyah* and studied independently. There he also educated many students in grammar and medicine.[64] Having carefully examined the historical data one can conclude that at the beginning of the year 609 A.H., i.e. 1212 A.D., an important event took place in Damascus. This event was the marriage between prince al-Malik al-Ẓāhir, the third Ayyūbid Sultan of Aleppo and his cousin Ḍaifah Khātūn bint al-ʻĀdil. The marriage pact was made in the month of *Muḥarram*, which is June 1212 A.D. In his *K. al-Sulūk li-maʻrifat duwal al-mulūk*, the historian al-Maqrīzī presents us with a fine description of the festivities which took place in that month:

> This year Ibn-Shaddād arrived in Damascus from Aleppo bringing a large sum of money and robes of honor for the celebration of the marriage between Ḍayfah, daughter of al-ʻĀdil, and her cousin al-Ẓāhir, prince of Aleppo. All the emirs and notables of the city went out to meet him. The marriage pact was made in the month of Muḥarram, on a dowry of 50,000 dīnārs. Pieces of gold were distributed in Muḥarram to the people in the citadel at Damascus. The princess was then equipped to go with great splendour to her spouse in Aleppo; among the things that went were cloths, instruments, and manufactured goods, borne on fifty mules, two hundred Bactrian camels, and three hundred (ordinary or one-humped) camels. Attendant maidens travelled on litters on a hundred camels, among them one hundred singers who could play a variety of musical instruments, and another hundred who could execute the most remarkable handicrafts. The day of her entry into Aleppo was a great occasion. Al-Ẓāhir presented her with his gifts, which included five strings of jewels that cost 150,000 dīnārs, a diadem of gems without equal, five amber necklaces ornamented with gold and five without

---

61 Manfred Ullmann, *Islamic Medicine* (Edinburgh 1978), at 80.

62 Toorawa, *Travel in the medieval Islamic world*, 63-64.

63 Toorawa, *Travel in the medieval Islamic world*, 55-59. Shawkat Toorawa has given the following definition of patronage: "Patronage is the support (financial and political), encouragement (moral, social and economic) and championing of an individual or group engaged in an activity without which they would otherwise have difficulty performing that activity".

64 Toorawa, *Travel in the medieval Islamic world*, 63.

such, 170 gold and silver objects, twenty linen bags filled with vestments, twenty handmaidens, and ten slaves.[65]

The historian Jamāl al-Dīn ibn Wāṣil more or less recorded the same story in his *Mufarrij al-kurūb fī akhbār Banī Ayyūb*, but his version also contains a short addition.[66]

The aforementioned Ibn Shaddād, who once was Ṣalāḥ al-Dīn's military judge, moved in 1195 A.D. from Damascus where he was in the service of al-Afḍal ʻAlī to enter that of another son of Ṣalāḥ al-Dīn, prince al-Malik al-Ẓāhir Ghāzī ibn Yūsuf at Aleppo. In Aleppo, he again served as *qāḍī* and exercised very wide authority.[67] The exchange of authoritative persons within the governing administration is a usual occurrence and a common practice within the system of patronage. ʻAbd al-Laṭīf found himself also under the patronage of Ṣalāḥ al-Dīn. Later he fell under the patronage of al-Malik al-Afḍal and al-Malik al-ʻAzīz in Damascus and Cairo and under al-Malik al-Ẓāhir in Aleppo. We can draw the conclusion that due to the system of patronage within the Ayyūbid dynasty ʻAbd al-Laṭīf journeyed to Aleppo in the month of *Muḥarram* 609 A.H. (i.e. June 1212 A.D.) as a consequence of the marriage between his new patron prince al-Malik al-Ẓāhir and Ḍaifah Khātūn bint al-ʻĀdil.

As an addition to the foregoing statement we need to take a closer look at the official position which both these men, ʻAbd al-Laṭīf and Joseph ben Judah, may have held at the court of the prince in Aleppo. It should, however, be put first and foremost that the Ayyūbid rulers and their predecessors the Fatimids did not knowingly promote the training and schooling of physicians, although they stimulated the private study of medicine and showed a great interest in it.[68] The study of medicine, which formed part of the foreign or ancient sciences, was not funded by the state, but financed through patronage. The major point of interest for the rulers was without a doubt the promotion of the study of the Islamic and the ancillary sciences. From ʻAbd al-Laṭīf's *Book of the Two Pieces of Advice* we understand that the Jewish physician Joseph ben Judah had a lot of influence over the other doctors which were present at the court in Aleppo. He for instance persuaded them to avoid bleeding the prince during his last sickness, and to resort to a different treatment. It has also been stated that he had control over the other doctors and could order them to do whatever he pleased. When Judah al-Ḥarizi visited Aleppo in the beginning of the year 1217 A.D., he moreover found Joseph

---

65 Ronald J.C. Broadhurst, *A History of the Ayyūbid Sultans of Egypt* (Boston 1980), 156-57.

66 Yasser Tabbaa, *Constructions of Power and Piety in Medieval Aleppo* (University Park/Penn. 1997), 48: 'When she entered the court of al-Malik al-Ẓāhir, he got up and took several steps towards her and showed her great respect'.

67 Donald Sidney Richards, *The Rare and Excellent History of Saladin or al-Nawādir al-Sulṭāniyya wa'l-Maḥāsin al-Yūsufiyya by Bahā' al-Dīn Ibn Shaddād translated by (...)* (Aldershot/Burlington 2002), 2.

68 Bärbel Köhler, *Die Wissenschaft unter den ägyptischen Fatimiden* (Hildesheim/Zürich/New York 1994), 131-33.

ben Judah at the peak of his professional glory. All this makes it plausible that Joseph ben Judah took a prominent position at the court. Perhaps he even may have held the post of chief physician (*ra'īs al-aṭibbā'* or *ra'īs sā'ir al-aṭibbā'*) or a similar position.

The Fatimids, for example, had a great liking for as many as possible titles. Besides a chief physician, who served the inhabitants of the palace, they knew the rank of a specialist (*al-khawāṣṣ* or *ṭabīb al-khāṣṣ*) who served the caliph only. Above the rank of specialist we find the private servants of the caliph (*ustādhūn*), who were in charge of the caliph's personal well-being and fulfilled special tasks for him.[69]

If we dig a little deeper and look at the medical profession in 12th century Byzantium, we also find a well-defined and well-developed hierarchical structure especially with regard to the staff of the *Pantokrator Xenon*. At the head of this legendary hospital were two *primmikerioi*, who outranked two *protomenitai*. Two physicians (*iatroi*) attended each of the five sections in the hospital. They were aided by three ordained medical assistants (*hypourgoi embathmoi*), two extra medical assistants (*hypourgoi perissoi*), and two servants (*hyperetai*) in each of the four sections for men. Apart from this, there were many other extra physicians amongst others for outdoor patients. The women's ward moreover had a hierarchical structure of its own.[70]

If we likewise attempt to take a closer look at 'Abd al-Laṭīf's rank as a physician we need to acknowledge Samira Jadon's observation that 'Abd al-Laṭīf served Ṣalāḥ al-Dīn as a teacher of medicine.[71] The latter is said to have provided 'Abd al-Laṭīf with a salary of 30 *dinars* a month, which was supplemented by Ṣalāḥ al-Dīn's sons to a total of 100 *dinars*. However, there is in my view no sound proof that he already taught medicine at that particular stage of his life, i.e. before the year 1193 A.D. It is much more credible to maintain that he was then a teacher of Islamic and ancillary sciences. Later on, in Cairo (1196-1202/03 A.D.) we find him teaching the Islamic sciences at the Azhar Mosque during the morning hours.[72] Mid-day, he would tutor students who wished to study medicine and other subjects at his house. From 1202/03-1204 A.D. he taught at the Aqṣā Mosque in Jerusalem 'on a variety of subjects'. In Damascus (1204-1212 A.D.) he taught law, grammar and medicine and studied independently.

---

69 Cf. Köhler, *Die Wissenschaft*, 119-123.

70 Timothy S. Miller, *The Birth of the Hospital in the Byzantine Empire* (Baltimore and London 1985, revised edition 1997), 15-16.

71 Samira Jadon, 'The Physicians of Syria during the Reign of Ṣalāḥ al-Dīn 570-589 A.H. 1174-1193 A.D.', *JHMAS* 25 (1970), 323-340, esp. 334.

72 This is according to a report by the chronicler Ibn abī Uṣaybi'a. The same Ibn abī Uṣaybi'a reported elsewhere that at that time the Azhar Mosque was supposed to have been closed by the Ayyūbids for ideological reasons, cf. Gary Leiser, 'Medical Education in Islamic Lands from the Seventh to the Fourteenth Century', *JHMAS* 38 (1983), 48-75, especially 55 (cf. there at footnote 29).

The salary of one hundred *dinars*, which 'Abd al-Laṭīf would receive for his services every month, equals the monthly wages of a private servant (*ustādh*) at the Fatimid court. A specialist at the Fatimid court was counted of less importance and would receive 50 *dinars*; a chief physician earned between 10 and 30 *dinars*. These amounts are more or less comparable to the wages that were paid at the Ayyūbid court. 'Abd al-Laṭīf held a post at the court in Aleppo which was similar qua job description to that of an *ustādh* at the Fatimid court.

However, 'Abd al-Laṭīf was an *ustādh* in the broadest sense of the word. Besides being a teacher of medicine and a sounding board for the physicians at court, he was also the confidant of the prince, a loyal servant who would do everything to keep his patron from harm and mischief. 'Abd al-Laṭīf's main treatise on alchemy, the *Risāla fī Mujādalat al-ḥakīmayn al-kīmiyā'ī wa-l-naẓarī*, lends weight to this argument and presents us with the information that he apparently had access to the private documents of prince al-Malik al-Ẓāhir,[73] while at the end of 'Abd al-Laṭīf's minor treatise on alchemy, the *Risāla fī l-Ma'ādin wa-ibṭāl al-kīmiyā'*, it is held that an alchemist asked for an introduction from 'Abd al-Laṭīf to his patron: al-Malik 'Alā' al-Dīn Dāwūd ibn Bahrām (Dāwūd Shāh), the governor of the Anatolian city of Erzinjān.[74] Here 'Abd al-Laṭīf acts as a mediator between a third party and the ruler, which seems to underline the important and influential position he held at the different courts. The death of prince al-Malik al-Ẓāhir did of course not much good to the already conked out relation of 'Abd al-Laṭīf and Joseph ben Judah. In the *Book of the Two Pieces of Advice* it is recounted that each one of the physicians who sat at the bedside of the prince gathered for a meeting to discuss and give an account of the ins and outs of the fatal treatment.

In these days it was common practice that the staff of physicians, present at a sultan's deathbed, would issue an official medical bulletin after he had succumbed to his disease.[75] In case of an 'ordinary' patient, the doctors would keep detailed notes on their patients, and, should someone in their care die, a chief physician, who usually would reside in town, would collect and examine these notes and decide whether the physician had been negligent and had to pay blood money.[76] In the case under consideration, it appears that a bulletin was issued, but for whom? Was it released for the public in general, or did a second bulletin also exist: an internal report, for physicians only? The text of the *Book of the Two Pieces of Advice* does

---

73 Franz Allemann, *'Abdallaṭīf al-Baġdādī: Ris. fī Mudjādalat al-ḥakīmain al-kīmiyā'ī wan-naẓarī ("Das Streitgespräch zwischen dem Alchemisten und dem theoretischen Philosophen"). Eine textkritische Bearbeitung der Handschrift: Bursa, Hüseyin Çelebi 823, fol. 100-123 mit Übersetzung und Kommentar*, [diss.] (Bern 1988), 120-21.

74 Stern, *A Collection of Treatises*, 67.

75 Felix Klein-Franke, 'What was the Fatal Disease of al-Malik al-Ṣāliḥ Najm al-Dīn Ayyūb?', in: Moshe Sharon (editor): *Studies in Islamic History and Civilization in Honour of Professor David Ayalon* (Jerusalem/Leiden 1986), 153-57, esp. 153.

76 Pormann, *The Physician and the Other*, 210; Martin Levey, 'Fourteenth Century Muslim Medicine and the Ḥisba', in: *Medical History* VII (1963), 176-182, at 177.

not give a decisive answer about it, although the latter is suspected of being the case.

It might well be that when Judah al-Ḥarizi visited Aleppo in the beginning of the year 1217 A.D., an enquiry was still being held on the questionable death of prince al-Malik al-Ẓāhir. This may explain al-Ḥarizi's observation that the physician (i.e. Joseph ben Judah) was in a state of distress, because one of his disciples had shown ingratitude towards him in a rather cruel and spiteful way. That Joseph ben Judah (through Judah al-Ḥarizi's report) addressed the anonymous person as a 'disciple' or a 'student' was perhaps prompted by the fact that it was not a done thing to wilfully disclose someone's identity.

'Abd al-Laṭīf, for his part, as well does not mention Joseph ben Judah by name and merely addresses him by a contemptuous term. Patronage had, besides huge advantages, its downside too. Insulting or accusing someone's protégé falsely could easily lead to very serious consequences for both the offender and his patron. The injured one and his benefactor would occasionally claim satisfaction from a third party by making use of brutal and drastic methods, which would actually serve no one.

In conclusion, we can state that although the two physicians, 'Abd al-Laṭīf al-Baghdādī and Joseph ben Judah, personally disliked each other, they were considered by the prince al-Malik al-Ẓāhir as professional craftsmen and caring and loyal subjects.

After the death of the prince, 'Abd al-Laṭīf stayed at the Court-Citadel in Aleppo until at least the year 1220 A.D. and then left the city.

The travelling poet Judah al-Ḥarizi visited Joseph ben Judah in Aleppo in the beginning of the year 1217 A.D. and found him at the pinnacle of his success. Proof of enquiries or inquisitions regarding the prince's death is not available to us. The documents which we possess, remain completely silent about the issue. The exact nature and circumstances of the prince's death therefore stay a mystery, and in consequence we are still unsure whether or not the prince al-Malik al-Ẓāhir Ghāzī ibn Yūsuf of Aleppo died of a natural cause or whether there were more lugubrious events, which contributed to his demise. Was there a conspiracy or perhaps a hush-hush policy? Only further evidence may help us to solve this rare conundrum in the future.

‘Abd al-Laṭīf al-Baghdādī and his Relation to Alchemy

In ‘Abd al-Laṭīf al-Baghdādī's day and age, long before the Paracelsian revolution took place,[77] alchemy or rather alchemical experimentation did not yet stand at the fundaments of theoretical and practical medical development, and therefore it could not be considered an *ancilla medicinae*. As a consequence, the relation between alchemy and medicine was just an external one: a stimulation or cross-pollination did not take place between these two fields of knowledge.

‘Abd al-Laṭīf engaged with alchemy for a short while only to abandon the art completely by rejecting not just its practice, but also its theory. He composed two passionate pamphlets against the vile art, but hardly touches upon it in his *Kitāb al-Naṣīḥatayn* or *Book of the Two Pieces of Advice*. In ‘Abd al-Laṭīf's view alchemy could not be placed in the system of the sciences, and its false presumptions and pretensions must be distinguished from true scientific knowledge which can be given a rational basis, such as mathematics, mineralogy, zoology, botany and of course also medicine.

It goes, however, without saying that the medical section of the *Kitāb al-Naṣīḥatayn* was composed as a so-called mirror: it would extol the noble art of medicine as practised by well-educated and dedicated physicians, and reject the practice of the abhorrent art of alchemy as practised by crooks, impostors, quacks and mountebanks. For this reason, it would perhaps be instructive or even instrumental, to seek the attention for ‘Abd al-Laṭīf's views on the art of alchemy here.

Unfortunately not much is known about the relationship of the polymath ‘Abd al-Laṭīf al-Baghdādī to the art of alchemy, and as a logical consequence the information that is available about his views on alchemy and its practitioners remains rather scarce. However, one must keep in mind that although it is far from easy to put oneself in the position of an historical figure who lived in bygone ages, it is certainly not an impossible task to reconstruct his world and milieu on the basis of the sources that are at our disposal, and about which we will report here on the best authority.

In 1962, with Samuel Miklos Stern's extensive description of the so-called Bursa manuscript,[78] the scholarly world became acquainted with the existence of ten thus far unknown treatises on a variety of subjects by ‘Abd al-Laṭīf and with one treatise (no. 9) by Alexander of Aphrodisias on the *differentia specifica*. Two of these treatises (no. 6 and no. 7) deal with the 'art' or 'craft' of alchemy. A good two years later, the German scholar Albert Dietrich released an edition and German translation of Bursa no. 9: the *Risāla lil-Iskandar fī l-faṣl khāṣṣatan wa-mā huwa* by Alexander of Aphrodisias, to which Dietrich also added a description of the entire

---

77 Charles Webster, *Paracelsus: Medicine, Magic and Mission at the End of Time* (New Haven and London 2008).

78 Stern, *A Collection of Treatises*, 53-70.

Bursa manuscript.[79] In the year 1972 Paul Ghalioungui and Said Abdou presented us with a detailed description of the Bursa manuscript in the Arabic language,[80] and in 1993 Seyfullah Sevim published a short essay on ‘Abd al-Laṭīf's views on alchemy and chemistry in the Turkish language.[81] But the by far most elaborate publication on the subject came to us in 1988 through the unpublished Ph.D. dissertation of the Swiss scholar Franz Allemann.[82]

Allemann prepared a critical edition of Bursa no. 6, to which he added a German translation and an extensive commentary apart from some very useful appendices. Unfortunately, Allemann could not hold the limelight and accordingly his fascinating dissertation did not receive the attention it so well deserved. In fact, it almost became forgotten, which has created a rather undesirable and unjust situation, because the work under consideration gives us an excellent insight into the author ‘Abd al-Laṭīf al-Baghdādī, his material, his sources and his social *Umfeld.* A brief introduction to ‘Abd al-Laṭīf al-Baghdādī's views on alchemy and all its transgressions was published in the year 2008 by the present author.[83]

The author Muwaffaq al-Dīn ‘Abd al-Laṭīf ibn Yūsuf al-Baghdādī (*557A.H. - †12 *Muḥarram* 629 A.H./*1162 A.D. - †9 November 1231 A.D.) dealt with the subject of alchemy in two tractates. The first tractate (no. 6), which bears the title *Risāla fī Muǧādalat al-ḥakīmayn al-kīmiyā’ī wa-l-naẓarī* ('a dispute between an adherent of alchemy and an adherent of theoretical philosophy') and has been preserved in the unique manuscript Bursa, Hüseyin Çelebi 823, fol. 100b-123b, has aroused our interest to a large extent. The treatise has been written during ‘Abd al-Laṭīf's first visit to Aleppo (609-617 A.H./1212-1220 A.D.) and was most probably revised in Erzinjān in the year 622 A.H. by the author himself.

The literary form of the tractate is that of the debate. ‘Abd al-Laṭīf applied an ornate and exceptionally varied style which is frequently adorned and embellished with rhyming prose of a very forceful, nonetheless elegant nature. There are two parties in the discussion: the alchemist and the philosopher. Both the parties to the discussion are not mentioned by name, but if we take a closer look at the scientific development of the author and his relation to alchemy, it goes without saying that the philosopher stands for ‘Abd al-Laṭīf himself. The figure of the alchemist has probably been composed of several persons. It is unlikely that the tractate presents

---

[79] Dietrich, *Die arabische Version*, 85-148.

[80] Ghalioungui and Abdou, *Maqālatān fī l-Ḫawāss*, 27-35.

[81] Seyfeddin (Seyfullah) Sevim, 'Abdüllâtif Bağdadi'nin Kimya-Simya Hakkindaki Görüşleri', in: Ahmet Hulūsi Köker: *Abdüllātif Bağdādi*, Kayseri: Erciyes Üniversitesi Matbaasi, Turkey [Erciyes Üniversitesi Gevher Nesibe Tip Tarihi Enstitüsü; Yayin No: 14 – Gevher Nesibe Sultan Anisina Düzenlenen Abdüllātif Bağdādī Kongresi tebliğleri 14 Mart 1992 Kayseri] (Kayseri 1993), 57-67.

[82] Allemann, *Ris. fī Muǧādalat.*

[83] N. Peter Joosse, "Unmasking the Craft': ‘Abd al-Laṭīf al-Baghdādī's Views on Alchemy and Alchemists', in: Anna A. Akasoy and Wim Raven (eds.): *Islamic Thought in the Middle Ages. Studies in Text, Transmission and Translation, in Honour of Hans Daiber* (Leiden/Boston 2008), 301-17.

us with a record of a debate which took place in reality. The external structure of the dispute is most likely fiction although it must be partly based on discussions between ‘Abd al-Laṭīf and his former advisors and mentors like for example Ibn at-Tātalī, or between him and vague acquaintances like for instance Yāsīn as-Sīmiyā’ī (Yāsīn, the word magician, or rather the letter magician).[84] There are two distinctive encounters between ‘Abd al-Laṭīf and Ibn at-Tātalī. The first one takes place in Baghdād in the year 577 A.H./1181 A.D. The second meeting is roughly nine years later in Damascus. The Almoravid Ibn at-Tātalī is supposed to be a Moroccan wandering tutor who left the Maghrib upon the accession of the Almohad 'caliph' ‘Abd al-Mu’min b. ‘Alī b. ‘Alwī in 524 A.H./1130 A.D.[85] When Ibn at-Tātalī, a man of imposing appearance who dressed in the robe of the Sufis, arrived in Baghdād he impressed everyone with his eloquence, erudition and charisma. A number of notables gathered around him to profit from his teachings, and he is supposed to have received influential men like Raḍī al-Dīn al-Qazwīnī and Ibn Sakīna. Ibn at-Tātalī was an authority on the works of Jābir ibn Ḥayyān (or Latin: Geber) and Ibn Waḥshīya and studied their books on alchemy and talismanic magic very thoroughly. Initially, he also did not fail to impress ‘Abd al-Laṭīf and thus filled the latter's heart with 'a desire to know all the sciences' (*shawqan li l-‘ulūm kullihā*), but in retrospect he questions Ibn at-Tātalī's knowledge and accuses him of having had a rather superficial awareness of the subject-matter of his teachings.

When Ibn at-Tātalī left to join the caliph Nāṣir li-dīn Allāh (575/1180-622/1233), ‘Abd al-Laṭīf settled down to assiduous study and applied himself with ardour to the analysis of the works of al-Ghazālī, Jābir ibn Ḥayyān and Ibn Waḥshīyah. He also read all the works of Ibn Sīnā and got hold of a copy the *K. al-Taḥṣīl* of Bahmanyār ibn al-Marzubān, a disciple of Ibn Sīnā.[86] Moreover, he started reading works on arithmetic and comprehended Euclid's *K. al-Uṣūl* (*Elements*).

In the year 586 A.H./1190 A.D. ‘Abd al-Laṭīf and Ibn at-Tātalī met anew.[87] At the time, Ibn at-Tātalī was living in the *Ma’dhana al-Gharbīya*, the western minaret, in Damascus where he lectured on alchemy and hermetic philosophy. He had become the subject of controversy and had two factions around him, one in

---

84 Allemann, *Ris. fī Muğādalat*, 62-3; cf. also Pierre Lory, *La science des lettres en islam* (Paris 2004), who considers *sīmiyā'* an art much similar to alchemy, in which the transmutation of the letter or word was practised instead of the transmutation of matter. Dictionaries of modern standard Arabic (MSA), like for instance that of Hans Wehr, usually render the term with 'natural magic'.

85 Shawkat Mahmood Toorawa, 'The Educational Background of ‘Abd al-Laṭīf al-Baghdādī', in: *Muslim Education Quarterly* 13 (1996), 35-53, especially 41; Allemann, *Ris. fī Muğādalat*, 13-15.

86 Jules Janssens, 'Bahmanyār Ibn Marzubān: A Faithful Disciple of Ibn Sīnā?', in: David C. Reisman (ed.): *Before and After Avicenna. Proceedings of the First Conference of the Avicenna Study Group* (Leiden and Boston 2003), 177-197.

87 Toorawa, *The Educational Background*, 44; *idem*, *The Autobiography of ‘Abd al-Laṭīf al-Baghdādī (1162-1231)*, 156-164, especially 160; Allemann, *Ris. fī Muğādalat*, 17-18.

favour of him and the other against him; the latter included the preacher and scholar in the domain of *fiqh* al-Khaṭīb al-Dawla'ī. When 'Abd al-Laṭīf found out that Ibn at-Tātalī ruined himself in an intellectual as well as in a materialistic sense, he scolded him badly and reproached him for delving into alchemy and hermetic philosophy in such a superficial way, and strongly advised him to abandon these deceiving sciences permanently. Ibn at-Tātalī did not follow up 'Abd al-Laṭīf's well-meant advice and left for the camp of Ṣalāḥ al-Dīn before Acre, to complain to him of the behaviour of al-Khaṭīb al-Dawla'ī and perhaps also of 'Abd al-Laṭīf's bad conduct. After Ibn at-Tātalī left, 'Abd al-Laṭīf realized that his tutor was not the man he imagined him to be. He pondered over his state and was warned by his evil end, which made him give up the craft of alchemy, but not entirely! The past student had become the master by now. In Baghdād, 'Abd al-Laṭīf still stood in awe of his master Ibn at-Tātalī and was keen to know all the sciences (including alchemy) taught by him, while in Damascus 'Abd al-Laṭīf formed a bad opinion of his master and tried to pull him way from the evil influences of alchemy and related sciences.

Toorawa does not mention Ibn at-Tātalī, but opts for the alternate reading of 'Abdallāh ibn Nā'ilī.[88] I do not see any reason to follow Toorawa's example here since both names cannot be identified in a conclusive manner. The name 'Abdallāh ibn Nā'ilī of course reminds us of that of Abū 'Abdallāh an-Nātilī, who was one of the first tutors of Ibn Sīnā. Ibn Sīnā considered him a person who possessed only a slight and shallow understanding of the various sciences he taught and who was not able to conduct a proper analysis of the works he studied. The wandering philosopher an-Nātilī is known as a reviser of Dioscorides's book on medicinal plants (*Materia Medica*). Together with an-Nātilī, Ibn Sīnā studied Porphyry's *Eisagoge*, Ptolemy's *Almagest* and Euclid's *Elements*.[89]

If we would compare the autobiographies of Ibn Sīnā and 'Abd al-Laṭīf we would find out that both scholars were in search for mentors and tutors in many different branches of science. Ibn Sīnā already gave up looking for suitable teachers at a tender age, after his unsatisfactory meeting with an-Nātilī, and then managed to study and master all the sciences by himself. At the age of sixteen, he excelled in the study of medicine, to the point that distinguished physicians began to read the science of medicine under him. He regarded medicine as one of the easy sciences (*wa-'ilm aṭ-ṭibb laysa huwa min al-'ulūm al-ṣa'ba*).[90] When he reached the age of eighteen he was finished with all the sciences and considered himself fully-qualified in them.[91]

'Abd al-Laṭīf, on the other hand, believed that he had to persevere in the search for good teachers although he felt –not unlike Ibn Sīnā– that the majority of his

---

88 Toorawa, *The Educational Background*, 41-42 and 44.

89 Gotthard Strohmaier, *Avicenna* (München 1999), 21-23 and 97-98; William E. Gohlman, *The Life of Ibn Sina. A Critical Edition and Annotated Translation* (Albany/New York 1974), 21-25.

90 Gohlman, *Life of Ibn Sina*, 24-25.

91 Gohlman, *Life of Ibn Sina*, 36-37.

teachers were not capable of imparting knowledge to him, and that he conceptualized the subject matter better than his masters. ʻAbd al-Laṭīf's search for the perfect master only ended on the day he encountered the wise Shaykh Abū al-Qāsim al-Shāriʻī during his prolonged stay in Cairo.

The alchemist Ibn at-Tātalī has been mentioned only in Ibn abī Uṣaybiʻa's autobiographical portrait of ʻAbd al-Laṭīf.[92] Information regarding him is lacking in the *K. al-Naṣīḥatayn* and the other autobiographical fragments.

ʻAbd al-Laṭīf briefly refers to the alchemist and magician Yāsīn as-Sīmiyā'ī (or perhaps: al-Kīmiyā'ī) in both the autobiographical reports.[93] The idea has been suggested that Yāsīn was Abū al-Ṭāhir Ismāʻīl b. Ṣāliḥ b. Yāsīn al-Sāʻī of the *Shadharāt.*[94] However, it is a more likely, although not a conclusive, option to assume that Yāsīn as-Sīmiyā'ī is a pseudonym for Abū al-Qāsim Muḥammad b. Aḥmad al-Simāwī, known as al-ʻIrāqī.[95] Al-Simāwī is said to be the author of several books on the cultivation of gold (e.g. *K. al-ʻIlm al-muktasab fī zirāʻat adh-dhahab*; *K. Zubda aṭ-ṭalab fī zarʻ adh-dhahab*[96]), and on the knowledge of the elixir (e.g. *K. ʻArf al-abīr fī ʻilm al-iksīr*).[97] Apart from that, he also wrote two other alchemical works: *K. al-Aqālīm al-sabʻa*, "The Book of the Seven Climes"; and *K. al-Kanz al-afkhar*, "The Most Glorious Treasure". All these books contain a curious mixture of alchemical processes, lists of alchemical *Decknamen*,[98] drawings of alchemical equipment and operations, alchemical legends, sayings of famous persons from the past as for instance Plato, Aristotle, Hermes, Pythagoras, Mary the Copt, Zosimos and many others, and much trivial matter which was obviously

---

92 That is, in August Müller's edition, but not in Nizār Riḍā's edition. In the latter edition, we find the name Ibn Nā'ilī.

93 Allemann, *Ris. fī Muğādalat*, 18 and 117; Ibn abī Uṣaybiʻa, *K. ʻUyūn al-anbā' fī ṭabaqāt al-aṭibbā'*, ed. Imru'ulqais b. aṭ-Ṭaḥḥān (August Müller), Djuz' 1.2. (Cairo-Königsberg 1299 A.H./1882 A.D.), Vol. 2, 205, line 24-29; Toorawa, *The Autobiography of ʻAbd al-Laṭīf al-Baghdādī (1162-1231)*, 161; H.A.R. Gibb, 'Life of Muwaffiq Ad-Din Abd al-Latif of Baghdad by Ibn Abi Usaybiya [Translated from the Persian, and for the first time rendered into English]', in: R.H. Saunders (editor), *Healing through Spirit Agency by the Great Persian Physician Abduhl Latif ("The Man of Baghdad") and information concerning The Life Hereafter of the deepest interest to all enquirers and students of Psychic phenomena* (London 1927), 75.

94 Toorawa, *The Educational Background*, 45.

95 Cf. *Kitāb al-ʻIlm al-muktasab fī zirāʻat adh-dhahab. Book of Knowledge Acquired Concerning the Cultivation of Gold by Abu 'l-Qāsim Muḥammad ibn Aḥmad al-'Irāqī*, ed. and tr. by Erik John Holmyard (Paris 1923). [cf. also Manfred Ullmann, *Die Natur- und Geheimwissenschaften im Islam* (Handbuch der Orientalistik, I. Abt., Erg.-Bd. VI, 2) (Leiden/Köln 1972), 235-37; Toorawa, *The Educational Background*, 45; *idem, A Portrait*, 91-109, especially 104; Holmyard, 'Abu' l-Qāsim al-'Irāqī', in: *Isis* VIII (1926), 403-26].

96 Apparently this book is not extant, cf. Holmyard, *Abu' l-Qāsim al-'Irāqī*, 412, note 21.

97 Apparently this book is likewise not extant, cf. Holmyard, *Abu' l-Qāsim al-'Irāqī*, 413, note 28.

98 Cf. Alfred Siggel, *Decknamen in der arabischen alchemistischen Literatur* (Berlin 1951).

meant as some kind of jest.[99] Moreover, he is also known as the author of a couple of books on magic: the *K. al-Ishārāt al-juz'īya* and the *K. 'Uyūn al-ḥaqā'iq wa-īḍāḥ aṭ-ṭarā'iq*, "The Sources of Initiation and the Clarification of [magic] Methods".[100]

The actual debate between the alchemist and the philosopher has been embedded in a frame story. The author is invited by a person -who is simply addressed as "you"- to relate about the dispute. The author belongs himself to the circle of listeners and joins in on the conversation only once and moreover in a non-direct way. Apart from this, he merely acts as a minute-keeper, who from time to time sketches the mood of the participants in the discussion. At the beginning and at the end of the debate, he adds the distinctly instructive passages while focussing on the main points of the discussion. The debate takes place on two different days, during two separate sessions. In the first session the philosopher refutes alchemy in no uncertain terms. Surprisingly, the alchemist has no reply to the verbiage and in fact is not able to get a word in at all. 'Abd al-Laṭīf although mentions in his preface that both the philosopher and the alchemist were outstanding representatives of their respective branches of science. In the second session the alchemist appears as someone who has just been chastened by the philosophical wisdom which his opponent scattered over him. He abandons and renounces "the abominable craft" and out of gratitude towards God and the philosopher, he decides to destroy all his own works on alchemy and finally gives up alchemy altogether. Moreover, it soon becomes clear from the narrative that the theoretical or speculative philosopher (*ḥakīm al-naẓarī*) also represents 'Abd al-Laṭīf's *alter ego*.

The definition of the genre presents us with a serious problem. Following the perusal of the previous version of this chapter by some of my honoured colleagues, it was suggested to me that the anecdotes, which form the major part of the tractate, were merely composed to serve as amusement or jest. It was stated that these anecdotes were to correspond qua contents and style with the communications of al-Jaubarī on quacks and charlatans and that they could be interpreted in two different ways. However, this is far removed from the truth in view of the fact that amusement has the connotation of entertainment. These forbidding, dismal and sinister anecdotes are hardly entertaining and qua atmosphere they on no account show similarities to the rather light-hearted stories of al-Jaubarī.[101] Moreover, there

---

[99] Holmyard, *Abu' l-Qāsim al-'Irāqī*, 417: "Another amusement: If you would like to amuse yourself at the expense of a dog, by making him leap and bound with delight, make a small cake of bread kneaded up with cinnamon and pepper. When the dog eats it he will go out of his mind on account of the excessive joy and excitement which he experiences".

[100] Cf. Ullmann, *Die Natur- und Geheimwissenschaften*, 391-92. Ullmann has rendered *'Uyūn al-ḥaqā'iq* as "Die Quellen der Wahrheiten", but most likely *ḥaqīqa* is used here in the mystical sense of "initiation". Cf. also Holmyard, *Abu' l-Qāsim al-'Irāqī*, 413, note 27.

[101] Eilhard Wiedemann 'Über Charlatane bei den Muslimen nach al-Gaubarī', in: *Sitzungsberichte der Physikalisch-medizinischen Sozietät zu Erlangen*, Erlangen, Bd. 43 (1911), 206-232. [Reprint in: Eilhard Wiedemann, *Aufsätze zur arabischen*

is no question of ambiguity here, so that they can only be interpreted in one way. They have to be considered a grave and stern warning against the concealment of so-called "unspeakable things" and against the dangerous increase of utter simplicity and gullibility among the masses in the author's time. The author genuinely feared that the rise and spread of alchemy, astrology and magic would threaten rational thought, especially because these false arts were looked upon as true sciences by the great majority of the population, and even by quite a few scholars.

In the words of J. Christoph Bürgel, it is stated that these pseudo-sciences were hothouses of irrationalism, the rational disguise making them only more harmful.[102]

'Abd al-Laṭīf considered them extremely dangerous and believed them to be a menace to science in general and in particular to rational medicine, i.e. Galenic medicine.

Allemann proposed to classify the tractate under the heading *Die Kontroversliteratur über die Wahrheit der Alchemie.*[103] But because in this specific type of literature the discussion takes place on the basis of premises, which can neither be proved nor disproved, a solution or a step forward in the discussion can never be realized.[104] At the first glance, the treatise in question indeed seems to focus on the discussion of the truth, the value and the scientific character of alchemy. However, it soon becomes clear that its actual goal is to brand alchemy as a complete fraud and to show its evil and immoral nature. Therefore, it is not too hard to predict that in the given dialogue the alchemist is defeated by the philosopher, who in the course of his speech quotes a number of anecdotes of contemporary cases of fraudulent alchemists, con-artists and foolish dupes.

We are also in favour of a classification of our tractate under the header *Kontroversliteratur*, but believe that this classification is not sufficient to give a comprehensive overview of the genre. In order to give a more detailed and well-considered picture of the genre, a sub-division should be introduced. Thus it goes without saying that our tractate should be classified under a new header, which may be defined as *Paränetische Literatur* (paranetic literature), a type of literature in which the author intends to warn against the pitfalls of the ideologies, aims and objectives of false alchemists/physicians/philosophers, charlatans and quacks as well as to provide a holistic understanding that should he not warn the people, the communities would suffer untold harm. In short, should his warnings not be taken to heart, the masses would not be protected against the false ideologies, motives and pretences propounded by the deceivers of this world.

Alchemy is of a twofold nature, an outward or exoteric and a hidden or esoteric.

Wissenschaftsgeschichte I (Collectanea VI/1) mit einem Vorwort und Indices herausgegeben von Wolfdietrich Fischer (Hildesheim/New York 1970), 749-775]; cf. also Lawrence M. Principe, *The Secrets of Alchemy* (Chicago/London 2013), at 49-50.

102 Bürgel, *Secular and Religious Features*, 44-62, especially 54.

103 Allemann, *Ris. fī Muǧādalat*, 1 and 64; cf. also Ullmann, *Die Natur- und Geheimwissenschaften*, 249-55.

104 Cf. Ullmann, *Die Natur- und Geheimwissenschaften*, 249.

Exoteric alchemy is concerned with the attempts to produce a substance known as the elixir or the tincture, which was sometimes also called by the name "Philosophers' stone" or "sublime stone". The main goal of these false alchemists was to prepare such an elixir or tincture. They believed in the substantial transmutation of metals and thought that the *differentia specifica* of metals could be produced during an artificial process, which in the end would always lead to the transformation of the base metals lead, tin, copper, iron, and mercury into the precious metals gold and silver.[105] The true alchemists, or rather chemists, were more interested in the colouring or dying of metals and in producing alloys. They rejected the substantial transmutation of metals vehemently.[106]

Esoteric alchemy or mystical alchemy was developed through the belief that the elixir could only be obtained by divine grace. The transformation of metals became merely symbolic of the transformation of a sinful man into a perfect being through prayer and submission to God's will.[107]

Both in exoteric alchemy as well as in esoteric alchemy, the alchemists used to describe their theories, materials, and operations in a cryptic language full of allegories, allusions, analogies, metaphors, and riddles.[108] This was on occasion done for reasons of safety, but often selfish motives predominated. There was, however, not always a clear-cut division between the two types of alchemy. The language of exoteric alchemy was for instance frequently used in esoteric treatises for the sole purpose of expressing theological, philosophical, or mystical beliefs and views.[109]

Before entering at some length into the stories itself, it might perhaps be fitting here to call the attention once more to the author Muwaffaq al-Dīn ʻAbd al-Laṭīf ibn Yūsuf al-Baghdādī, who is also known as Ibn al-Labbād, the son of the felt-maker, by briefly introducing him in 'what lies beneath'.

In his *Paradise of Wisdom*, the 9th century Arab physician ʻAlī ibn Rabbān aṭ-Ṭabarī laconically observes that one should not live in a country in which four things do not occur: a sound government, running water, useful medicine and a cultivated and skilful physician. The educated physician, the *ḥakīm*, became one of the idealized pictures of medieval Arab society.[110] Having had no proper education

---

105 That this idea is wide-spread shows its frequent occurrence in works of fiction; cf. for instance Marten Toonder, 'De loodhervormer', in: *Een groot denkraam* (Amsterdam 1972; separate edition: Amsterdam 2005), 185-245; cf. also Joanne Kathleen Rowling, *Harry Potter and the Philosopher's Stone* (London 1997).

106 Allemann, *Ris. fī Muğādalat*, 42-44; Ullmann, *Die Natur- und Geheimwissenschaften*, 257-61.

107 Holmyard, *Alchemy. The story of the fascination of gold and the attempts of chemists, mystics, and charlatans to find the Philosophers' Stone* (Harmondsworth 1957), 13-14.

108 Holmyard, *Alchemy*, 14; Allison Coudert, *Alchemy: the Philosopher's stone* (Boulder (Colorado), 1980), Ch.III, 62-79.

109 Holmyard, *ibid.*, 14.

110 Heinrich Schipperges, 'Zum Bildungsweg eines arabischen Arztes', in: *Orvostörténeti Közlemények* 60-61 (1971), 13-31, especially 13.

from a famous teacher caused one's honour to be at stake, was considered a very shameful matter and could bring harm to one's future career.[111] 'Abd al-Laṭīf's father, Yūsuf, a devoted scholar in the field of the religious law and by no means a felt-maker, must have been extremely aware of this problem. He must have encouraged his son from a young age to learn from a multitude of teachers. Ibn abī Uṣaybi'a has quoted extensively from the autograph notes of 'Abd al-Laṭīf. The following text –apparently written by 'Abd al-Laṭīf at a ripe age– contains his well-meant advice to students in the form of a collection of aphorisms:

I commend you not to learn your sciences from books unaided, even though you may trust your ability to understand. Resort to professors for each science you seek to acquire; and should your professor be limited in his knowledge take all that he can offer, until you find another more accomplished than he. You must hold him in the highest regard and respect him; and if you can render him assistance from your worldly goods, do so; if not, then do so by word of mouth, singing his praises.[112]

It is most awkward to learn that 'Abd al-Laṭīf gave such pedantic educational advice to (his) students, primarily because he very often did not seem to have practised what he preached himself. He was moreover not the paragon of virtue which Ibn abī Uṣaybi'a wants to make of him here. Although Ibn abī Uṣaybi'a reports to have taken the sayings from 'Abd al-Laṭīf's own handwriting, it is strange to observe that its contents are sharply in contrast with the autobiographical fragments and many of 'Abd al-Laṭīf's other writings qua tenor and tone. An exception too is perhaps his work *K. al-Ṭibb min al-kitāb wa l-sunna*,[113] 'Abd al-Laṭīf's alleged book on the medicine of the prophet, which contains a combination of religious and medical information, providing advice and guidance on the two aims of medicine, i.e. the preservation and the restoration of health, in careful conformity with the teachings of Islam as laid down in the Koran and the prophetic traditions.

The demonstration and elucidation of the -intricate and at times not so intricate-relationship between different fields (and themes) of science holds an important position in 'Abd al-Laṭīf's works. Most of the time, this was done by him in a very attractive and captivating, although far from light-hearted style. The book on prophetic medicine is, however, written in a rather scholastic, uncomfortable and unattractive style: it is rigid and wooden and happens to be interspersed with an almost non-natural piousness that is quite indistinctive and uncharacteristic of our author. One sincerely may want to question 'Abd al-Laṭīf's authorship of this work on prophetic medicine, which apparently formed the nucleus for Ibn Qaiyim al-Jawzīya's *Medicine of the Prophet* (*al-Ṭibb al-nabawī*). The latter work is said to

---

111 Schipperges, *Zum Bildungsweg*, 16.

112 George Makdisi, *The Rise of Colleges. Institutions of Learning in Islam and the West* (Edinburgh 1981), 89; Gibb, *Life of Muwaffiq Ad-Din Abd al-Latif of Baghdad by Ibn Abi Usaybiya*, 83-84; Ibn abī Uṣaybi'a, *K. 'Uyūn al-anbā' fī-ṭabaqāt al-aṭibbā'*, ed. Imru'ulqais b. aṭ-Ṭaḥḥān (August Müller), Vol. 2, 208-209.

113 'Abd al-Mu'ṭī Amīn Qal'ajī (editor), *Al-Ṭibb min al-kitāb wa l-sunna* (by [Pseudo-] Muwaffaq al-Dīn 'Abd al-Laṭīf al-Baghdādī), (Beirut 1406/1986).

have followed 'Abd al-Laṭīf's(?) example step by step.[114] I arrived at this negative conclusion primarily on the basis of stylistic features. However, as it appears now, the Finnish scholar Irmeli Perho many years ago already provided solid proof for the arguments against it being a composition by 'Abd al-Laṭīf.[115] Perho attributed the work with good reasons, i.e. on the basis of chronology, to the 13th century Damascene scholar Shams al-Dīn al-Dhahabī.[116] The mistake of attributing the text to 'Abd al-Laṭīf may be based on the fact that he, or actually one of his students Muḥammad ibn Yūsuf al-Birzālī (d. 636/1239), had written a book on the Prophet's medicine under the title *al-Arba'īn al-ṭibbīya al-mustakhraja min sunan Ibn Māja*. This book was apparently used extensively as a source for *al-Ṭibb al-nabawī*.[117]

Because the biographical and autobiographical *curriculum vitae* of 'Abd al-Laṭīf is fairly broad and readily available to many, it does not make good sense to treat it here in full detail. Instead of it, I shall present in a more or less chronological order, some examples of the development of 'Abd al-Laṭīf's attitude towards his teachers and mentors and towards the ones intended by him to become his teachers and mentors.[118] At an early age 'Abd al-Laṭīf was put under the care of Kamāl al-Dīn 'Abd ar-Raḥmān al-Anbārī: 'Abd al-Laṭīf couldn't understand any of his continuous and considerable jabber, although he states that Kamāl al-Dīn's other students seemed pleased enough with it. However, Kamāl al-Dīn did not like to teach children and sent the young 'Abd al-Laṭīf to his pupil Abū Bakr al-Wajīh al-Wāsiṭī of whom 'Abd al-Laṭīf afterwards would say that he outstripped him in powers of memory and understanding. 'Abd al-Laṭīf used al-Wajīh to get ahead. He surpassed him and enjoyed the double advantage of al-Wajīh's and Kamāl al-Dīn's initiatory company. (Raḍī al-Dawla Abū Naṣr) Ibn Hibat Allāh b. Ṣā'id taught 'Abd al-Laṭīf in medicine. 'Abd al-Laṭīf calls the son of the celebrated physician Ibn at-Tilmīdh in his *K. al-Naṣīḥatayn* the only person who, in the true sense of the word, is worthy enough to be called a (true) physician.[119]

Ibn abī Uṣaybi'a, however, states in his *'Uyūn* that Ibn Hibat Allāh b. Ṣā'id was not of such high merit and that 'Abd al-Laṭīf only praised him so highly because of his extreme partiality for the Iraqis. Apart from Ibn at-Tilmīdh there is only one

---

114 Cf. Qal'ajī, *Al-Ṭibb*, 53; Ibn Qaiyim al-Jawzīya, *Medicine of the Prophet* (*Ṭibb al-nabawī*), translated by Penelope Johnstone (Cambridge 1998). Ibn Qaiyim's *Ṭibb al-nabawī* forms part of his larger work the *Zād al-Ma'ād* or *The Victuals of Pilgrimage*.

115 Irmeli Perho, *The Prophet's Medicine: A Creation of the Muslim Traditionalist Scholars* (Helsinki 1995), 36-40; cf. also Peter E. Pormann and Emilie Savage-Smith, *Medieval Islamic Medicine* (Edinburgh 2007), 73-74, and 79: note 64.

116 Perho, *The Prophet's Medicine*, 36-40; Pormann and Savage-Smith, *Medieval Islamic Medicine*, 73-74, and 79: note 63.

117 Perho, *The Prophet's Medicine*, 39 and 56.

118 Cf. among others: Toorawa, *The Educational Background*, 35-53; Makdisi, *Rise of Colleges*, 84-91; Ibn abī Uṣaybi'a, *K. 'Uyūn al-anbā' fī-ṭabaqāt al-aṭibbā'*, ed. Imru'ulqais b. aṭ-Ṭaḥḥān (August Müller), Vol. 2, 201-13.

119 Cf. Stern, *A Collection of Treatises*, 64; Allemann, *Ris. fī Muğādalat*, 13; Ms. Bursa, Hüseyin Çelebi 823, fol. 89v, line 17-89r, line 1.

other physician to receive the same amount of credits from ‘Abd al-Laṭīf. This person is Abū Ja‘far Aḥmad b. abī l-Ash‘ath (died ca. 360 A.H./970 A.D.). ‘Abd al-Laṭīf puts him on a par with Hippocrates and Galen and calls him the last physician in the Islamic period, worthy to be counted among these "Ancients".[120] ‘Abd al-Laṭīf is reported to have written a compendium of Ibn abī l-Ash‘ath's *K. al-Ḥayawān* ("The Book of Animals") and of his *K. al-Qūlanj* ("The Book of Colic"). His compendium of the *K. al-Ḥayawān* is expected to be the source of the many Ibn abī l-Ash‘ath-quotations found in later works.[121]

Ibn at-Tātalī (or: Ibn Nā’ilī, or: al-Bābilī) initially filled ‘Abd al-Laṭīf's heart with a yearning for all knowledge, but in retrospect he calls him a dabbler who attached value to "procedures" thought contemptible and trivial. One day ‘Abd al-Laṭīf addressed him in the following way:

If you had devoted the time you have wasted in the pursuit of the craft to some of the Islamic or rational sciences you would today be without equal, waited on hand and foot. This alchemy nonsense simply does not have the answers you seek.

In search of a new master ‘Abd al-Laṭīf went from Baghdād to Mosul. He was disappointed there, although he did meet al-Kamāl ibn Yūnus (1156-1242 A.D.),[122] who was an expert in mathematics and jurisprudence, but only partially learned in the other branches of knowledge and unfortunately much misguided. His love of alchemy and his work in connection with it, so absorbed his mind and his time that he thought little of anything else. It has been said that as a young man, al-Kamāl ibn Yūnus had philosophical/theological discussions with Michael the Syrian, the West-Syrian Patriarch of Antioch (d. A.D. 1199).[123] Later in life, he became the renowned

---

[120] Cf. Stern, *A Collection of Treatises*, 62; Ms. Bursa, Hüseyin Çelebi 823, fol. 73v, line 17.

[121] Kruk, *Ibn abī l-Ash‘ath's Kitāb al-Ḥayawān*, 119-168, especially 162-63.

[122] Cf. Toorawa, *The Educational Background*, 43: "...Fortunately for him, he came across such scholars as al-Kamāl b. Yūnus". This remark does not fully justify ‘Abd al-Laṭīf's impression of al-Kamāl ibn Yūnus. ‘Abd al-Laṭīf's meeting with al-Kamāl cannot be called 'fortunate' at all, because ‘Abd al-Laṭīf apparently did not learn much from the famous scholar. According to ‘Abd al-Laṭīf, al-Kamāl's love of alchemy and its practice had so drowned his intellect and his time that he dismissed and disdained everything else (cf. Toorawa, *The Autobiography of ‘Abd al-Laṭīf al-Baghdādī (1162-1231)*, 159).

[123] Francis E. Peters, *Aristotle and the Arabs: The Aristotelian Tradition in Islam* (New York/London 1968), 277; cf. also Dorothea Weltecke, *Die «Beschreibung der Zeiten» von Mōr Michael dem Grossen (1126-1199). Eine Studie zu ihrem historischen und historiographie-geschichtlichen Kontext* (Louvain-la-Neuve 2003), 108, 118. [= CSCO Vol. 594, Subsidia Tomus 110]. Weltecke mentions the presence of the Persian philosopher Kemal ad-Dīn from the court of the Rūm Saljūq Sultan Qilij Arslan II Ibn Mas‘ūd, who in the year 1182 A.D. accompanied the Sultan and Patriarch Michael on their trip from Melitene, and contributed to their discussions on the Christian faith. Was the Persian philosopher Kemal ad-Dīn actually al-Kamāl ibn Yūnus al-Mawsilī, who was otherwise known as Kamāl ad-Dīn ibn Mana? See for the latter: Ibn Khallikān, *K. Wafayāt al-a‘yān wa-anbā' abnā' al-zamān*, [E] tr. Baron W. McGuckin de Slane, *Ibn Khallikan's Biographical Dictionary*, 4 vols. (Paris-London 1842-1871) [Reprint: Beirut 1970], III, 466-474.

exegete of Fakhr al-Dīn al-Rāzī, and the teacher of both the Syriac scholar Severus Jacob bar Shakko (d. A.D. 1240/1241) and the famous Persian scholar Naṣīr al-Dīn al-Ṭūsī (d. A.D. 1274).[124]

Then, he heard of the fame of Shihāb al-Dīn al-Suhrawardī (al-Maqtūl) and wanted to visit him in Diyār Bakr, but fortunately he read some of Suhrawardī's books before commencing his journey. Suhrawardī proved to be a deluded fool. ʻAbd al-Laṭīf considered his own marginal and supplementary notes with which he was not satisfied better than the arguments of this sot, and he found in his works a clear proof for the ignorance of his contemporaries. Suhrawardī afterwards became the personal astrologer and alchemist of the prince al-Malik al-Ghāzī, the middle son of Ṣalāḥ ad-Dīn. Suhrawardī appeared to have lost his senses by then. He was recognized as a wandering *ṣūfī* and became a self-declared prophet. It has been said that he was dirty in appearance and never cut his nails or hair. He was a walking flea-circus and lice crept over his face and clothes. Whosoever saw him tried to outflank him or ran away from him! Ṣalāḥ ad-Dīn ordered his death, apparently under the pressure of the local *ʻulamā'*. It has been said that Suhrawardī isolated himself and then died from hunger at the age of barely thirty-six.[125] Other sources, however, maintain that Suhrawardī was executed publicly.[126]

ʻAbd al-Laṭīf left for Damascus in 586 A.H./1190 A.D. where he studied under al-Kindī al-Baghdādī al-Naḥwī. ʻAbd al-Laṭīf describes him as a fine-looking sheik with a keen wit, but very self-satisfied and troublesome and offensive to his associates. ʻAbd al-Laṭīf surpassed him on many topics and soon left his side. After that, ʻAbd al-Laṭīf set out for Jerusalem and Acre (or: Akka) in order to join up with Ṣalāḥ ad-Dīn's camp. There he asked al-Qādī al-Fāḍil, Ṣalāḥ ad-Dīn's chief counsellor and director of his chancellery, to be sent to Cairo. He obtained permission to go and a letter of introduction was given to him.

In Cairo ʻAbd al-Laṭīf sought for three persons. The first one he met was the aforementioned word (or rather letter) magician Yāsīn as-Sīmiyā'ī. ʻAbd al-Laṭīf often had lengthy discussions with Yāsīn, a self-proclaimed holy man, on the subject of that, what was fair and foul, or allowed and forbidden, and had to endure some very strange stories, which exposed Yāsīn's confused lines of thought and brought to light his dubious methods. ʻAbd al-Laṭīf found him utterly absurd, a liar, a conjuring cheat and a charlatan. It was said of him that he could do things even the prophet Moses was unable to do, that he could produce minted gold whenever he wished, and of any quantity he wished, and that he could turn the waters of the river Nile into a tent in which he would then sit and chat with his friends. Sometimes Yāsīn's loony companion ash-Shāqānī attended these meetings.[127] Both Yāsīn and ash-Shāqānī fostered the misconception that they had a monopoly on wisdom. They stood by each other through thick and thin: Yāsīn used to testify to

---

124 Peters, *Aristotle and the Arabs*, 107, 196-97.

125 Samira Jadon, *The Physicians of Syria*, 323-340, especially at 338-39.

126 Hossein Ziai, art. "Al-Suhrawardī", in: *EI²*: vol. IX (1997), 782a-784b.

127 See the hilarious anecdote on ash-Shāqānī below (cf. at 52-3).

ash-Shāqānī's knowledge of alchemy, while ash-Shāqānī used to testify to Yāsīn's knowledge of magic.

The Jewish scholar Moses Maimonides (Mūsā ibn Maymūn) was the second person 'Abd al-Laṭīf met in Cairo. He was a man of the highest merit, but overcome with the love of leadership and a courtier of those in high station. He wrote a book with the title *K. al-Dalāla* ["The Guide for the Perplexed"] and cursed anyone who transcribed it into anything but Hebrew script. 'Abd al-Laṭīf looked through it and found it to be an evil book that corrupted the articles of Faith and Law with elements the author thought would reform them. One of his works was on medicine, based on the sixteen books by Galen and on five books by others. He took it upon himself not to alter a single word unless it was an "and" or a "so", and, as a matter of fact, copied sections in their entirety.

Finally, 'Abd al-Laṭīf encountered Abū al-Qāsim al-Shāri'ī.[128] It is only in this person that 'Abd al-Laṭīf finds the fulfilment of his desire: "It is you I seek!" (*iyyāka aṭlub*), he cries out when meeting Abū al-Qāsim for the very first time in Cairo. Abū al-Qāsim introduced 'Abd al-Laṭīf, among others, to the works of Alexander of Aphrodisias and Abū Naṣr al-Fārābī. 'Abd al-Laṭīf later declares that he had no belief in these authors, because he used to think that the whole of philosophy had been comprehended by Ibn Sīnā and commented upon in his works. Abū al-Qāsim tamed 'Abd al-Laṭīf's defiance, and wore down his natural intractability, until he inclined to his side, putting one foot forward and the other back. The discussions with Abū al-Qāsim caused 'Abd al-Laṭīf to renounce the vile craft of alchemy entirely. Abū al-Qāsim would surpass 'Abd al-Laṭīf in producing proofs and in the strength of his argument, whereas 'Abd al-Laṭīf would surpass him in disputation and use of language. They remained constant companions and were inseparable morning till night. Their harmonious relationship only ended with the master's death. After Abū al-Qāsim only masters *extraordinaires* would do, namely rulers: Ṣalāḥ al-Dīn, al-Malik al-Afḍal, al-Malik al-'Azīz, al-Malik al-Ẓāhir, 'Alā' al-Dīn Dāwūd ibn Bahrām and Shihāb al-Dīn Ṭughril Atabeg.

According to George Makdisi in his *The Rise of Colleges*, looking at the curriculum followed by 'Abd al-Laṭīf we get some insight into one of the best and most successful products of the Muslim educational system at the time.[129] Shawkat Mahmood Toorawa adds to this, that in the medieval Arabic autobiographical and biographical *curriculum vitae*, such success is not measured only by works

---

[128] Abū al-Qāsim al-Shāri'ī has been identified by Toorawa as Abū al-Qāsim Hibat Allāh ibn 'Alī al-Anṣārī al-Buṣayrī (506-598 A.H./1112-1201 A.D.), cf. Toorawa, *The Educational Background*, 46 under p; However, Dietrich, *Die arabische Version*, 110, holds a completely different view: 'Dieser Šāri'ī war also ein dezidierter Philosoph und mit Sicherheit nicht identisch mit dem von de Sacy zweifelnd beigezogenen Abū al-Qāsim Hibat Allāh b. 'Alī b. Mas'ūd al-Munastīrī al-Būṣīrī, der ausschließlich als Traditionarier bekannt war'.

[129] Makdisi, *Rise of Colleges*, 84.

authored, but also by debates won and masters surpassed.[130] In this context, Toorawa speaks about a homosocial bond, a bond of mastery and subordination in which a desire for the object of other men's desire, here: knowledge, is predominating.[131] The nature and development of this mastery and subordination role-play may, according to Toorawa, be seen clearly in the trajectory of ʻAbd al-Laṭīf's attitude towards his teachers and mentors and the unfolding of his success. It is quite tempting to follow Toorawa's ideas on this particular subject. They are quite enlightening and provide one with much food for thought, but at the same time create a serious dilemma for the present author due to the latter's unfamiliarity with the specific jargon used in Toorawa's essay. However, it has become perfectly clear by now that Abū al-Qāsim is not only the perfect companion to ʻAbd al-Laṭīf, but also his perfect rival.

A new ʻAbd al-Laṭīf, cleansed and purified, arises. Because he is rejuvenated after the fruitful and mutually complimentary relationship with Abū al-Qāsim, ʻAbd al-Laṭīf gets more and more convinced of the superiority of the books of the "Ancients" and of the works of al-Fārābī over the writings of Ibn Sīnā. Although ʻAbd al-Laṭīf from now on mainly focuses on the science of logic, there is still that voice in his head which tells him to rebel against the deceiving craft of alchemy and to deal with it in a final way. After all, ʻAbd al-Laṭīf was in his younger days a convinced adherent of alchemy. He studied books by Jābir ibn Ḥayyān and Ibn Waḥshīya on alchemical transformation and experimentation. In the *ʻUyūn* it is told that he started to practice the illusory art and made frivolous experiments of error. The most potent of the influences that led him astray was, however, that of Ibn Sīnā, by his "Book on the Art (of Alchemy)" (*K. aṣ-Ṣināʻa* or *Ṣanʻa*), in which his philosophy is said to have attained completion. According to ʻAbd al-Laṭīf, this completion added nothing to philosophy, but rather derogated from it. Therefore, he considered Ibn Sīnā a false philosopher with a bad moral character and ended up feeling only contempt for the man and his *oeuvre* since Ibn Sīnā drank wine, kept the company of prostitutes and composed his work under the influence of alcohol and other stimulants. But as a matter of fact, Ibn Sīnā expressed himself very clearly on this subject. He was unfavourably disposed towards alchemy and alchemists, rejected the substantial transmutation of metals, and merely wrote about the possibility of accidental transformation of metals.[132] According to Ibn Sīnā, the idea of a substantial transmutation of metals was not just unimaginable, but also a sheer impossibility, because the specific differences of the individual substances were unknown to man,[133] whereby the combination of their elements could not be split up

---

[130] Shawkat Mahmood Toorawa, 'Language and Male Homosocial Desire in the Autobiography of ʻAbd al-Laṭīf al-Baghdādī (d. 629/1231)', in: *Edebiyât* NS Volume 7, Number 2 (1997), 251-265, 256.

[131] Toorawa, *Homosocial Desire*, esp. 251-53.

[132] Allemann, *Ris. fī Muǧādalat*, 35-51; Holmyard, *Alchemy*, 88-95.

[133] Allemann, *Ris. fī Muǧādalat*, 40; Holmyard, *Alchemy*, 93, quotes from a medieval Latin translation of the section on alchemy in the *K. al-Shifā'*, which has long been known under the title *Liber de mineralibus Aristotelis*: "Those properties that are perceived by

without causing a disruption of the continuity. Therefore, he held the view that the individual species of the types of metals were not just separated from each other by accidental [characteristic] features as most alchemists believed, but also by substantial [characteristic] features or so-called specific differences. The mere facts that one wanted to split up a substance into its individual elements by way of alchemical methods and directly join them together with another substance, contradicted according to Ibn Sīnā the Aristotelian principle of the continuity in nature i.e., that natural processes always run in a continuous and not in an erratic way.[134] On the one hand, Ibn Sīnā rejected the transmutation of metals on the basis of arguments from the Aristotelian natural sciences. On the other hand, he based himself on the religious-philosophical axiom of God as the sole creator of all things. He believed that what God had created with the instrument of nature could not be imitated by man in an artificial manner.[135] Sometimes his theories were inconsistent and disagreed with each other, but nowhere had he defended the possibility of actual transmutation of base metals into precious metals.[136] In his view, alchemists would never be able to bring about any true change of the metallic species. The essential nature of metals would always remain unchanged. They could, however, produce excellent imitations, whitening a red metal so that it closely resembled silver, or tinting it yellow so that it closely resembled gold.[137]

In his works (e.g.: *Risālat al-Iksīr*; *Ishāra ilā 'ilm fasād aḥkām an-nujūm*; *Risāla fī aṣ-Ṣinā'a al-'āliya*; *K. al-Shifā'*: *K. al-Ma'ādin wa l-āthār*) which treat the subject of alchemy, Ibn Sīnā mainly focused on the colouring and cleansing of metals and the production of alloys. Occasionally he offered recipes for the colouring of metals with a tincture of sulphur and mercury.[138]

Ibn Sīnā's illustrious "Book on the Art (of Alchemy)" is not known to us. It has been suggested that it might have belonged to a series of Shiite-mystical tractates known collectively as *ḥikma mashriqīya/mushriqīya* (or: Eastern wisdom/Radiant wisdom). According to Allemann, 'Abd al-Laṭīf was a notorious opponent of Ibn Sīnā's philosophical teachings and of the so-called *ḥikmat al-ishrāq* (or: Philosophy of Illumination), and especially took a dislike to his visionary recitals: the trilogy *Risālat aṭ-Ṭayr*, *Ḥayy ibn Yaqẓān* and *Salāmān wa-Absāl*, apparently because he did not want to understand or could not understand the symbolic language of this specific group of scholars any longer.[139]

---

the senses are probably not the differences which distinguish one metallic species from another, but rather accidents or consequences, the essential specific differences being unknown. And if a thing is unknown, how is it possible for any one to endeavour to produce it or to destroy it?".

134 Allemann, *Ris. fī Muǧādalat,* 40-41.

135 Allemann, *Ris. fī Muǧādalat*, 42 and 44; Strohmaier, *Avicenna*, 104.

136 Strohmaier, *Avicenna*, 104; For an overview of Avicenna's views on alchemy, cf. Principe, *Secrets*, 47-8.

137 Holmyard, *Alchemy*, 92.

138 Allemann, *Ris. fī Muǧādalat*, 35-51.

139 Allemann, *Ris. fī Muǧādalat*, 16 and 45-46.

It is very difficult to confirm Allemann's assumption because ‘Abd al-Laṭīf does not once mention the *ḥikmat al-ishrāq* or the Avicennian trilogy in his works, although one cannot deny that ‘Abd al-Laṭīf must have developed a strong aversion for the language of exoteric alchemy with its allegories, assumed names, codes, metaphors and allusions. Moreover, the Avicennian trilogy does not reveal any factual traces of alchemical symbolism. The latter can, however, be found in a different version of the *Qiṣṣat Salāmān wa-Absāl*. In this pseudepigraphical recital the language of exoteric alchemy has been used to describe the different phases of spiritual transmutation (i.e. of esoteric alchemy). This is the fully developed conception of alchemy, which by no means excludes the reality of the operations performed by the adept, the electus, but which gives them essentially the meaning of a liturgy or a projection of his inner ascetism.[140]

It may be a much more plausible option to range Ibn Sīnā's "Book on the Art (of Alchemy)" under the heading of pseudo epigraphic writings or falsifications.[141] It is known that quite a few books on alchemistical theory and practice were brought into circulation under Ibn Sīnā's name. Some of them were composed in such an ingenious way that even the famous author himself would have had difficulties to distinguish between an authentic work and a bogus one.[142]

It is otherwise most significant that al-Fārābī, who was honoured greatly by ‘Abd al-Laṭīf, actually believed in the possibility of the substantial transmutation of metals, but only explained this possibility in theory. He did not present us with records of experiments or recipes and hardly ever mentioned the elixir in his writings.[143]

However, the father of the false science of alchemy is, according to ‘Abd al-Laṭīf, Jābir ibn Ḥayyān, a scoundrel of the first water, who led astray many of the great scholars of subsequent generations like for instance Abū Bakr ar-Rāzī (or Latin: Rhazes) and Ibn Miskawayh. "All the blood, that was shed because of this art, all the money that vanished, every sin that was committed, all the great minds that went to ruin, and every person who because of alchemy dwelled from the straight path, is chargeable to Jābir. It is his sin", recapitulates ‘Abd al-Laṭīf bitterly. He goes on by saying that if a thousand persons like him spent their whole lives to try and efface the traces of alchemy they could not erase the slightest part of it, for Jābir wrote four thousand books, that these books are spread in the entire world and stuff bookcases, that a single purge cannot cleanse the impurities of the world and that one farmer cannot uproot the weeds of a thousand gardens, unless he were a

---

140 Henry Corbin, *Avicenna and the Visionary Recital* (Princeton 1960), 209; N. Peter Joosse, 'An Example of Medieval Arabic Pseudo-Hermetism: The Tale of Salāmān and Absāl', in: *JSS* 38/2 (1993), 279-293.

141 Ibn Sīnā's "Book on the Art (of Alchemy)" is most likely the *De anima in artis chemicae principes, Avicenna atque Geber* (Basel 1572), which is a Latin translation of an Arabic forgery attributed to Avicenna, of which the Arabic original is lost, cf. *infra* footnote 187 at 58.

142 Strohmaier, *Avicenna*, 105.

143 Allemann, *Ris. fī Muǧādalat*, 52-57.

prophet. Jābir's words are pretences, misrepresentations and fabrications and are just as dangerous to the people as the teeth and claws of barking jackals and wild boars who rout up the earth.

Overcome by hatred now for the false art, ʿAbd al-Laṭīf began to express his feelings in two treatises, the aforementioned *Risāla fī Muǧādalat al-ḥakīmayn* and another one, the *Risāla fī l-Maʿādin wa-ibṭāl al-kīmiyāʾ*. Below we shall present some of the anecdotes which ʿAbd al-Laṭīf collected for his first treatise. The second treatise mainly deals with the formation of minerals and distinguishes between genuine and useful chemical operations and the procedures of the false alchemists.

Let us first explore the scene and the scenery a bit: ʿAbd al-Laṭīf sketches a desolate, chaotic picture of his social and geographical environment – briefly that means the triangle Aleppo-Baghdād-Damascus. However, it is not the Near East as we like to picture it. ʿAbd al-Laṭīf pictures an unholy no man's land which on the outside might resemble a landscape as painted by Pieter Brueghel the Elder.[144] In it, grotesque gruesomeness and sinister situations are coupled with an almost complete absence of upholding the law. The atmospheric description roughly approximates that of a gold-rush *avant la lettre*, a gold fever without gold and is similar qua monstrosity and atrocity to ʿAbd al-Laṭīf's description of the famine in Egypt during the years 597-98 A.H. (1200-02 A.D.) in which we encounter such realistic, or rather surrealistic, tales of cannibalism. The image of roasted or boiled little children is vividly present in the mind's eye and the anecdote of the fat lady who was killed, cut and sliced, and converted into a human flesh stew with vinegar, the *sikbāj*,[145] still makes the flesh creep![146] Medical doctors were also greatly in

---

[144] Cf. for instance Brueghel's painting "Victory of Death". In an engraving by the same artist, entitled "An Alchemist at Work" a raggedly-dressed alchemist sits near his fire, surrounded by broken alembics, flasks and pots. Nearby his distressed wife shakes an empty purse. Two hungry children scrounge vainly in the cupboard for scraps to eat. Through a window in the background one sees the inevitable ending of the drama: the alchemist and his family are welcomed into a poorhouse, cf. Coudert, *Alchemy: the Philosopher's stone*, 202.

[145] From Middle Persian sik: 'vinegar' and bāg: 'stew'. A recipe for *sikbāj* with ordinary meat can for instance be found in the *K. al-Ṭabīkh* (*The Book of Dishes*) by the 13th century Arabic author Muḥammad b. al-Ḥasan b. Muḥammad b. al-Karīm al-Baghdādī, cf. *A Baghdad Cookery Book. The Book of Dishes* (*Kitāb al-Ṭabīkh*). Newly translated by Charles Perry (Totnes 2005), 30-31.

[146] Kamal Hafuth Zand and John A. and Ivy E. Videan, The Eastern Key: *Kitāb al-Ifādah wa'l-iʿtibār of ʿAbd al-Laṭīf al-Baghdādi* (The Book of Instruction and Admonition…Translated into English by…) (Cairo/London 1204/1964), esp. 223-255. It is still a difficult matter to decide on whether these horror stories are an eye-witness account by ʿAbd al-Laṭīf al-Baghdādī or represent a *topos*, a literary stereotype. The 15th century author al-Maqrīzī (766-845 A.H./1364-1442 A.D.) quotes a slightly different version of the story of the fat lady in his *K. al-Mawāʿiẓ wa l-iʿtibār fī dhikr al-khiṭāṭ wa l-āthār* and likewise in his *K. Ittiʿāẓ al-ḥunafāʾ*. Apparently he does not seem to refer to the Egyptian famine of 1200-1202 A.D., but to the famine during the "great crisis": *ash-*

demand, especially general practitioners. Not because they tasted so good, but chiefly because they were considered easy prey. The hunters just laid in wait until the house-calls were made and then they pounced.

Blacksmiths, bakers and millers desert their work abruptly, notable citizens (judges, legal experts, notaries) neglect municipal administration, only to devote themselves fully to the production of the elixir, a schoolmaster leaves his pupils in the lurch just to execute gross experiments, judges let themselves be cheated and deceived by sly and pretentious swindlers, people who belong to the nobility and are elected for the office of vizier wholly run aground, are obliged to sell all their assets and finally end up in jail, merely for the fact that they became the victims of these false alchemists.

According to ʻAbd al-Laṭīf, the sole person who was able to stand up against all the bickering around him and who could see through the lists of the alchemists, was Ṣalāḥ al-Dīn.[147] ʻAbd al-Laṭīf does him great honour by saying: "I have never seen in my life a cleverer and smoother ruler than this man. He is loved by righteous men and evil-doers, Muslims and unbelievers". Here and elsewhere, the honour which ʻAbd al-Laṭīf bestows on Ṣalāḥ al-Dīn is obviously sincere, for Ṣalāḥ al-Dīn appeared to have had a good reputation among both parties. However, we should by no means forget that eulogies to worldly- and religious leaders and other dignitaries are often uttered for the sake of lip-service and do unfortunately not come straight from the heart. My scepticism is not completely unfounded as may become clear from the following story. When Ṣalāḥ al-Dīn made a truce with the Franks and returned to Jerusalem, ʻAbd al-Laṭīf joined him for a while. Ṣalāḥ al-Dīn assigned

---

shidda al-ʻuẓmā: 457 A.H./1065 A.D.-464 A.H./1072 A.D. Al-Maqrīzī, however, quoted the story of the fat lady directly from the *K. an-Nuqaṭ li-muʻjam mā ushkila (ʻalayhi) min al-khiṭāṭ* by the 12th century author Muḥammad ibn Asʻad al-Jawwānī, cf. Johannes den Heijer, 'Muḥammad b. Asʻad al-Ǧawwānī and his report on cannibalism. A study in source criticism', in: Frederik de Jong (editor): *Miscellanea Arabica et Islamica. Dissertationes in Academia Ultrajectina prolatae anno MCMXC* (Leuven 1993), 255-266. Stories which involve famines and as a consequence thereof cannibalism, can for instance also be found in Byzantine literature, for example in the *Historia et laudes SS. Sabae et Macarii*, ed. G. Cozza-Luzy (Roma 1893), 13, para 6 (written at the beginning of the eleventh century). It is not unrealistic to maintain that ʻAbd al-Laṭīf al-Baghdādī's oeuvre consists of three parts of unequal measurements: truth, half-truth and *topos*. The *topoi* in his work are duly noticed. Without a doubt, their amount shall increase when we manage to obtain a better and more detailed picture of his entire oeuvre. It needs to be stressed here though that the *topos* often causes data to be added to an existing text. At the same time, the *topos* can also cause data to be omitted from an existing text, but most of the time it does justice to a text without changing the facts too severely. Therefore, we must realize that a *topos* is merely an indicator for the existence of a problem which, in the eyes of an author, deserves to be dealt with in the most serious way. That a myth springs from truth, is a truth in itself, cf. Joosse, *ʻAbd al-Laṭīf al-Baghdādī as a Philosopher and a Physician*, especially at 38-40.

147 See also ʻAbd al-Laṭīf's anecdote on Ṣalāḥ ad-Dīn's acumen and shrewdness *infra* at 51-2.

him a monthly stipend of thirty dinars, and Ṣalāḥ al-Dīn's sons added sums of their own, bringing the total monthly stipend to one hundred. This amount, at the time, was approximately ten times the normal monthly stipend of a college professor of law and it made ʻAbd al-Laṭīf by far one of the best paid physicians, employed by Ṣalāḥ al-Dīn and his family. His duty was, however, to teach medicine, not to treat patients! The best paid physician at Ṣalāḥ al-Dīn's court was, without a doubt, Asʻad ibn al-Muṭrān, a Christian who converted to Islam, who was Ṣalāḥ al-Dīn's private physician and at the same time his chamberlain (*ḥājib*). Ṣalāḥ al-Dīn gave him one of his wives' handmaids in marriage and thus he gained great wealth both from his work as a physician and through his wife who brought with her jewels and valuable gifts from Ṣalāḥ al-Dīn's wife. Apart from this, there were times when he treated acutely ill patients at the *Bīmāristān al-Nūrī* in Damascus and sometimes he travelled outside Damascus at the request of sick dignitaries, who competed with one another for his services and rewarded him with large sums of money.[148]

However, we should return to the anecdotes! Are they exaggerated? Most probably! Is there a germ of truth in them? Without a doubt![149] Much of the action in the majority of these anecdotes took place during the Crusades. Poverty and famine reigned everywhere and Ṣalāḥ al-Dīn was, during this period, entangled in fatiguing attempts to consolidate his newly acquired power in Egypt, while at the same time, he was fighting against the crusaders for the possession of Jerusalem. There was chaos (*fitna*) and confusion all over and in all ranks: among the rural population and among the city-dwellers; among the rich and the poor; among the dignitaries; among the military; and certainly also among the scholars in- and outside the institutes of learning, the *madāris*.[150] Faris mentions that the constant

---

148 Jadon, *Physicians of Syria*, 330-32; cf. also Jadon, 'A Comparison of the Wealth, Prestige, and Medical Works of the Physicians of Ṣalāḥ Al-Dīn in Egypt and Syria', in: *BHM* 44 (1970), 64-75, esp. 68-69.

149 In recent studies it has been considered in the context of Islamic literary styles of the medieval period that the technique of providing extreme and gruesome examples to embellish a text was in common usage at that particular time in almost all topics that received literary attention; cf. Lawrence I. Conrad, 'Usāma ibn Munqidh and other witnesses to Frankish and Islamic medicine in the era of the crusades', in: Zohar Amar, Efraim Lev and Joseph Schwartz (editors): *Medicine in Jerusalem Throughout the Ages* (Tel Aviv 1999), 27-52; Piers D. Mitchell, *Medicine in the Crusades. Warfare, Wounds and the Medieval Surgeon* (Cambridge 2004), 213-14. It is, however, far too simplistic to state that these examples were provided merely for the adornment and the embellishment of a text. These extreme examples of course were often also meant to highlight an issue and could for instance be viewed as a severe warning, in order to make the readers and/or listeners aware of the real problems in their community and in society as a whole. The authors of such texts believed that society was in danger of being caught off guard and thereby not focusing on the fundamental issues threatening it!

150 Nabih Amin Faris, 'Arab Culture in the Twelfth Century', in: Norman P. Zacour and Harry W. Hazard (editors): *A History of the Crusades* (general editor: Kenneth Meyer Setton), Volume V: *The Impact of the Crusades on the Near East* (Madison, Wisconsin

warfare was disruptive, not only politically, but also socially and economically. Manpower was depleted, farmers left their land uncultivated rather than have their crops pillaged, public security broke down, and because of a rising wave of brigandage and crime the populace often took the law into its own hands, organizing itself into special units for self-defence (*al-aḥdāth*). Furthermore, epidemics, droughts, famines were of regular occurrence and decimated large areas.[151] The forced neglect of agriculture caused people to leave their homes and roam the countryside in search of food and other means for their sustenance.

Since there was no actual prospect of jobs, the rumour must have spread that it would be a genuine possibility to produce gold out of base materials and even out of blood, urine and faeces. Many people must have believed in this cruel myth: an environment of extreme violence and poverty is likely to blur or to exceed the boundaries of decency, humanity and normality. In spite of the effects of war and political instability, the urban centres -especially Aleppo and Damascus- retained a fairly high measure of prosperity.[152] For the rural areas it must have been a completely different situation, although a traveller like Ibn Jubayr, who visited the region at the end of the 12th century, describes the life and the conditions in the area in his *Riḥla*, and notes "thriving villages and fertile lands abounding with rich crops and palm groves".[153]

Damascus and Aleppo give the impression of having been prosperous cities according to eye-witness reports of contemporary travellers. The only legitimate argument to explain this apparent prosperity of the urban region is, without a single doubt, the incontestable fact that the rural area had become largely unfit for habitation, and was difficult to access. The city Baghdād of the 12th century appears to be an exception because it very distinctly reflects the reverse side of prosperity. It had two parts, one on each side of the river Tigris. The newer part, on the east bank, looked shambled, run down and neglected. The older part, on the west bank, was in ruins.[154] 'Abd al-Laṭīf confirms in his *Risāla fī Muğādalat al-ḥakīmayn al-kīmiyā'ī wa-l-naẓarī* that Baghdād, under the caliph al-Mustaḍī' ibn al-Mustanjid bi-amri-llāh (1170-1180 A.D.), was in an advanced state of neglect. The prices of commodities, merchandise and daily shopping were shooting up, and the population lived on the verge of starvation.[155] The deplorable state in which Baghdād found itself has also been eye-witnessed by the Jewish poet, translator and traveller Judah al-Ḥarizi (1165-1225) who visited the Abbāsid capital, which then was under the reign of the caliph an-Nāṣir ibn al-Mustaḍī', in the year 1217 A.D. or shortly after that date:

1985), Chapter I, 6; Michael Chamberlain, *Knowledge and social practice in medieval Damascus, 1190-1350* (Cambridge 1994), 91-107.

[151] Faris, *Arab Culture*, 6.

[152] For the example of Aleppo, see: Tabbaa, *Constructions of Power and Piety*; cf. also Gérard Degeorge and Jean-Claude David, *Alep* (Paris 2002).

[153] Faris, *Arab Culture*, 9-10.

[154] Faris, *Arab Culture*, 11.

[155] Allemann, *Ris. fī Muğādalat*, 113; Ms. Bursa, Hüseyin Çelebi 823, fol. 118v.

Today, however, it stands bereft: its elders have departed; only raw youths are left. The wheat is gone, the chaff stays on, Virtue has vanished without a trace, Vileness has seized her place; the lions are all dead and foxes roam the hills instead, fouling the ruins of Giving's hall and tower. I sought but found no vower; no, not one endower.[156]

Politically, the area was plagued by instability and unrest: there were struggles between Muslims and Franks, between Sunnites and Shiites, between Sunnite princes in the various urban centres and in the outlying districts, between ambitious dynasts and greedy viziers, and between the mass of the population, mostly Arabs, and the foreign elements, mostly Turks. Each of these struggles was sufficient to disrupt the normal course of life and to ravage the general good of society. Together they wrought havoc throughout the empire, rendered communications unsafe, increased lawlessness,[157] and gave rise to various forms of brigandage.[158] A situation like that must have been a fertile soil for the coming into existence of such grim and gruesome anecdotes. Alchemy in all its weird and wonderful manifestations may apparently have provided a favourable outlet for angst, chaos, confusion, dissension, ignorance and poverty; although one of course cannot deny that a passion for gold, a love for quick gain, evidently was the principal motive for many individuals among the common people and the upper-crust to start practicing the craft.

Many people also held the conviction that the "sublime stone" was the blood. ʻAbd al-Laṭīf mentions his meeting with the *qāḍī* (judge) of Baalbek (*ba'labakk*) who buried ten Damascene *raṭl* (= circa 18 kg and 50 pounds) of blood in secret places. When ʻAbd al-Laṭīf asked him if he fulfilled the acts necessary for the processes of distillation, purification, coagulation, solution and fixation, the *qāḍī* replied: "do not talk nonsense, man. That is useless stuff. I can do without it!". A few days later the *qāḍī* showed ʻAbd al-Laṭīf a silver dirham, which supposedly was created out of blood through a secret procedure, which the *qāḍī* preferred to keep to himself. Of course, the dirham was genuine and made of pure silver, but the *qāḍī* did not want to look like a fool in front of ʻAbd al-Laṭīf and pretended that he produced the coin himself.[159] This example clearly illustrates how far people were willing to go in their self-deception and in the deception of others. The same *qāḍī* was once approached by an Egyptian man, who made him believe that urine was the "Philosophers' stone". They co-operated and obtained the urine from the eunuchs, who often held the position of superintendents of the public baths, and in this way collected seven hundred earthenware jugs of the specific liquid for the special price of five jugs for one dirham. They placed the urine in large containers and left these in the sun to bake until the urine became thick. Because of the ghastly stench, the neighbours came out of their houses and scolded the *qāḍī* and his new friend badly. Therefore, the Egyptian proposed to bring the "concentrated" urine to his house, but

---

156 Judah al-Ḥarizi, *The Book of Taḥkemoni*, 354-55.

157 Cf. Faris, *Arab Culture*, 4-5: "Perhaps the most terrifying form of lawlessness, however, was the rise of the Ismāʿīlī Assassins...".

158 Faris, *Arab Culture*, 4.

159 Allemann, *Ris. fī Muğādalat*, 85; Ms. Bursa, Hüseyin Çelebi 823, fol. 107v.

the *qāḍī* would not hear of this plan, being afraid that the Egyptian would take off without giving him his share of the gold. They haggled about it for weeks and finally split up, being completely estranged from each other.[160] Unfortunately, 'Abd al-Laṭīf does not clear up what was done with the urine afterwards.[161]

A similar event took place (at a deserted site) on the outskirts of Baghdād. A man, who endeavoured to produce the elixir, created a long-necked bottle out of glass and filled it with a mixture of body-juices (most likely: blood, urine and sperm). He possibly also stirred in some watery stool and buried the lot for a period of seven days in decaying manure. Then he dug it out again and opened the bottle. But, out of sheer greed, he opened it too hastily and a pillar of fire rose up, which made him fall to the ground. The bottle fell on the floor and broke into pieces, which enabled the stench to spread. Somebody found him lying there on the ground and brought him to town. The people recognized him and carried him home. He was ill for eight months, but did not make a good recovery, for the accident caused him to become a mentally disturbed person.[162]

Something that happened in the *al-Khātūnīya* area of Baghdād is that a teacher sold his property, sent his pupils home, and from then on, occupied himself only with the execution of alchemistical experiments. He collected blood and egg yolks and deliberately caused it to rot. After many difficult years filled with countless setbacks, he finally got lucky and by means of putrefaction, worms and maggots were generated spontaneously. Unfortunately, the creatures started eating each other up and in the end only one worm survived. It became mighty big because the false alchemist fed it twice daily with freshly cupped blood. When the alchemist ultimately reached the point where he could feed the worm with the amalgam, a metal mixed with quicksilver (mercury), which had to change into an elixir in the worm's stomach, he had to expose the worm to intense heat. Hardly had he started to place the animal on a leaf in the burning sun, when a pussycat grabbed it and quickly ran away with it. The alchemist jumped up like a mother whose baby had just been snatched from under her eyes and went after the naughty cat, panic-stricken, like a headless chicken. He climbed from roof to roof, falling down every time and hurting himself, but the pussycat disappeared without leaving a single trace![163] These experiences must have had the effect of a nightmare on the unfortunate alchemist. Perhaps the pussycat's name was *qābūs*!

Another story from Baghdād is the following titillating tale: In the middle of summer, twenty town dignitaries had gathered in an unoccupied house in a dead-

---

160 Allemann, *Ris. fī Muǧādalat*, 85-86; Ms. Bursa, Hüseyin Çelebi 823, fol. 107v-107r.

161 On the stories and tales about alchemists and their greed and lust for money, see likewise: Johann Christoph Bürgel, *The Feather of Simurgh. The "Licit Magic" of the Arts in Medieval Islam* (New York/London 1988), 45-7; cf. also Joosse, *Unmasking the Craft*, 309-15.

162 Allemann, *Ris. fī Muǧādalat*, 86; Ms. Bursa, Hüseyin Çelebi 823, fol. 107r.

163 Allemann, *Ris. fī Muǧādalat*, 86-87; Ms. Bursa, Hüseyin Çelebi 823, fol. 107r; cf. also Johann Christoph Bürgel, *Allmacht und Mächtigkeit. Religion und Welt im Islam* (München 1991), 205.

end street. They had met there to execute a specific chemical process called *bāb ḥabs al-zi'baq* (= the process of the secret -lit. holding back- of the quicksilver).[164] They double locked the door of the house, dug a deep pit, filled it up with dung and buried in it a bulbous iron container, a kind of *qumqum*, which was filled with quicksilver and sealed several times with the so-called *ṭīn al-ḥikma*, "the clay of wisdom", which is fermented clay mixed with a little dung, cut animal-hair and salt. They lighted the fire under the container, but this threw out such an intense heat that they had to take off their clothes and sit around the fire naked. Telling stories and having a lot of fun, the good gentlemen forgot to observe the fire so that all of a sudden the container started to make a terrible noise and exploded in their faces. They landed on the roof of the house, fell on the floor, jumped up again and hurried for the outer-door. Twenty naked and barefooted old and young men with baldheads and long beards came out of the house all at once so that the women, who were spinning in the oriel rooms, believed that the *djinn*, the demons, had come to the surface in broad daylight. Soon the men were chased by the whole town and even the police were hot on their trail and eager to throw them in jail (The Arabic reads here *bāb ḥabs al-luṣūṣ* = the door to the cell of thieves).[165]

In one of his anecdotes, 'Abd al-Laṭīf tells us that one day a Yemeni man turned up in Damascus who claimed that he reached "the ultimate goal" through the craft of alchemy. He asked permission to visit al-Mubāriz al-Mu'tamid, the governor of the city.[166] The latter came to him and invited him to his palace where he stayed for seventeen days. During this period al-Mubāriz al-Mu'tamid tried to win the Yemeni man over to his side by making him all kinds of tempting proposals. But when he finally saw, that his plans were doomed to fail, he decided to hand over the Yemeni to a more powerful individual. So he introduced him to Sultan Ṣalāḥ ad-Dīn, who at the time was fighting against the Franks who were besieging the city of Acre. Ṣalāḥ ad-Dīn said to al-Mubāriz al-Mu'tamid: "What brings you to me in these difficult

---

164 Cf. Coudert, *Alchemy: the Philosopher's stone*, 20. What is described here is the so-called 'death-process' or 'mortification of the quicksilver'. The notion that death must precede birth is a constant alchemical theme and explains why the first stage of the alchemist's work, in which a substance is deprived of its form and reduced to prime matter, is referred to as the 'death', 'putrefaction' or 'mortification' of the impure substance which will later turn to gold, cf. also Roger Bacon (c. 1220-92), *Secretum secretorum, in: Opera hactenus inedita Rogeri Baconi*, Vol. 5, ed. Robert Steele (Oxford 1920); cf. P.G. Maxwell-Stuart (ed./tr.), *The Occult in Mediaeval Europe, 500-1500. A Documentary History* (London/New York 2005), 217.

165 Allemann, *Ris. fī Muğādalat*, 87-88; Ms. Bursa, Hüseyin Çelebi 823, fol. 108v-108r; cf. also Bürgel, *Allmacht*, 205.

166 Allemann, *Ris. fī Muğādalat*, 143, note 114 and idem, *Ris. fī Muğādalat*, 119; Ms. Bursa, Hüseyin Çelebi 823, fol. 120v. In 'Abd al-Laṭīf's autobiography [AUT 1] we are also told that al-Mu'tamid was a 'friend' of alchemy and the alchemists. After the death of Ibn at-Tātalī, 'Abd al-Laṭīf's former mentor and alchemy teacher, al-Mu'tamid took all of his books; cf. Ibn abī Uṣaybi'a, *K. 'Uyūn al-anbā' fī-ṭabaqāt al-aṭibbā'*, (ed. A. Müller), Vol. 2, 205; cf. Gibb, *Life of Muwaffiq Ad-Din Abd al-Latif of Baghdad by Ibn Abi Usaybiya*, 74.

times? And under whose protection did you leave Damascus?" He answered: "I found out that the Sultan finds himself in an unfortunate position because of this enemy, that he needs credits and has to request for loans. This man here, which I took along with me, can fill your treasure-chest with gold and silver, so that you can conquer the whole inhabited world with it". Thereupon Ṣalāḥ ad-Dīn asked: "Dear *faqīr*, can you really do that?" The Yemeni replied: "Yes", to which Ṣalāḥ ad-Dīn responded: "Leave [*imḍi*], go out of my sight. Make it (i.e. the gold and the silver) for yourself!" Also al-Mubāriz al-Mu'tamid was chased away under a volley of curses and was given the command, to give the Yemeni his marching orders, and to return, to defend the city of Acre. 'Abd al-Laṭīf interrupts the narrative here by stating that he has never seen a more intelligent ruler than Ṣalāḥ ad-Dīn. Later 'Abd al-Laṭīf met the Yemeni again and asked him why he stayed so merciless towards al-Mu'tamid and showed so much cooperativeness towards Ṣalāḥ ad-Dīn:

"Al-Mu'tamid is an avaricious man and a swindler"; he [the Yemeni] said, "if I would have given him a negative answer, when he asked me whether or not I was able to produce gold and silver, he would have sent me away. Therefore, I fed his greediness, so that he would beg me to stay with him. When I met Ṣalāḥ ad-Dīn I immediately noticed that he bore the signs of intelligence and wisdom; if I would have lied, he would have become very suspicious and distrustful. (I believe) that Ṣalāḥ ad-Dīn -due to the loftiness of his power and sovereignty- was either too proud to admit that he needed a *faqīr* like me when I gave him a positive answer, or that he already knew that it would be an impossible task to produce gold and silver through the craft of alchemy; in both cases the virtue stayed with him and did not leave his side" [*lam ta'dūhu al-faḍīla*].[167]

'Abd al-Laṭīf reports the following on the aforementioned ash-Shāqānī, a *ṣūfī* from the convent in Cairo:

He was a noisy and obtrusive windbag and a friend of the charlatan Yāsīn as-Sīmiyā'ī; ash-Shāqānī was intellectually poorly developed: When I told him a true story, he did not believe me; when I told him a false story, he would accept it and kiss my hand. In fact, he would ask me to write it down for him, and would express his heartfelt gratitude to me. But when I gave him some real good advice and told him the truth, he would reprimand me and complain about me to others. He was expelled from Egypt to Syria, because he raised a complaint in court against the notorious Ibn Shukr.[168] In Syria, he was put in the trust and under the power of al-Malik al-'Ādil, who had his ears boxed and banished him (also) from Syria. Ash-Shāqānī now started to travel around and terrorized the peoples of Irbil, Mosul, Diyār Bakr and Arzan. It has been said that he set traps for them in a very cunning and sly manner, and that he left behind an imperfect elixir everywhere he went. At the time, the governor of Arzan was al-Malik 'Izz al-Dīn Kaikhusrau, a young man full of energy and zest for action. The charlatans tried to convince him with a great deal of cunning, that only the discoveries of

---

167 Allemann, *Ris. fī Muğādalat*, 89-91; Ms. Bursa, Hüseyin Çelebi 823, fol. 108r-109a.

168 Allemann, *Ris. fī Muğādalat*, 140, note 92. Ibn Shukr was first of all appointed as vizier under Sultan al-Malik al-'Ādil. When prince al-Malik al-Kāmil became the supervisor of the Egyptian (Ayyūbid) administration, he carried out radical changes, fired Ibn Shukr, and appointed Ibn Shukr's stepfather al-Qāḍī al-A'azz Fakhr al-Dīn Abū 'Abdallāh Miqdām ibn Aḥmad ibn Shukr as head of all the treasuries. But after the death of al-'Ādil, al-Malik al-Kāmil assumed power and reinstalled Ibn Shukr as vizier of the entire Ayyūbid government in Egypt.

the craft (of alchemy) would give him power and supremacy, and that Alexander (the Great) had only been capable of ruling the world through these discoveries. As a result of these (lies), he began to invite the practitioners of the craft to his palace and the ones, who came of their own accord, he gave a warm welcome. Ash-Shāqānī also turned up. The governor kissed him and (apparently without a moment's thought) handed-over his duties to him. Ash-Shāqānī only passed strange judgements and led a very peculiar life. However, in the end Allāh -may his name be praised- received him mercifully. Once, ash-Shāqānī told me a few of his many odd stories, which includes the following one: In Sicily the dead arise, stumble over the crockery and the tableware in the houses and smash it to pieces. When they catch someone in the house, they will kill that person; but when the latter would read the Koran in their presence, the living dead (or: zombies), would calm down, and the house and its inhabitants would be spared from their havoc and devastation. Such nonsense it is which that man spoke; and at the same time he had such a wise and intelligent appearance![169]

At the present time, a man known under the name of Ibn Munqidh[170] lives in Hama; he is supposed to be a dissolute human being. Certain important persons and legal scholars, however, agreed with each other on the fact that he reached his goal and produced and applied the tincture (i.e. the elixir) in their presence and with their aid. The ruler of Hama had him send for, so he came and manufactured artificial gold for him. The ruler, however, threw it away and said: "I want Egyptian gold![171] For the man in the street, (this alchemist here) produces the Egyptian, but for us he only makes the artificial stuff!" And the pride of rulers and the regal dignity arose in him: thus he had Ibn Munqidh clamped in heavy irons and thrown in a cramped dungeon, where he is still to be found.[172]

However, an-Najīb al-Hamadhānī was one of the most curious characters of his time. He studied theology and law in Mosul and claimed that he was a philosopher. Once a meeting was summoned for him in Qaisarīya in order to allow him to participate in a philosophical disputation. At that meeting, he cursed the *qāḍī* (of the city) and exploded with fury. The Sultan tried to appease him by dismissing the *qāḍī* from his duties, while at the same time conferring upon him the juridical teaching at the local *madrasa*. That decision caused al-Hamadhānī to earn more than a thousand dinars on a yearly basis. He created a tremendous amount of havoc, displayed damned impertinent conduct, and behaved like the Pharaohs[173] until he

---

169 Allemann, *Ris. fī Muğādalat*, 117-18; Ms. Bursa, Hüseyin Çelebi 823, fol. 119v-119r.

170 This Ibn Munqidh should not be confused with the Syrian prince Usāma ibn Munqidh (1095-1188 A.D.), although the person mentioned here may have been a scion of the famous Banū Munqidh, the lords of Shayzar, a city with an impressive and inaccessible stronghold to the north of Hama in Syria.

171 Egyptian gold is real, pure, gold, cf. Allemann, *Ris. fī Muğādalat*, 143, note 112.

172 Allemann, *Ris. fī Muğādalat*, 89; Ms. Bursa, Hüseyin Çelebi 823, fol. 108r.

173 That is, he behaved inordinately proud and extravagant, or corrupt, or unbelieving; cf. Edward William Lane, *Maddu-l Kamoos, an Arabic-English Lexicon derived from the best and the most copious Eastern sources…*, Parts 1-5 (London 1863-1874), Parts 6-8: edited by Stanley Lane Poole (London 1877-1893) [Reprint: 2 vols., Cambridge 1984], II, 2380-81.

finally also gave the nobility of the city a really hard time. For this, he was executed in a particularly disgraceful way.[174]

Because alchemy, or rather experimenting with chemicals, was in popular demand at every level of society, many impostors saw their way clear to make big money out of it. And thus, we should also mention Ja'far, the alchemist here. He liked to play games with people with a high social status and loved to ridicule them. One fine day he conceived a plan to do an experiment with human excrements. So, he asked three well-off citizens, who were not averse to gold, to join him at his house for an extended period. While they stayed with him, he only fed them on honey, eggs and unleavened bread and denied them the pleasure of all exquisite foods. Moreover, he ordered them to collect their excrements for a period of forty days and commanded them to distil, filter, contract, liquefy and harden it again. In every phase he let them taste and smell their own excrements and most certainly also that of the others and asked them after their sensory perception. This experiment took six months to conduct and during this period the three men presented Ja'far with the finest wines [*sic*!] and also helped him to indulge in wild excesses, although they were known to bear an irreproachable character.[175] Of course, this Ja'far was a major crook and unfortunately he had an unusual preference for offering his "victims" faeces!

It is also told that in the city of Mosul a Moroccan alchemist, a damned devil and a godforsaken rebel, made the streets unsafe. He used to sweet-talk and butter up the municipal elite and the town dignitaries, so that they left their wives, sons and daughters in his care. He committed outrageous and shameful acts and among others practiced anal sex with barefaced boys and told them that the "sublime stone" was his sperm. He abused them for three long years until finally his deception and lies came to light. Then, he was executed in public in a particularly nasty and humiliating way.[176]

Worthwhile to relate may also be the story of one of the companions of as-Suhrawardī (al-Maqtūl), an emir of the Saljūqs of Anatolia, known as the Rūm Saljūqs, whose opinion it was that the eyes were the "Philosophers' stone". For a while, he took great pains to collect the eyes of sheep and goats, but when once 12.000 Franks were butchered near Acre, he and a few of his friends headed for the battlefield and cut out the eyes of the dead soldiers, whereas other practitioners of the craft took away their gall-bladders.[177] 'Abd al-Laṭīf refers here to the chronicler

---

174 Allemann, *Ris. fī Muğādalat*, 119; Ms. Bursa, Hüseyin Çelebi 823, fol. 120v.

175 Allemann, *Ris. fī Muğādalat*, 88-89; Ms. Bursa, Hüseyin Çelebi 823, fol. 108r; cf. also Bürgel, *Allmacht*, 205.

176 Allemann, *Ris. fī Muğādalat*, 111; Ms. Bursa, Hüseyin Çelebi 823, fol. 117v.

177 A recent example of mutilation and cannibalism in times of war is evidenced by the Syrian civil war (2011-2014 so far). It happened near the Syrian town of Al-Qusayr on the border with Lebanon. According to Sky News and many other broadcast media all over the world on the 14th of May 2013, a Sunni commander of the Syrian opposition against the Bashār al-Asad government, Abū Sakkar (of the independent Islamist 'Omar al-Fārouq Brigade), was seen on a videoclip carving out the heart and one of the lungs of

and personal secretary to Ṣalāḥ al-Dīn, 'Imād al-Dīn al-Kātib al-Iṣfahānī, who appeared to have been an eye-witness to these atrocities. From the ambiguous and vague way in which 'Abd al-Laṭīf relates the story, one gets an eerie feeling as if more is meant than meets the eye. Did al-Kātib al-Iṣfahānī also contribute to the "stealing" of the eyes or was he just an innocent bystander? Some false alchemists took the view that the perfect elixir could be produced only with the eyes of a strong, healthy human being: blond, blue-eyed and of fair complexion. Occasionally, they bought a slave for that purpose, but now and then they also set a trap to catch people who were fully unaware of the danger they found themselves in. The alchemists tied their hands and feet and pulled out their eyes with a type of fishhook, but they did it in such a violent manner that they often teared off a piece of flesh which was attached to the brain.[178]

'Abd al-Laṭīf informs us that Suhrawardī's followers mainly consisted of common people and riff-raff. They were either singers and flute-players or owners of public houses and inns in which vulgar amusement ran rampant. A highwayman was once hanged on the gallows in Aleppo; a few alchemists agreed on stealing his eyes. They promised one from within their midst a dinar if he could get hold of the hanged person's eyes. The chosen one came at midnight, gripped the dead man's neck and cut the rope which was bound around his throat. Because the blood and the wind in his abdomen were pressed together, strange croaking sounds escaped from his throat. It was as if the dead man had said something very nasty or pronounced a curse. The alchemist became frightened out of his wits and passed out on the spot.[179]

There must have flourished a lucrative, yet illicit and illegal, trade in body parts in these days and in that area during a relatively short period if we take it as a fact that alchemy was widespread and practiced by many.[180] However, reports of

---

a regime soldier and placing the heart in his mouth, thereby saying: "I swear to Allāh, you soldiers of Bashār, you dogs, we will eat from your hearts and livers! O heroes of Baba Amr, you slaughter the Alawites and take out their hearts to eat them!" For a similar account of mutilation and cannibalism in war times during the medieval period in Syria, cf. Joosse, *'Abd al-Laṭīf al-Baghdādī as a Philosopher and a Physician*, at 39. There are, however, significant differences between the two. The latter merely is an account of survival cannibalism, whereas the former is situated in a sectarian milieu and is instigated by a deep-seated hatred for the enemy that is coupled with strong feelings of revenge and retaliation.

178 Allemann, *Ris. fī Muğādalat*, 109-110; Ms. Bursa, Hüseyin Çelebi 823, fol. 116r; cf. also Bürgel, *Allmacht*, 205-06.

179 Allemann, *Ris. fī Muğādalat*, 110; Ms. Bursa, Hüseyin Çelebi 823, fol. 116r.

180 The collection of human body parts, with the aim of using them as an ingredient in an elixir is a motive rarely attested in Arabic literature. 'Abd al-Laṭīf is to my knowledge the only Arabic author to speak so freely about this controversial topic, which without any hesitation may be counted among the so-called "unspeakable things". An example of the usage of human blood (and of the possible usage of human body parts) in an alchemical operation is to be found in the work *Secretum secretorum* of the English Franciscan scholar Roger Bacon (c. 1214 or 1220-c.1292 A.D.), in: *Opera hactenus inedita Rogeri*

interference by the local governments (or the central government) or any specific jurisprudence (*fiqh*) with regard to a prohibition of these evil and objectionable practices seem to be fully absent, which is perhaps caused by the fact that the whole area was in such a gigantic turmoil during the Crusades. The rulers could not cope with the situation and as a consequence public security all but collapsed. Decisions on any matter whatsoever were put on a back burner or postponed indefinitely during this period of chaos and confusion. Thus by the time the peace had been restored, the boom of alchemy with all its undesirable side effects past its peak and declined, so that the officials did not feel the necessity to amend or to change the laws.

Because traditions have developed independently of each other and history has the propensity to reinvent itself all the time in a more or less cyclical mode, it is definitely not out of the ordinary that the trade in body parts, with the aim of using them as an ingredient in an elixir, a medicine, a (magic) potion or an ointment, is not restricted to a particular geographical area or a specific period in time. Even now, in modern-day South Africa, there occurs the phenomenon of murder for the use of human body parts in the making of potions, the so-called *muti* murder. The *muti* traders often attack young and healthy children. Not so long ago, a 6-year-old boy and a 10-year-old boy were killed for their body parts. In the first case, the boy's head was cut off and kept in a fridge in expectation of prospective customers to come. In the latter case, the boy died in hospital more than a week after attackers had hacked off his hands, ears and penis.[181] Some clients are willing to pay the trader huge amounts of money for "strong" *muti*. The trade in strong *muti* has led to some people raiding mortuaries and stealing body parts from corpses and selling them to *inyangas* (diviners, traditional healers). It has to be emphasized here strongly that *muti* murder has nothing in common with that which is sometimes erroneously called bush medicine, in which plant matter and occasionally parts of

---

Baconi, Vol. 5, ed. Robert Steele (Oxford 1920); cf. P.G. Maxwell-Stuart (ed./tr.), *The Occult in Mediaeval Europe*, 217; cf. also William R. Newman, 'An Overview of Roger Bacon's Alchemy', in: Jeremiah Hackett (editor): *Roger Bacon and the Sciences. Commemorative Essays* (Leiden/New York/Köln 1997), 317-336, esp. 329-332. In Pseudo-Avicenna's *De anima* (see: *infra* footnote 187 at 58) the "stone which is not a stone", the philosophical egg of the *Secret of Secrets*, is openly equated with human blood, cf. Newman, *Overview*, 330. Bacon was intimately acquainted with this pseudo epigraph, which contains extensive recipes for separating the four elements from a variety of products; cf. Newman, *Overview*, 321.

Of course, Bacon's *Secretum secretorum* is the famous *Secret of Secrets* (Arabic: *K. Sirr al-asrār)* by Pseudo-Aristotle, the apocryphal correspondence between Aristotle and his former pupil Alexander the Great. It was a work that Bacon held in the highest regard and even glossed. It was initially translated from the Arabic into the Latin language in a partial version by John of Seville ca. 1130 A.D., and approximately one hundred years later it appeared in a complete version through the efforts of Philip of Tripoli, cf. Steven J. Williams, 'Roger Bacon and the *Secret of Secrets*', in: Jeremiah Hackett (editor): *Roger Bacon and the Sciences*, 365-393, especially 365.

181 Report from the South African newspaper the 'Cape Argus' of Saturday 21/08/2004.

animals are being used for potions and ointments etcetera. *Muti* murder or medicine murder is also distinctly different from ritual murder, when a victim is sacrificed in public for the "benefit" of the whole community. *Muti* murder is committed by individuals and for selfish motives. It is a criminal act strongly tied to the beliefs in the power and benefits of human body parts and to certain beliefs in witchcraft. It is highly remarkable that also in this situation any specific jurisprudence with regard to these dreadful offences is lacking. The South African government (by means of The Ralushai Commission) proposed and drafted a new Act: The Witchcraft Control Act. In it, related issues such as *muti* murder shall almost certainly be addressed, because this type of murder is ever-increasing and not yet covered by any existing Act.[182]

According to Ullmann, the relationship between alchemy and medicine is merely an external one.[183] Although the Greek physician Galen is also considered an alchemist in the eyes of the Arabs, this classification must be seen as a myth and does not prove anything concerning Galen's possible influence on the doctrine of alchemy. Even in the case of Rhazes, who was thought of as an outstanding physician and an eminent chemist, there is no concrete evidence for the assumption that both fields of knowledge, alchemy and medicine, stimulated- and cross-pollinated each other. The same situation arises in the case of pharmaceutics: in the preparation of mineral drugs entirely different principles are applied than those used in alchemy. However, as in alchemy, distillation stills are being used in the production of perfumes.[184] In the *Corpus Jabirianum* it is reported that the elixir is able to cure illnesses and poisonings. We must consider this to be a legend of magic; a statement without a real factual basis which cannot be empirically proved. Alchemy and medicine are strictly separated in their fundamentals and in their methods i.e. in theory and in practice.[185] For this reason, alchemy cannot be

---

182 Anthony Minnaar, 'Legislative and legal challenges to combating witch purging and *muti* murder in South Africa', in: John Hund (editor): *Witchcraft Violence and the Law in South Africa* (Pretoria 2003), 73-92. The phenomenon of *muti* murder, with its distinct but highly unsavory relation to AIDS and HIV, has become one of the most serious and heinous issues of present-day society in Southern Africa. The subject has now luckily also pervaded the modern fictional literature of/on Southern Africa, see for instance part one of the award-winning series *The No. 1 Ladies' Detective Agency* [dealing with the adventures of the African (Botswanan) "Miss Marple" Precious Ramotswe] by the Scottish professor of medical law Alexander McCall Smith (London 1998).

183 Ullmann, *Die Natur- und Geheimwissenschaften*, 150, note 3; However, Owsei Temkin ('Medicine and Graeco-Arabic Alchemy', in: *BHM* 29 (1955), 134-153, especially 148-49) states that at the end of the 9th century A.D. the elixir had become endowed with medicinal properties, and thus an approach from alchemy to medicine was affected. Temkin endorses the view that the connection between alchemy and medicine was as yet a tenuous one in its practical effects, but at the same time he believes that the establishment of this connection paved the way for further developments in the fields of medicine and (medical) chemistry.

184 In the production of perfumes pharmaceutical –not alchemical– methods are applied.

185 Ullmann, *Die Natur- und Geheimwissenschaften*, 150, note 3.

considered an auxiliary science of medicine. But in the European Middle Ages people thought differently about this particular subject, as the following textual fragments might prove. In the first text *De erroribus medicorum* by the 13th century English Franciscan author Roger Bacon it is explicitly stated that alchemy is valuable for practical medicine, and that its working is extremely useful for the theory of medicine. The author sees alchemy as a necessary part of theoretical medicine, in that it investigates how things come into being, and in that it examines the special properties of their individual characters:

...The fifth fault [among physicians] is their ignorance of alchemy and agriculture, because almost all herbal medicines are derived from these two branches of knowledge, as is perfectly obvious. They prescribe the wrong things particularly because of their ignorance of alchemy. Since the art of medicine presupposes that the working properties of medicines are accepted as valid without the presence of a material substance, and since on innumerable occasions this must happen, because the substances used are gross, earthy, and harmful, one cannot give a detailed description of them except by referring to the methods used in alchemy which is the only branch of knowledge which teaches us how to extract the working properties from anything. In things used for healing, solutions and separations of one thing must be produced from another, something which cannot happen without the power of alchemy which teaches us how to condense one thing out of another....[186]

Bacon envisages two roles for alchemy in medicine, both related to the technology contained in alchemical texts, especially the distillation-technology of pseudo-Avicenna's *De anima*.[187] The first role consists in purifying ordinary pharmaceuticals. The second role concerns the prolongation of human life to its utmost, with the help of substances that have been "reduced to equality" with the aid of alchemy.[188] The second text *Practica vera alkimica* (c. 1386) by the author Ortulanus or rather Hortulanus deals with the realization of the perfect medicine out of an alchemical process:

...This is perfected aqueous alcohol and a sound medicine for the body, a more valuable medicine than those of Galen, Avicenna, Hippocrates, and any other doctor, having the power to pluck out, uproot, purge, and expel all infirmities from the human body. Even if the infirmity has lasted for hundred years, it will be completely cured in one month; and if it has lasted for fifty years, it will be completely cured within a fortnight. If some infirmity has lasted for twenty years, it will be completely cured within eight days; and if some infirmity has lasted in the human body for seven years, it will be cured within three days; and if some infirmity has lasted for one year, it will be cured in a single day. This is quite obviously the secret of the secrets. Its powers cannot be bought, and it is rightly called 'the blessed stone'

---

186 Roger Bacon, *De erroribus medicorum*, in: *Opera hactenus inedita Rogeri Baconi*, Vol. 9, ed. A.G. Little and E. Withington (Oxford 1928), cf. P.G. Maxwell-Stuart (ed./tr.), *The Occult in Mediaeval Europe*, 220-21.

187 *De anima in artis chemicae principes, Avicenna atque Geber* (Basel 1572). This is a Latin translation of an Arabic forgery attributed to Avicenna, which should not be confused with the genuine *De anima* or *Liber sextus de naturalibus*, cf. Newman, *Overview*, 321.

188 Newman, *Overview*, 324.

because there has not been anything which Almighty God has given humankind, which is more precious....[189]

Alchemy and medicine also meet when questions of sickness and health are raised, and especially when a causal relation between them is assumed. The influence of lead and other metals on the human body is rarely spoken of in the vast Arabic medical literature that has come to light. The pursuit of alchemy by shadowy alchemists and charlatans who worked in poor and unprofessional circumstances, and who fooled around with chemicals without fully understanding their properties, caused them to be in real physical danger.[190] The frequent use of lead and other harmful substances may therefore have contributed to a massive increase of lead poisoning during the middle ages. Avicenna was cognizant of the dire consequences of medicinal lead and also warned for the use of leaden pipes to transport water. Moses Maimonides counted *martak* or its synonym *murdarsanj* (hydrated lead monoxide)[191] and *saccharum saturni* or *lithargyros* first among the deadly mineral poisons.[192] Also Rhazes knew of the good and bad properties of lead.[193] The symptoms of lead poisoning were the topic of discussion between a doctor and his patient in Dioscorides's *Materia Medica*, a Greek work, from the first century B.C., which was translated into Arabic in the 9th century, and copied many times during the centuries to come.[194] The traditional distinctive and protracted symptoms of lead poisoning were colic (excruciating abdominal pains/cramps) followed by palsy (paralysis) and gout (or: similar diseases of the joints).[195] Only recently it has been proven that lead poisoning, due to occupational lead exposure, may cause delayed effects on the brain (damage of the central- and peripheral nerve-system) and kidneys (lead nephropathy).[196] That lead poisoning was commonplace in the

---

189 Ortulanus, *Practica vera alkimica*, in: *Theatrum Chemicum* Vol. 4 (Strasborg 1659), cf. P.G. Maxwell-Stuart (ed./tr.), *The Occult in Mediaeval Europe*, 219.

190 Coudert, *Alchemy: the Philosopher's stone*, 154.

191 Bassam I. El-Eswed, 'Lead and Tin in Arabic Alchemy', in: *Arabic sciences and philosophy*. A historical journal 12: 1 (2002), 139-153, especially 148-49 and 152-53.

192 Richard P. Wedeen, *Poison in the Pot. The Legacy of Lead* (Carbondale and Edwardsville 1984), 15.

193 Wedeen, *Poison*, 51.

194 These copies were often beautifully illustrated; cf. *Aramco World Magazine*, January-February 1989, in which a 13th century copy made in Iraq is displayed. It shows among others a physician and a patient discussing vitrified lead poisoning.

195 Cf. for instance the poem *The Canonization* by John Donne (1572-1631): "For Godsake hold your tongue, and let me love, Or chide my palsie, or my gout, My five gray haires, or ruin'd fortune flout...". See also some of Donne's other poems in which he refers to the "Elixir Vitae" (*Love's Alchymie*), to "poisonous minerals" (*Holy Sonnets: Divine Meditation No. 5*), to "quicksilver" (*The Apparition*), and to "the equal mixing, the balance, of the four humours" (*The Good-Morrow*), cf. Helen Gardner (ed.), *The Metaphysical Poets* (Harmondsworth -revised edition-1972), 58, 61, 70, 73, 85.

196 Especially among workers in the lead industry; those who manufacture solder to be used for electrical connections; those who prepare solder creams by converting molten lead into powder; those who manufacture batteries, cf. Wedeen, *Poison*, 1-9.

medieval Near East is difficult to prove, but can hardly be denied on the analogy of similar cases from the rest of the medieval world. Its symptoms and consequences were at least very well known and many people indeed must have suffered from this painful disease. In medieval and renaissance Europe the situation was different. The differential diagnosis of colic was totally obscure and there was no possibility at all to distinguish dysentery from obstructed bowel or lead colic.[197] European physicians had forgotten the lessons of the ancients and during this particular period Arabic physicians filled the gap and became the repository for Greek and Roman medical knowledge, and hence brought sophistication and illumination upon what is often designated as the European Dark Ages.[198] That lead poisoning was nevertheless commonplace in medieval and renaissance Europe is evident from the recurring laws requiring the elimination of lead from alcoholic beverages.[199] Coudert pointed out that the death rate among Chinese alchemists and their patrons seems to have been significantly higher than among their Western fellow craftsmen. Unlike the majority of the Western and Middle- and Near Eastern alchemists, their Chinese pendants were constantly trying to eat, drink or breathe immortality in one form or another, which of course very often caused a deadly mercury, arsenic or lead poisoning.[200] Like alchemists in the West the Chinese believed in the possibility of transmuting base metals into gold, but it was not the gold itself they were after.[201] They used gold to prepare elixirs or as an ingredient in many different strange foods and brews. Recipes for nibbling melted gold were numerous.[202] Elixir addicts among alchemists often were the rule rather than the exception.[203] The quest for immortality under Arabic alchemists was existent too and played an important role, although it needs to be assumed that the search for the "Elixir of Life", by which life could be indefinitely prolonged, was above all fashionable under early Arabic alchemists such as Jābir ibn Ḥayyān and his school, and under those who

---

197 Wedeen, *Poison*, 15.

198 Referred to is the important discussion whether or not the so-called European Dark Ages were truly Dark Ages in which no progression or enlightenment was visible. In a four-part documentary television series (BBC 4: The Dark Ages: An Age of Light, 2012) - written, directed, and presented by art critic Waldemar Januszczak- the art and architecture of the (European) Dark Ages is overviewed, and the conclusion drawn is that the era is shown to be an age of enlightenment or renaissance. There is a strong element of truth in this vision. Medieval European medicine with its Greek-Roman foundations was on the brink of decline and sinking to the level of quacks, mountebanks, herb-doctors and soothsayers, and therefore very close to a total collapse. The emergence of Islam brought new medical achievements to medieval Europe and paved the way for further medical and scientific discoveries.

199 Wedeen, *Poison*, 16.

200 Coudert, *Alchemy: the Philosopher's stone*, 184.

201 Coudert, *Alchemy: the Philosopher's stone*, 161.

202 Coudert, *Alchemy: the Philosopher's stone*, 173.

203 Coudert, *Alchemy: the Philosopher's stone*, cf. Ch. 7: Chinese Elixir Addicts, 161-191; cf. likewise Ping Yu Ho & Joseph Needham, 'Elixir Poisoning in Medieval China', in: *Janus* 48 (1959), 221ff.

continued the tradition of Jābir. This search for the "Water of Life" or any other form of immortality seems to have been an alien element in Arabic alchemical thought, which perhaps came into being under the influence of models from the Far East. However, alongside with the hunger for genuine chemical experimentation, the profit motive, the thirst after easy gain, might have been predominant and must have played a key role among workers in the field of Arabic alchemy.

During the rest of his life, ʻAbd al-Laṭīf did not desist from taking the strife against alchemy very seriously. In the tractates which are devoted to combating the 'false art', we are able to observe a sincere anger, which is almost always attended by a genuine astonishment of the fact that completely honourable persons may be so easily beguiled by something that is so obviously humbug. This is once more demonstrated by the subsequent fragments, which are taken from the aforementioned *Risāla fī Muǧādalat al-ḥakīmayn al-kīmiyāʼī wa-l-naẓarī*:

The first fragment deals with a letter which ʻAbd al-Laṭīf (or rather: his common alter-ego 'the theoretical philosopher') had found in an archive at the Ayyūbid palace in Aleppo shortly after the death of prince al-Malik al-Ẓāhir Ghāzī ibn Yūsuf in the month October of the year 1216 A.D. In this letter, which was sent from the city of Ḥarrān by the former teacher of prince al-Malik al-Ashraf, one of Ṣalāḥ ad-Dīn's other sons, the writer incites prince al-Malik al-Ẓāhir to rely and hold on to a certain Mr. X (who appears to be al-Qāḍī al-Aʻazz Fakhr al-Dīn Abū ʻAbdallāh Miqdām ibn Aḥmad ibn Shukr, the stepfather of the dismissed vizier Ibn Shukr) who had just come from Jerusalem to Aleppo and had been mentioned as a candidate for the post of vizier of the entire Egyptian (Ayyūbid) administration.[204] The former teacher of al-Malik al-Ashraf then states the following:

When I would have been given the opportunity to stay with him, we would have produced the perfect elixir, changed lead into the finest gold and filled the treasuries of the Sultan with gold and silver. Because of this, we would have been in the position to mass new troops which would have conquered the lands of the Franks and the Armenians and subjected the unbelievers to the Sultan's rule; the sphere of his influence (then) would have been extended immensely and his fame would have immortalized him. (ʻAbd al-Laṭīf then says): Such rhetoric from the mouth of this man does not sound as sly plotting and scheming, swindling and passionate desire. No, it is rather rooted in firm belief and (is meant) as sincere advice.[205] However, such must be the result from a flaw in his intellect and a malfunction of the powers of his imagination, for this man also composed works of poetry and prose. He particularly professed his commitment to the teachings of Ibn Umail and hardly payed attention to al-Rāzī and Jābir.[206] His house was intended only for (practising) the 'art': any old works and

[204] Allemann, *Ris. fī Muǧādalat*, 139, note 86: 'In den Anekdoten (…) nennt 'Abdallaṭīf –aus verständlichen Gründen– sehr oft keine Namen (…) 'Abdallaṭīf wollte ja sehr oft sicher nicht "Personen", sondern "Amtsinhaber" blosstellen'.

[205] Allemann, *Ris. fī Muǧādalat*, 153, note 219: 'Wahrscheinlich behandelt 'Abdallaṭīf diesen Alchemisten aus Ḥarrān auch deshalb so nachsichtig, weil er einerseits seine Kunst in den Dienst der Eroberung der Frankenländer stellen wollte, andererseits aber der Lehrer eines Sohnes von Saladin gewesen war'.

[206] For Ibn Umail at-Tamīmī, cf. Allemann, *Ris. fī Muǧādalat*, 153, note 220.

procedures were going on there incessantly. Deep inside (this man) did not doubt that he had come closer to the actual goal than all the other people (who inhabit) the earth.
But it is strange, how he can explain, that he wanted to join forces with this man (in particular), and that (he felt that) he was equal to him (i.e. to prince al-Malik al-Ẓāhir).[207]

In the second fragment ʻAbd al-Laṭīf informs us that:

This candidate for the post of vizier also resided for a short while in Ḥarrān under the auspices of al-Malik al-Ashraf, and still hoped for the office of vizier. Meanwhile, he devoted himself, together with a group of people, to the "art" and put the (alchemistical) procedure (called) *bāb al-manāra* to the test. Envious persons (around him), however, planned a conspiracy against him and slandered him in the eyes of the Sultan, (for they claimed) that he forged money. Then, they raided his house, cleaned it out, arrested his comrades, tied them to the whipping-post and imprisoned them. He, however, (escaped) and moved to Hama; there again he practised the "art", without coming to his senses, just as the impertinent lover (would behave).[208]

At the end of ʻAbd al-Laṭīf's second treatise on alchemy (no. 7: the *Risāla fī l-Maʻādin wa-ibṭāl al-kīmiyā'*) we find an addition. In it, ʻAbd al-Laṭīf advises us that he was just re-reading his work in Erzinjān in the year 622 A.H., when by a curious coincidence a visitor was announced who turned out to be an alchemist and who asked for an introduction from ʻAbd al-Laṭīf to al-Malik ʻAlā' al-Dīn Dāwūd ibn Bahrām, the ruler of the city, so that he might use the body of a slave or a condemned criminal for the preparation of his elixir![209] Having learned a little bit more about ʻAbd al-Laṭīf's flamboyant personality, his use of often abrasive and excessive language, his at times unwarranted prejudice and his slight but undeniable inclination towards exaggeration, one can only begin to imagine what ʻAbd al-Laṭīf's reply to the poor alchemist must have been like. Still we gain the impression that all his display is justifiable and evidently not without a reason. It merely functioned as a means to an end. ʻAbd al-Laṭīf al-Baghdādī was indeed a rebellious intellectual, but unmistakably a rebel with a cause.

---

207 Allemann, *Ris. fī Muǧādalat*, 120-21 (§ 95); Ms. Bursa, Hüseyin Çelebi 823, fol. 120v-120r.

208 Allemann, *Ris. fī Muǧādalat*, 121 (§ 96); Ms. Bursa, Hüseyin Çelebi 823, fol. 120r; for another anecdote regarding this candidate for the office of vizier, cf. Allemann, *Ris. fī Muǧādalat*, 84 (§ 31); Ms. Bursa, Hüseyin Çelebi 823, fol. 106r-107v and 83 (§ 29); fol. 106v.

209 Stern, *A Collection of Treatises*, 67; Allemann, *Ris. fī Muǧādalat*, 26; Ms. Bursa, Hüseyin Çelebi 823, fol. 131v, line 8-132v, line 7.

The *Book of the Two Pieces of Advice* or *Kitāb al-Naṣīḥatayn* by ʻAbd al-Laṭīf ibn Yūsuf al-Baghdādī (1162-1231): Annotated Translation of the Medical Section - Ms. Bursa (Turkey): Hüseyin Çelebi 823 (fol. 62r-78r)

(62r) The *Book of the Two Pieces of Advice* by ʻAbd al-Laṭīf, the son of Yūsuf, to the public at large.

(62v) In the name of God, the Merciful, the Compassionate.

This is a book, which (in its strive) to gain favor with the Creator, may he be praised and hallowed, takes pains to abstain from sin by giving sincere advice and by bringing guidance to its loyal adherents and devotees who are divided over the towns and who are wandering in the villages and the big cities. Moreover, it (strives to)[210] give sincere advice and to bring guidance to kings of faraway regions,[211] governors and princes, and furthermore to everyone who wishes the best for himself, and desires happiness. To all these people it [this book] brings love, solidarity, rejection of blind authority and fanaticism, by way of using insight, contemplation and consideration. But the first thing one should commence with, is to praise the glorious God who is the key towards all the good, to pray to him who is the guide towards every noble deed, and give him the praise he is worthy of. Thereupon, blessings have to be bestowed upon the prophet of mercy, because the leader of the community, the savior from every error and affliction, the guide towards the paths of salvation and bliss is Muḥammad, the Prophet, the one who could neither read nor write. Blessings have to be bestowed also upon his family, upon the pure-hearted, and upon the saints, the martyrs and the just. Furthermore, gratitude has to be shown to the great sages who followed the example of the prophets to the extent of their power, in the sense that they improved themselves first and thereupon gave advice to the masses of that which was composed by them regarding the outstanding sciences and the useful crafts. They made wisdom the goal of their fleeting lives and their provision towards the gate of the hereafter. They devoted their time and their effort in acquiring knowledge and were in no need of transitory acquisitions and perishable accidental qualities. With regard to

[210] Please note that round brackets denote an addition to the text. Square brackets denote an explanation of the text, whereas squiggly or curly brackets denote a doubtful reading.

[211] The wording *mulūk al-aṭrāf* may either have the meaning 'kings of faraway regions' or 'learned and noble kings'.

their bodily needs, they restricted themselves to that which would lead them to the exalted and sublime place, and to that which would not distract them from the aspired goal. They became averse

(63r) to everything but wisdom and perceived that acquiring knowledge would bring them closer to the one and only, the sempiternal, the unique, the subsistent, the everlasting Judge. They devoted the benefit of their wisdom to that which would bring advantage, with regard to the souls and the bodies of the masses. And they propagated among them various sorts of useful sciences and crafts with regard to their earthly life and afterlife, of which the vestiges deserve acknowledgment and the external actions are commendable: particularly medicine, astronomy, agriculture, navigation, arithmetic, engineering, and geometry. And everyone who came after them, and who led their assembly by the example (of these sages), followed their pattern, and took their method as a model, was limited in number and could be counted on the fingers of one hand. Such an individual would receive a reward like theirs and would deserve praise and thanks in the measure of his capability and the sincerity of his intention. And those kings in charge, who would help with this, would receive a double reward and an additional, enhanced merit, because (most) people tend to follow the authority of the ruler and compare themselves with him, (although they also could) hatch a plot against him and seek to depose him. This is, however, imbedded in their innate nature and (deeply) rooted in their character. Suchlike (behavior) can be seen through the youth who imitates the habits of his parents and his educators, as a result of which the parents may witness greed and fear by the child. A person who does not take note of (his own behavior) may (therefore) receive an equivalent of the evil consequence of his deed. But when his good deeds (virtues) are placed opposite to his bad deeds (vices), the reward for his good deeds (virtues) must be increased. My aim in this book to my loyal adherents, may God guide them well and grant them success, is to give (them) advice and to arouse them from the sleep of negligence and (to liberate them) from familiar and habitual customs and practices and to warn them for the afflictions which are propagated (everywhere) and whose harm is prevailing over all the souls and bodies and to put them on their guard against falling into harmful situations (like these). For he who knows that what I say is correct, his devotion and faith shall increase. And he who does not know this,

(63v) I wish for him that he shall acquire knowledge (about it). And if one of those who possess knowledge (about it) takes what I say as an example, then that person would satisfy me through the reward which he would be given, whereas the glory which he would receive, would suffice me. The wrong of this (specific) affliction in riffraff and (other) scum pales by the side of the wrong (of this affliction) in kings and powerful people; that is, the harm caused by the latter [i.e. the elite] is more disgusting than that caused by those who do not possess (sound) knowledge [i.e. the ignorant]. And if you would pose me (a question) and would say to me: 'which harm is more significant than that of not possessing the (true) wisdom', then I would answer you: 'listen, understand and learn from me that the acquisition of false knowledge is more harmful and more damaging than not being in possession of the true wisdom'. And if a leader does not possess wisdom (at all), and realizes that he is free from it, void of it, and in need of it, then he must yearn for it, try to obtain it, and ardently aspire to acquire it. Someone who possesses false wisdom may believe that he is rich, while actually he belongs to the poorest of the poor. He is scared to educate himself and improve himself and is (thus) in want of (proper) instruction and (crucial) development. Moreover, someone who does not possess religion at all hastens himself more towards compliancy than someone who possesses the false religion. But someone who includes a flaw in his faith is harder to comply than someone who has no faith (at all). Therefore, the common people can be quickly educated and are more pliable than those who possess the false faith. (For example), how much is (the difference) between a white leaf and another leaf which is filled with corrupt and false writings? The holy prophecy already pointed at this notion with the following utterance: 'every child comes into the world with a natural disposition until both his parents decide for him whether he shall become a Christian, a Jew, or a Mazdean'.[212] Plato said in his *Book on Politics* [= *Politeia, The Republic*]: 'for evil is of course more contrary to good than to what is not [lacks] good'. Plato also said: 'knowledge colors the soul, but the object which receives the color shall not shine until it is cleansed of its impurities'.

(64r) The greatest affliction of all and the greatest calamity of all, for which I try to seek recompense by bringing the attention to it, takes place in medicine with regard to the issue of liberating the bodies from illnesses, and in philosophy with regard to the issue of liberating the souls from the pain of ignorance, and guiding them towards a sound knowledge and a correct understanding of the truth. First of all, we shall comment on the factual afflictions with respect to medicine, the more so because its evil is prevalent among the general public, and because everyone will receive a share of its evil, since everyone is concerned with the liberation of his body from suffering, but not everyone is concerned with the liberation of his soul from ignorance.

But we will commence by stating that the art of medicine is an honorable and respectable art, the merits of which are acknowledged by the general public. The people set aside their differences, made a covenant and came together to legitimate the art of medicine, so that the need for it became greater. In the art of medicine we are able to find revelation, divine inspiration, and authentic visions which were attributed to the prophets, peace be upon them, and the divine sages. The art of medicine was brought about during sleep by those who were closest to God, may he be praised and glorified. The one who made an effort in the art of medicine was not denied his (high) rank of glory and his praise was not withheld from him by all (other) parties. Verily, (all of) this reveals the merits, benefits and deeds of the art of medicine, which resembles magic.

---

212 For this famous *ḥadīth*, cf. Arent Jan Wensinck *et alii*, *Concordance et Indices de la Tradition Musulmane*, VI (Leiden 1967), 174. This strong *ḥadīth* is related by al-Bukhārī, Muslim and Ibn Ḥanbal.

However, those (spongers), who asked, or demanded *rizq* [subsistence i.e. just to make profits and gains] (without having earned it, or giving something in return) extinguished the light of the art of medicine, made its memory vanish, obliterated its merits, slandered its good reputation, lowered its rank, and caused it to fail and have shortcomings. When the conditions [*shurūṭ*] of the medical art are fully adhered to, then it never makes a mistake. The skillful physician only errs occasionally, but gets things right a hundred times, as Galen said. Moreover, his miss will be neither small [decisive], nor great nor far removed from a hit [= from what is correct].

(64v) One can compare him to an expert in archery who hits the target in most cases, and when he misses the target, then (his arrow) will not be very far off from it [the target], but rather it will land near it [the specific target]. But in the event of the arrow falling entirely in the opposite direction, then (this is on a par with) a physician who commits an error. We have already stated that the art of medicine knows no mistakes and that the skillful physician only makes few mistakes and is mostly correct (in his decisions). For the arts which are concerned with matter are subject to many conditions because of the form, and many conditions because of the matter. This has to do with the universal and the particular. To the universal (things) belong teaching and learning. The particular, i.e. individual things [i.e. concrete patients and diseases] cannot (all) be discussed here. Only a character which endeavors to assiduously obtain it [the particular], is the one which (can) conjecture it and approach it. A certain tolerance [i.e. margin of error] is (only) natural; it does not matter and it can be rectified, especially in the case of diseases which are not especially acute and dangerous.

I shall give you as an example the surface of the circle or a square root such as that of (the number) ten.[213] Someone skilled in this art determines this (irrational number) as closely as possible, and will tolerate (only) the smallest part (of error) the difference of which is not apparent to sense-perception; however, it is not equivalent to a small difference for the intellect [i.e. the error cannot be perceived by the eye, but by the intellect]. Such a judgment is deemed to be correct, even if a certain tolerance is present in it, inasmuch as it (only slightly) exceeds a part [i.e. an amount] which basically does not count. As long as the part which one tolerates [i.e. the margin of error] is small, the judgment is quite correct, and the person arriving at it is quite skilled. Therefore, artful conjecturing in medicine is similar [*bi-hāḏihī l-manzilati*]. Yet what is different to this (small amount of error) is evidently a (full

---

[213] 'Abd al-Laṭīf here likens the inexactness of medicine to that of mathematics. Just as the latter can only give approximations of irrational numbers as π and $\sqrt{10}$, so medicine, when concerned with particulars [i.e. patients and diseases] can only provide estimates, see: N. Peter Joosse and Peter E. Pormann, 'Archery, mathematics, and conceptualising inaccuracies in medicine in 13th century Iraq and Syria'. Available from: www.jameslindlibrary.org (Sir Iain Chalmers and Jan P. Vandenbroucke (editors). [Republished as: 'Archery, mathematics, and conceptualizing inaccuracies in medicine in 13th century Iraq and Syria', in: *Journal of the Royal Society of Medicine* 101 (2008), 425-27].

fledged) error, and those who commit it are not deemed to belong to those exercising the art (of medicine). Likewise, if someone says that the square root of ten equals three, he cannot be counted as an arithmetician, and his words cannot be accepted.

(65r) This is also valid for those who are in the same situation, namely those who claim to master the art of medicine, without (actually) being a physician. It is desirable that one stays away from them and avoids being in their presence.
One should be on his guard against them, more than one should be on his guard against predatory animals, who cry out with hunger and against venoms that would necessarily (cause) death [= lethal poisons] and against all the calamities which could befall the people. The result being, that becoming infected with all of this, is the worst thing one has to withstand and for which one needs to be on one's guard. Where the ignorant physician is concerned, he is clearly an enemy disguised as a friend, and a poison disguised as an antidote [or: theriac]. He makes use of common, widely known drugs and is capable of killing (somebody) with them if he does not happen to find the (right) place (and time) to administer them. For this reason the ignorant physician should be considered a deadly poison (himself). And if the drinking of a potion at the wrong time or without (certain) preconditions can already kill (a person), then one should leave off (administering) poisonous purgatives such as *sanā* [Cassia senna], *basfā'īj* [Polypodium vulgare L.],[214] *turbid* [Ipomoea turpethum L.], *shaḥm al-ḥanẓal* [Pulpa colocynthidis], *saqmūnīyā* [Convonvulus scammonia L.], and similar ones like those which are either a (genuine) poison or (slightly) poisonous. Whenever the disease reaches its most aggressive and most serious stage, then the harm caused by the error of the physician shall be the greatest, so that it may happen that a patient who was cured by a potion shall die when the potion is taken away from him, and that another patient who was not given the potion shall die when he is given the potion. But in none of the given situations should the error of the physician be regarded with contempt, for (you should consider that) a small error (committed by a doctor) can have major consequences, and an error (committed by a doctor) which at first sight may seem insignificant, can have an enormous impact. Hippocrates has already said that when the physician employs the (medical) names which the quacks employ as well, then the vulgar cannot make a distinction between the genuine practitioner and the quack, that is to say, the physician employs the medical names at the right moment and the quack employs them at the wrong moment. The vulgar people do not understand the meaning of this. Hippocrates has already said something similar in the introduction of his *Book on regimen in acute diseases* [*K. al-Amrāḍ al-ḥādda*].[215] He also composed a *Book on the rules of conduct and manners of*

---

[214] Cf. Reinhart Dozy, *Supplément aux dictionnaires arabes*, 2 vols. (Leiden 1881) [reprint: Beirut 1981], vol. 1, at 86-87.

[215] Cf. Fuat Sezgin, *GAS*, III, 33-34.

doctors [*K. fī Adab aṭ-ṭabīb*][216] and another one on the qualities and characteristics of doctors (bearing the title):

(65v) *Kayfa yanbaghī an yakūna* [*How it is appropriate (for a doctor) to act and (be)have*].[217] Galen wrote a *Book on the examination of the physician* [*K. fī Imtiḥān aṭ-ṭabīb*] which is an outstanding and essential work to become acquainted with, and which can be used as a guide by someone who is in need of consulting a physician.[218] One of the [many] things he said in this book is that although a lot of of the leaders and wealthy lords do not spend more time in occupying themselves with the art of medicine, they are still in need of doctors whenever diseases should befall them. The skilled physician takes away their pain, but the ignorant one causes them to suffer more pain and lets them fall into perdition. Galen wished that (certain) diagnostics (or: guidelines) could be (developed) by which people [the chiefs and the lords] could make a distinction between the genuine practitioner and the quack, and that they could examine their (own) conditions through these traits and (thus) prevent themselves from (possible) danger, so that (without taking any risks) they could turn over their lives to the other [= the physician]. Just as Galen wished for mankind that they would possess the skill to distinguish between poison and foodstuff, and that one (substance) would not be mistaken for another. He furthermore said that he wished that the one who claims to be a physician is attentively looked at and examined (thoroughly) on the topic of that to which he dedicated his time at the start of his career and (on the topic) of that to which he dedicates his time in his present condition, after first having found out about the goodness of his nature, the excellence of his disposition, the soundness of his reasoning and his intelligence with which he was endowed, from the day he was born. Thereupon, his faith, his integrity, his sense of honor and his ability to keep things a secret should be examined. All of these things should not fail to be found in his deeds and words. If everybody is pleased with his words and they all adorn the things which have become manifested in his deeds towards the people, then it has become necessary to examine the state of his solitariness [= his perusal and silent study of medical books], and to scrutinize that what has become perceptible of the safety of the person who submits himself to him [the physician]. Accordingly, his abstinence with regard to the belly [= food] and the pudenda [= sexual intercourse], and the measure of his desire in the attainment of the *dirham* [= greed] should be

---

216 This title cannot be found under this specific name within the Hippocratic Corpus; is it perhaps one of the *Waṣāyā*? - cf. Sezgin, *GAS*, III, 39 under no. 12.

217 This is most likely the *Yanbaghī li-man arāda an yakūna ṭabīban fāḍilan*, cf. Sezgin, *GAS*, III, 39.

218 Cf. Sezgin, *GAS*, III, 125: *K. fī Miḥnat afḍal al-aṭibbā'*; cf. likewise Albert Z. Iskandar, (ed.), *Galen on Examinations by Which the Best Physicians Are Recognized*, [= *Corpus Medicorum Graecorum* (*CMG*), Supplementum Orientale 4] (Berlin 1988); cf. also Manfred Ullmann: *Die Medizin im Islam* (Handbuch der Orientalistik, I. Abt., Erg.-Bd. VI, 1) (Leiden/Köln 1970), 52-53: *K. Miḥnat aṭ-ṭabīb* or *K. fī l-Miḥna allatī bihā ya'rifu l-insān afḍal al-aṭibbā'*.

put to the test. If he venerates all these things, then he is devoid of anything good, because an evil person is not expected to sell

(66r) his worldly existence and his life in the hereafter for one single *dirham* or for one single transgression. If his innate nature displays foolishness and if his natural disposition contains destructive elements, then do not expect (any) good from him, do not wait for virtue(s) from his side, abandon (all) hope for his success, and do not expect righteousness from him. It is not to be expected that he improves his exercise in the sciences, but (instead of this) he shall (probably) cause the increase of harm and immorality. Just as some poet said: 'knowledge is an addition to an intelligent man and a shortcoming to a foolish and thoughtless man, just as the day brightens the vision of man with its light, whereas the light of day dims the vision of the bat'. The following (words) are taken from the sayings of Plato: 'knowledge makes very evil persons even more evil, because knowledge serves as a substitute for the canine teeth and the claws of predatory animals'. But if he nevertheless possesses envy, adulation and avidity, then all the instruments of evil may already have assembled in him and may have formed a pact with the causes that may draw him towards evils and vicissitudes. And if falsehood and lack of devotion are added to this, then one should be very much on one's guard against him. However, if he can be characterized by outstanding intellect and sagacity, but started out the early days of his life in idleness and trade, then do not expect cleverness from him in the crafts and the arts, but do (also) not give up all hope on him. If he dedicates his present time to pleasures and delights, then he is just as far removed from the virtue as he is engrossed in the vice. Galen has already said in his *Book (on the examination of the physician)* [*K. fī Imtiḥān aṭ-ṭabīb*] that he likes to examine how a physician dedicates his time and (how he spends) his activities. If he devotes both of them [i.e. his time and his activities] during the night to amusement and the attainment of pleasures, and during the day to meet up with those in high station [i.e. the leaders], in order to do them honor and offer them lots of presents, then he has no good inside of him and does not possess virtue. But if he spends the night(s) and his spare time

(66v) on reading, studying, thinking, and acquiring additional knowledge, and if he dedicates the rest of his time to the benefit of the people and the healing of the sick, takes pains to serve them, liberates them from pains and illnesses, whilst (at the same time) he takes pleasure and delight in healing them and (thus) gets closer to the creator of everything and the one who is cognizant of the secrets of the hearts, then he should be considered a virtuous physician who likes (the people) to have confidence in his knowledge and wants them to rely upon his treatment and opinion. But his qualities should nevertheless entail that he is in possession of mercy and compassion, which are a far cry from harshness and cruelty. Moreover, his pleasure in diagnosing (the disease) rightly should weaken his joy of acquiring the *dirham* and the *dinar*. What good is it to an intelligent person to surrender his life to someone who is drunk at night and befuddled in the morning? For like this, are those who have a psychical and physical illness. For how can someone who is suffering from two diseases treat someone who is suffering from a single disease?

The condition of a person who is addicted to alcohol is dissimilar to the condition of someone who is learned and skilled. If the addict (to alcohol) is ill, then the compressed damp and moist vapors which are pressed together within the brain follow (each other) up in an uninterrupted succession, for they block the breathing holes of the body, cloud the breath of life, darken the senses, extinguish the light of life and the splendor of the soul, render the place of thinking inactive and destroy the seat of knowledge, sense and judgment. How can this be similar for someone who passes the night in devotion to study, thinking, researching and digging deep into science or knowledge in order to polish the mirror of his intellect, whet the sharp edge of his understanding, sharpen his faculties and stimulate his thoughts and ideas? His speculation will become a benefit for the people through his knowledge [= theory], his deeds [= practice], the way he puts into practice what he learned, and his intuition. Can such a person be similar to someone, whose ultimate aim is the (material) world,

(67r) and whose utmost concern is chasing dancing girl(s) and the pursuit of every *dirham*? Hence, the poets lowered their eyes to the ground in disapproval while criticizing the alcoholics: 'The sprinkling of wine protects from many imperfections, but be careful not to increase what causes foolishness, for no sensible person is satisfied with the squandering of his intellect for wine, for the latter robs one of one's reason'. Hippocrates and Galen and those who followed their path were skeptical about the ignorance of the physicians of their time. They questioned their poor knowledge and their high frequency of attacking one another. Hippocrates already often ridiculed them in his *Book on regimen in acute diseases* [*K. al-Amrāḍ al-ḥādda*]. Where Galen is concerned, he began the majority of his books by accusing the physicians of his time of having faults and vices and cautioned against them by revealing their shortcomings. Yet, he did of course not observe the time in which we now live, and he did not see what we have now seen and he did not pay attention to the matters to which we nowadays pay attention. Galen complained about the methodist sect [μεθοδικοί, *aṣḥāb al-ḥiyal*][219] and the empiricist sect [ἐμπειρικοί, *aṣḥāb al-tajārib*]. Even though they all generally fall short and are deficient, they have useful rules and principles, which it is best to acquire and learn, especially those of the empiricists. Galen reported many of their procedures (and inserted them) in his *K. al-Mayāmir*[220] [*On Compound Drugs according to Places*] and *K. al-Qaṭājānis*[221] [*On Compound Drugs according to Types*].

---

219 The Arabic term *aṣḥāb al-ḥiyal* is ambiguous. It literally means 'those using *ḥīla*,' the latter term denoting both "method" and "trick"; it is therefore a technical term for "methodists" (μεθοδικοί)', cf. Pormann, *The Physician and the Other*, at 196-97.

220 Cf. Sezgin, *GAS*, III, 70, 71, 73, 119, 222, 264, 316, 412. The *K. al-Mayāmir* or *K. (fī) Tarkīb al-adwiya bi-ḥasab al-mawāḍi' (al-ālima)* is the second part (ten *maqālāt*) of Galen's *K. fī Tarkīb al-adwiya* (cf. *GAS*, III, especially 118-120).

221 Cf. Sezgin, *GAS*, III, 119-120. The *K. al-Qaṭājānis* or *K. fī Tarkīb al-adwiya 'ala l-jumal wa-l-ajnās* or *bi-ḥasab ajnāsihā* is the first part (seven *maqālāt*) of Galen's *K. fī Tarkīb al-adwiya*.

Our contemporaries do not belong to any of the three sects which he (Galen) defined in his *Book on the Sects (for Beginners)* [*K. al-Firaq*],[222] but rather rely on luck and chance like a blind man shooting (an arrow) without knowing in which direction the target is. The sects of the methodists and empiricists know the target, but shoot (the arrow) without (first) examining its [the target's] exact position.

(67v) The masters of reason [the rationalists, δογματικοί, *aṣḥāb al-qiyās*] know the direction and the (exact) location of the target, directing their arrow there in the most perfect and correct fashion. The empiricists receive a manifestation [i.e. a non-essential characteristic] of the target, such as for instance its shadow, so that they deserve to hit the mark. The contemporary doctors, however, do not hit the target and do not find its direction. One is therefore surprised not by their making a mistake, but by their getting things right, whereas one is surprised by the mistake of the rationalists, and not their getting things right. For the latter get things mostly right – and essentially right at that [*wa-bi-l-dhāti*], whilst making mistakes only rarely – and accidentally [*bi-l-'araḍi*]. But these (spongers) rarely get things right, and only accidentally, whilst mostly making mistakes, and essentially at that.

We add the following as an explanation through an example which we posit. Take a man who suffers from fever. A physician of each of the sects comes to him. The methodist aims at loosening him [the patient] insofar as the fever arose out of stricture [*ikhtināq*]. The empiricist says: 'I have observed [*raṣadtu*] many times people suffering from such fever. I resorted to blood-letting, and extracted such-and-such a quantity of blood until he [the patient] fainted. Yet afterwards he [the patient] recovered from his fever in one fell swoop'. The rationalists will make the fever into a genus [*jins*], divide it by its essential differences [*fuṣūl dhātīya*] into three species [*anwā'*]. He [the rationalist] then looks at the fever of this man (to determine) of which of the three (species) it is. From the fever he determines the essence of the (disease) matter [*dhāt al-mādda*]. Then, he divides this fever into its species according to the (disease) matter, and determines that it [the fever] is bloody. He divides the bloody (fever) into the pure [*al-khāliṣa*] and the mixed [*al-mashūba*], and finds that it is pure. He divides the pure (bloody fever) further into that which has putrefied, and that which has begun to boil, and finds that it is that which has begun to boil. Then he considers the location, the age,

(68r) the present time, the habit, the past regimen, and other things of a nature to change the diagnosis [*al-ḥukm*]. From all these collected facts he derives a picture of the necessary regimen. Then he proceeds to let the blood (of the patient) until the latter fainted. I wished I knew who of these three physicians more accurately gets things right, and errs less frequently. Yet no intelligent man can choose anyone other than the rationalist, judging him to be skilful and wishing him victory and success [*al-ẓafar wa-l-falāḥ*].[223] And where each one of the contemporary

---

[222] Cf. Sezgin, *GAS*, III, 79-80, and 146. This is likely to be Galen's *K. Firaq aṭ-ṭibb li-l-muta'allimīn* or *K. Arāsīs* which is also mentioned under the name of *K. Firaq aṭ-ṭibb al-musammā Arāsīs*. Cf. also the edition of the Arabic translation by Muḥammad Salīm Sālim (Cairo 1977), *Kitāb Jālīnūs fī firaq al-ṭibb li-l-muta'allimīn*.

[223] Cf. Joosse and Pormann, *Decline and Decadence*, 8-12.

physicians is concerned, he would have come to see and examine (the patient). Thereupon, he would have bled him, or (on the other hand) would have prohibited the bloodletting (of the patient). He would have reached a conclusion on how to treat the patient without having had any knowledge of the established principles which are mentioned above, but he would have reached a conclusion according to that which he believed without having been skilled in the art. He would have made (mere) guess-work according to that, which his fantasy would bring forth, and not because of argument and proof, or because of experiment and observation. The majority of the contemporary physicians are like this, but the doctors who take some of the abovementioned conditions and stipulations into account do not stand alone. (Unfortunately), they only come one at a time. I believe that all the corruption with respect to the examination of physicians is attributable to the negligence of the princes and the other leaders. They sometimes give preference to a weak physician and raise him above the rank of an accomplished one, so that the latter's zeal and ambition (as well as that of other educated physicians) and their interest to guide themselves to the attainment of additional knowledge is thwarted. They [the physicians] thus come to the conclusion that the world bestows (its favors) through chance, and not merit, and fall short in their quest for them [the world's favors].

It is astonishing (to perceive) that a prince can be extremely careful with regard to someone whom he entrusts with his food and his beverages. He investigates and examines his affairs (with the same care) and he looks after his flock [his subjects] and his exclusive property in the same way, but he fails to consider the domain of medicine. Medicine is, however, more honorable, more important, more superior, more precious and weightier (than all other things). It deserves to be examined, observed and protected more than all those (other) things which we have already looked at, on the ground that the neglect of all those (other) things causes offense to the most pleasant and delightful matters (of life), but the neglect in the domain of medicine causes offense to life itself. It is to be desired that a prince

(68v) shall concern himself more (often) with medicine and physicians than with other matters. It is amazing (to perceive) that someone chooses the best and most skilled veterinarians for his donkey and his horse and accordingly surrenders his life to some person upon whose skills one cannot rely. It is (equally) amazing that someone who disallows the rabble to cook his food, to broil his meat and to bake his bread, disregards to contact the doctors and lets the doctors poke fun at life. It is also amazing that the *fiqh*-experts [= legal experts, experts in jurisprudence] neglect this domain. They guard the domain of property; for they only trust faithful and reliable persons to enter it. They only disburse the *dirham* to those of whom they have witnessed their honesty, but they accept the word of one of these quacks about life without examining his belief, his faith, his knowledge and his intellect. (Likewise), it is amazing to see that the expert in jurisprudence is about to reach, or has already reached, a rank by which he can form an independent judgment in legal questions, but that he surrenders his life to the man in the street who cannot memorize one (single) fascicle of a book on medicine. It is (equally) amazing to observe how they ignore this and do not act according to the word of the prophet, God bless him and grant him salvation: 'Whoever practices medicine[224] without formerly having had any acquaintance with it, and as a result kills a person, must be held responsible'.[225] It is an astonishing thing to learn that the masses have said about someone over whom the physicians have committed a mistake: 'he died at the appointed time, for God pronounced judgment over him'. Although they believe that all deeds of humans are created by God, may he be praised and exalted, they nevertheless murder a killer and take vengeance on a perpetrator. God, may he be praised, rather assumes the responsibility for the killing of someone over whom the physicians have committed a mistake without that person having had his throat slit and having had his head cut off. I have not heard about a community who in such a way guard the art of medicine, hold the doctors in esteem and stand by their doctors, as the (good) people of Constantinople. They do not enable anyone to practice medicine without him having been (properly) graded in the parts of medicine

(69r) and (without) him having had (proper) practice (in it). He had to pursue his studies for many years, after which he had to give testimony (of the subjects that he studied) to (a congregation of) elderly and venerable gentlemen. Thereupon, a meeting was summoned and in a gathering of these learned sheiks, he was put subject to a test in which a number of sick persons with different diseases were presented to him. He would make his rounds (and examine the patients) in the presence of these very excellent and very learned men. If they were satisfied with his deeds [practice], after first having been satisfied with his words [theory], they would impose the Hippocratic Oath on him, which he had to take in the presence of strangers, before they would reunite him with a group (of people) that would include (his) offspring and relatives. This was the situation (then) when the Byzantines (still) had control over the people of Constantinople, but in the current years the Franks made Constantinople their property. They changed many of the good (Byzantine) customs and abolished most of the old regulations. So I do not know how the situation of the people of Constantinople is today [i.e. I do not know whether or not examinations are still held there]. I saw the people of Baghdād take some care with regard to their physicians. This is the same with the people of Cairo: only someone, who possesses a certificate which is signed by the leading men of the profession, is at liberty to practice. The same situation can be found in Damascus.

---

224 The verb here is *taṭabbaba*, which according to the dictionaries has the meaning of 'to practice medicine' or 'to engage in the medical field'. However, the context could very well justify a meaning such as 'studied medicine a little' or 'studied medicine peripherally', cf. also Gutas, *Philosophy in the Twelfth Century*, at 13, with regard to the verb *taṭarrafa* in the meaning of 'studied them a little, peripherally'.

225 Cf. Wensinck *et alii*, *Concordance et Indices de la Tradition Musulmane*, III (Leiden 1955), 531. This *ḥadīth* is related by Abū Dāwūd (*Diyāt* 23), al-Nisā'ī (*Qasāma* 41) and Ibn Māja (*Ṭibb* 16), from *ḥadīth* of ʻAmr b. Shuʻayb, from his father, from his grandfather; cf. also Ibn Qayyim al-Jawziyya, *al-Ṭibb al-Nabawī* (*Medicine of the Prophet*), translated by Penelope Johnstone (Cambridge 1998), especially 103-107.

But, I have never witnessed greater neglect of the medical art (than) in the city of Aleppo. For their [the inhabitants'] behavior was extremely bad, and the ways of their physicians were in such a state of corruption that there was nothing viler than (this). No power compels them, no religion repels them, no knowledge guides them, no chief guides and scares them. They have one ambiguous method from which they rarely deviate, namely, if someone complains to them about a disease, they hasten to make him drink a purgative in order to collect quickly its price and take the maximum value for it; they pay no attention to whether it is well cooked, and neglect other conditions (necessary for preparing remedies). They apply (the potion) to someone about whom they had a report without actually seeing him. Their only worry is to pilfer the price of the purgative by crooked means. They obtain (its price) through all sorts of ruses, and do not care at all

(69v) how they kill through these means, and sell a man's life for the quarter of a *dirham*. I believe that the one who allotted these shameful deeds and despicable practices among them, was a *maghribī* [North African] sheik who had been converted to Islam, but returned to the Jewish religion outwardly – though they (the Jews themselves) firmly believed that he was neglectful with regard to their religion, thought little of observing their devotional duties, was careless in (his) obedience to (the regulations of) the *sharī'ah* [= the revealed or, canonical, law of Islam], and could not be believed at all (even) if he swore on the Torah and the Ten Commandments. He used to be a poor man who was traveling through the (different) countries in the service of merchants, and who (only) took a serious interest in the art of medicine at a (relatively) late age. He had a strong desire for worldly belongings and possessed the strength, tenacity and avidity of a dog, which made him annihilate human lives and attack human beings in the manner in which a lion attacks his prey. People agreed on the fact that he had no fear for the Creator or for (any) created being, and that he attached no importance whatsoever to the massacre of a thousand souls in one hour. They said that he took much pleasure in such things.

In the years 613 and 614 [A.H.] a group of noblemen and notable citizens passed away. I witnessed (the death of) a few of them, but information concerning (the death of) the others reached me through reports. Among those who passed on in the year 13 was the governor of the city [Aleppo], [the prince] al-Malik al-Ẓāhir Ghāzī ibn Yūsuf. He had become feverish on Saturday the 26th of (the month) *Jumādā* I of the year mentioned above. He was plump and overweight and had already surpassed the age of forty.[226] Thoughts and worries about the battle array of his army, (ways

[226] Two well-known medieval Arabic authors provided a description of 'Abd al-Laṭīf al-Baghdādī's physique. Ibn abī Uṣaybi'a depicted him as "thin-bodied and of moderate stature", whereas Ibn al-Qifṭī reported that 'Abd al-Laṭīf was "lean as a rake, short of stature, of a repulsive appearance, and had furrowed and sunken cheeks". Ibn al-Qifṭī likewise stated that 'Abd al-Laṭīf was given the nickname "the shrivelled one" because of his appearance. 'Abd al-Laṭīf, on the other hand, gave a rather unflattering description of two Ayyūbid princes. He called al-Malik al-Ẓāhir, his patron, "plump and overweight at the age of forty" and furthermore said that al-Malik al-'Ādil, Sultan Saladin's brother,

of) forcing (his) enemies to surrender [= battle strategies] and the costs of war had taken root in his mind, which caused him to abandon the drinking of fluids and to decrease the intake of food, whereas (at the same time) his insomnia increased and the thoughts kept spinning around in his head. Therefore, a physician who had embraced Islam (or: had become a Muslim) suggested bleeding him, to which all the (other) doctors unanimously agreed.

(70r) But this one damned devil prevented them [the other doctors] from bleeding him by saying to them in secret that bleeding him would cause the particular doctor to enjoy the favors and good graces (of the prince) and that he [the former] then would become their chief. Thus they avoided bleeding him. Accordingly, on the sixth day of his illness (this evil doctor) gave him [the prince] his (own) approved potion [= his purgative][227] to drink, (which was administered to the prince) before it had reached boiling-point and had received (the level of) maturity.[228] It made him [the prince] walk (run) to the latrine 24 times, but during the 24th time, his strength broke down, his body cooled off and his movements stopped for approximately 30 hours. They (continued) giving him medical treatment, but this damned devil sat there laughing and enforced his judgment on all those who were next in line to examine him [the prince]. A man, who was dedicated and experienced, stood up from their midst to examine (the prince's) strength. They closely watched him (examining the prince) and said (to him): 'Do you want to quicken the dead?,' to which he replied: 'There is still hope that he may live, the more so because the (reason for the) breakdown of his faculties is (due to) the treatment and not to the malignancy of the disease'. Once with great difficulty the prince had managed to open his mouth, they gave him a little chicken broth to drink.[229] Thereupon his pulse came back and he regained his strength and opened

---

was "a voracious overeater and an insatiable glutton who delighted in eating all different kinds and varieties of food. At night he would increase his intake of food and graze like a horse, and at bedtime he would suck one Damascene *raṭl* (circa 1.85 kg) of assorted sweets made out of dates and clarified butter (*khabīṣ al-sukkar*), which he consumed as a digestive (*jawarish*)". Whether he also designated the famous philosopher al-Ghazālī as "being obese" remains an open question (cf. Gutas, *Philosophy in the Twelfth Century*, at 23). One should keep in mind that because ʻAbd al-Laṭīf was obviously rather thin, he apparently made comparisions between others and himself and consequently considered many persons overweight. For the Arabic text of the second fragment, cf. Claude Cahen, "ʻAbdallaṭīf al-Baghdādī, Portraitiste et Historien de son Temps. Extrait inédits de ses Mémoires', in: *BEO* XXIII (1970), 101-128 at 111.

227 Lit. 'a (his) tested remedy'.

228 An optional rendering would read: 'before the illness [or: fever] reached its breaking point/crisis'. For the Galenic usage of the term *naḍj*, 'maturation', see: Oliver Kahl, *Yaʻqūb ibn Isḥāq al-Isrāʼīlī's "Treatise on the Errors of the Physicians in Damascus"*. A critical edition of the Arabic text together with an annotated English translation (Oxford 2000) [*JSS* Suppl. 10], 33, 53, and 67-8, note 43.

229 Apart from it being the only active treatment in this specific case, one should also bear in mind that chicken broth might have been a common sick-dish in ʻAbd al-Laṭīf's time. Chicken turns up very frequently in medieval sick-dish recipes. Terence Scully mentions

his eyes and spoke, after which he asked for water and food. He then rose up (from the bed) all by himself. The physicians all returned (to visit the patient), but this diabolical doctor saw that his arrow had not reached its target and thereupon he administered (to the prince) one enema after another [that is, by his anus], and in between every two enemas he (also) gave him multiple (soap-like) suppositories. Yet, the doctors, who were (also) attending him [the prince], held him back and prevented him from (undertaking further actions), which made his face turn gloomy before their very eyes. He abused them, called them idiots and said: 'My intention was rather to cleanse his body'. With (remarks like) this and with similar examples he tried to persuade the servants and the kinfolk (of the prince) to tie him [the prince] up and surrender him to fate.[230] Then, the retentive faculty [*al-qūwah al-māsika*][231] declined and flowed forth from him. Thereupon, they [these doctors] began to administer astringents in an excessive manner and believed the drugs to work by themselves without (the intervention) of a faculty within the body which would direct the drugs and would be able to influence them.[232] But I shall tell you that the drugs do not work by themselves, but rather are tools

(70v) for the bodily faculties. Whenever that which is governing the tools [the drugs] becomes corrupted, then the tool [the drugs] itself (also) becomes void, shall cease to function, and shall therefore not be of any use (anymore). But God's mercy upon (the prince) kept on flowing and did not cease until he passed away on the 24th day of his illness.[233] Each one of the physicians who had stayed with him gathered

---

that '(...) physicians and cooks resorted almost as a matter of course to chicken as an all-round problem-solver when it came to feeding the sick, sickly or convalescent', cf. Terence Scully, *The Art of Cookery in the Middle Ages* (Woodbridge 1995), especially chapter 8: *Foods for the Sick*, 185-195, 188; cf. also by the same author, 'The Sickdish in Early French Recipe Collections', in: Sheila Campbell, Bert Hall, David Klausner (editors) [Center for Mediaeval Studies, University of Toronto]: *Health, Disease and Healing in Medieval Culture* (Basingstoke and London 1992), 132-140; cf. also for the treatment with chicken bouillon: Kahl, *Ya'qūb ibn Isḥāq al-Isrā'īlī's "Treatise...*, 24-27, 47-48; cf. for the attempts of contemporary medicine to evaluate the effects of chicken soup in controlled trials: Kiumars Saketkhoo, Adolph Januszkiewicz, and Marvin A. Sackner, 'Effects of Drinking Hot Water, Cold Water, and Chicken Soup on Nasal Mucus Velocity and Nasal Airflow Resistance', in: *Chest*: the cardiopulmonary and critical care journal 74 (1978), 408-10. This study was not a controlled double blind study because the placebo could be distinguished by taste from chicken soup.

230 That is, the vicious doctor wanted to prevent the prince from rising up on his own accord! If the prince would have been already dead the translation would have read: 'to wrap (and shroud) him'.

231 For the different *quwan* (*māsika*; *nārīya*; *dāfi'a*; *jādhiba*), see: Thies, *Der Diabetestraktat*, at 190.

232 That is, the doctors first started administering purgatives and when these did not have the desired effect, they resorted to giving the patient the opposite, namely astringents!

233 If we would be willing to re-arrange the sequence of this phrase a little, an alternative translation would read: 'But the drugs kept on being administered until the prince –may

for a meeting and spoke out frankly that he [this wicked doctor] killed (the prince), and (thereupon) every one of them gave his own description of a specific aspect of the fatal treatment which he [this damned devil] pursued. One of the subtle tricks (which this damned devil employed) in (the course of) the disease, is that he made the one in charge of the servants, believe that the majority of the doctors was displeased with him (and hostile towards him). Thereupon, the doctors (who were allowed to stay at the prince's bedside) were limited to two (persons only). He [this deuced idiot] then suggested himself and an elderly, venerable gentleman who was intelligent, friendly and kind, and well-known for his good medical treatment. If he [the elderly doctor] would have been in the position to act as was his wont, then he would (certainly) have done so. However, he [the damned devil] and the elderly doctor, who was made subordinate to him, would stay alone with the prince, so that he [the devilish doctor] could diagnose (and treat) him [the prince] as he pleased, that is until the prince regained consciousness and demanded another doctor to keep him company.[234]

This person was a doctor of mature age, well-known for his sound treatment and his correct views. He (then) took over the medical attendance, but (soon) afterwards this damned devil was given precedence to (the other doctor) again, and thus surrendered the prince (to the fate of death). One of the many things that I have heard about this damned devil is that he wished to preserve health by means of (resorting to) the opposite and remove disease by applying something similar. In case of phlegmatic [= mucous] diseases, he gave (the patients) a fluid to drink which was made from the seeds of the cucumber, barley-water and rose syrup. In case of choleric, (melancholic), [= respectively black and yellow bilious] diseases and sanguinary [= blood-related] diseases and to those affected and weakened by the disease phthisis [or: consumption] he prescribed {pure and precious?} hot purgatives and warm(ing) aperients.[235] Some wise persons believed that he did all these things intentionally because he wanted to destroy human lives and took pleasure in the distortion of forms and shapes.

It has been told of [the grammarian Abū al-ʻAbbās] al-Mubarrad that he encountered a disciple of a religious brotherhood [i.e. of an order of dervishes] who spoke confusedly and improperly and with excessive grammatical mistakes. So, al-Mubarrad said to his companion: 'I think this person knows (quite) a bit of the Arabic language'. Thereupon, his companion replied: 'How do you know that'? To which al-Mubarrad answered: 'I noticed that the words which he pronounces correctly cannot be pronounced in such a well manner without him having a good understanding of the Arabic language'!

(71r) Thus, he stopped him and took him aside so that the (other) persons walking by dispersed themselves from him, and he asked him: 'Do you know any

---

God have mercy upon him– passed away on the 24th day of his illness'; cf. Joosse, *Pride and Prejudice, Praise and Blame*, at 134.

234 For an optional rendering of this difficult passage, cf. Joosse, *Pride and Prejudice, Praise and Blame*, at 135.

235 Dozy, *Supplément*, vol. 2, at 168: *maʻālin*: 'pure and precious', 'of superior quality'.

Arabic'? Thereupon, the man answered: 'Yes, but I rather turn away from the Arabic language lest not the ill-fatedness of fluency and eloquence descends upon me'![236] But we should now return to that what Hippocrates has said: 'letting nature take its course with regard to the diseases is better than surrendering the course of nature to a bad doctor (and having) it altered by him'. And [Abū Bakr] ar-Rāzī has said: 'who brings together (all) the doctors, is on the verge of collecting (all) their mistakes'. Where Galen is concerned, he has already filled up his books by warning against them [the bad doctors] and by barking at the sorts of mistakes they make. On the subject of this is his saying that the circumstances of the poor with regard to their diseases are better than the circumstances of the leaders and the prosperous people, because the poor do not have influence over the physician. Thus, the poor will continue to follow the course of nature, but the wealthy will assemble (all) the doctors around them. These doctors will pour out (all) kinds of medicaments, potions and varieties of erroneous medical remedies over them. Thus, they [these doctors] disturb and subdue the course of nature, avert from her, and leave her at loss (in the end). Thereupon Galen said: 'the poor people recover from their illnesses as often as the funeral procession of the rich people goes out. Sometimes the poor man escorts the funeral procession of the rich and pays the deceased the last honors'. Therefore, I say that the medicine of old women is better than that of those [physicians who killed the prince], for the old women only apply the things which they saw to be successful, and of which they have experienced its benefit. They are therefore close to the empirical sect. Those physicians, however, take risks because of false logical reasoning and defective opinions. Moreover, when the old women venture to use a strong and dangerous purgative drug -even if they venture to use (only) some of it- they do not insist on it nor do they overdo it. Rather, if they observe its success, they are confirmed (in their opinion), yet otherwise, they desist (from using it). But these (spongers), who asked, or demanded *rizq* [subsistence i.e. just to make profits and gains] (without having earned it, or giving something in return), promote irresponsibility and prescribe medicaments of which they do not know the quality. They did not test their strength nor did they witness their effect. I often ask each and every one of them about the simples of their drugs,

(71v) but they do not know the quality let alone the strength thereof. The most learned among them base themselves on a book and refer to a source, but do not have knowledge of the strength of simple drugs through test and experiment and (are also unfamiliar with) the strength of compound (drugs). If only these people would confine themselves to the (preparation) of compound drugs as it has been mentioned in books! However, they do not consult these books which would show them how to prepare the compound drugs. They do everything of their own accord and act without restriction when dealing with the qualities and the quantities of

---

[236] 'Abd al-Laṭīf included the story about the Arab grammarian Abū al-'Abbās Muḥammad b. Yazīd al-Azdī al-Mubarrad (d. 900 A.D.) to emphasize the similarity between the Jewish physician and the disciple of the religious brotherhood: they both refused to act for no apparent reason. That is, the Jewish physician wilfully did not heal the prince and the disciple of the religious brotherhood intentionally refused to speak proper Arabic.

these drugs. They are (extremely) ignorant about these things and about (the treatment) of the diseases which they pursue and encounter. Their intention is to cure a disease by means of its opposite, but they have no clue how to do this. They are (also) very ignorant with regard to (the determination of) the amount of distance between a disease and its opposite, and are very much in the dark about the differences between the species, not to speak of their ignorance with regard to the differences between individuals. A doctor cannot be content (only) with the correctness of a remedy through his knowledge of the differences between the species, but should also have knowledge of the differences between individuals. For a doctor rather treats individuals, not the species. Likewise is it the case with regard to the preservation of health by means of the similar. It is necessary for a doctor to be acquainted with the similarities between individuals, for he should pay attention to them and by no means devote himself (only) to the knowledge of the species. The latter is not sufficient, because it does not stand on its own and must be made subservient to the individual, so that knowledge of the species can be combined with knowledge of the individual.

I say that strangers who sell (their) potions in the middle of the highways are superior to these spongers. Firstly, because most people, and especially the elite, beware of them and do not hand themselves over to them.[237] Secondly, they give (the milky latex of) spurges [*yattū'āt*] and (the juice of) *bashbūsh*, that is colocynth leaves, to healthy people whose temperament can bear mistakes more than sick patients.

(72r) They mostly administer their drugs to peasants and (other) hard-working people, whose temperaments are able to endure strong drugs. Moreover, the strangers have tried and tested drugs and tried herbs which they gather and test themselves; and they tell each other what they know about them.[238]

It is the task of a skilled, intelligent and compassionate doctor to warn in the strongest manner those people who take purgative drugs.[239] The physician should

---

237 'Abd al-Laṭīf in fact tells us here that if he would have to make a choice between two evils, the highway physicians are to be preferred. They are less harmful than the spongers and the quacks, because only a small minority of the population makes use of their services. Moreover, these highway physicians appear to sell their drugs mainly to persons who are in a good physical condition, i.e. those who perform hard physical labor. They are closer to perfection than the spongers in the sense that they test unknown drugs and herbs and spread the knowledge about them, so that others can profit from their findings.

238 Cf. Joosse and Pormann, *Decline and Decadence*, 17-20.

239 Cf. also Maimonides, *On Poisons and the Protection against Lethal Drugs*. A New Parallel Arabic-English Translation by Gerrit Bos with Critical Editions of Medieval Hebrew Translations by Gerrit Bos and Medieval Latin Translations by Michael R. McVaugh (Provo, Utah 2009); cf. likewise Lena Ambjörn, *Qusṭā Ibn Lūqā (9th century A.D.) On Purgative Drugs And Purgation* (Frankfurt am Main 2004). [= Fuat Sezgin (editor), Publications of the Institute for the History of Arabic-Islamic Science: *Islamic Medicine*: Volume 100]; John M. Riddle, 'Fees and Feces: Laxatives in Ancient Medicine With Particular Emphasis on Pseudo-Mesue', in: John A.C. Greppin, Emilie Savage-

only give priority to the administering of purgative drugs when he is certain of their necessity, and in case there are ample requirements which make it necessary to administer them. He has to warn the ill people against purgatives more than he has to warn the healthy, for they are a more dangerous means of healing than blood-letting. Moreover, we should warn against purgatives because they purge (the constipated bowels) by means of a poisonous substance within them. However, nature (also) makes use of this poisonous substance to fight the poisonous elements which are at the root of disease. Thus, if it fits its aim, it is easy to undergo the poisonous elements of the drugs, the more so because the disease will be fought with a more poisonous substance than the drug itself, just as evil is fought with (stronger) evil and an enemy is fought with (a more formidable) adversary. Therefore, when the drug is given at the right time and administered in the right place, this will be appropriate for the nature (of man) and will facilitate the bearing of the consequences [= side-effects] of the drugs, so that the body will come to rest, and (everything) will follow as it should. When the drug is not administered in the right place, this will bring about damage, and then the afflictions (caused by the drug) will become many-fold. The sages have already said that if you imbibe the drugs which form an antidote [or: theriac][240] when there is poison in the body, their benefit becomes manifest. But if you imbibe them when the body is exempt of poison, then they will become poisonous (themselves). They [the sages] have said that the antidote [or: theriac] holds the middle ground between a pure poison and a genuine medicament. Hippocrates said in his *Book on Aphorisms* [*K. al-Fuṣūl*][241]: 'Persons who have a healthy body and receive purgative treatment, or become completely exhausted by (purgative) drugs, will quickly swoon. This is the same for a person who is nourished with spoilt food'.[242] Galen has (moreover) very seriously warned

(72v) against giving a purgative to drink to a person whose body is fully satiated. Galen has already explained this in his book on *The Stratagem of Healing* [*K. Ḥīlat al-bur'*][243] in which he recalled the mistakes of the physicians regarding those who possess this condition. In view of that, he indicated the treatment (for this

---

Smith and John L. Gueriguian (editors): *The Diffusion of Greco-Roman Medicine into the Middle East and the Caucasus* (Delmar/New York) 1999, 7-26.

240 The substance theriac was a compound of viper's flesh and other ingredients and was supposedly a universal antidote to poison as well as a remedy for diseases caused by an excess of melancholy and phlegm, see for this remedy for instance: Nancy G. Siraisi, *Medieval & Early Renaissance Medicine. An Introduction to Knowledge and Practice* (Chicago and London 1990), 118-19; Margreet Algera, *Mens en Medicijn. Geschiedenis van het geneesmiddel* (Amsterdam 2000), 84-85, 110, 148, 160, 192, 251, 260, 394.

241 Cf. Sezgin, *GAS*, III, 25, 28-32.

242 Hippocrates, *Aphorisms*, II, no. xxxvi: 'Persons in good health quickly lose their strength by taking purgative medicine or using bad food', cf. ed. William H.S. Jones, *Hippocrates with an English translation*, vol. iv (Cambridge, Mass. and London 1931 [reprint: 2005]), at 117.

243 Cf. Sezgin, *GAS*, III, 53, 96-98, 146.

condition) through vomiting by continuous rubbing [= massaging] in the right proportions, by embrocating the body (ointments), and by applying a specific class of compound remedies (oils) and to do this over and over again, so that (the patient) can become relieved of some (vomit) and can exude the rest. After that, it will become possible to purge or bleed (the patient), if there is (still) need for it. However, we have said that one should warn ill persons more seriously for the administering of purgatives than one should warn healthy persons for it, due to the fact that healthy persons have their full strength and possess healthy organs. A purgative can nevertheless weaken them, and can cause damage to them (even) when it is administered in the right place, let alone when it is not administered (in the right place). But what is one to think of ill persons whose strength has been weakened and whose principal organs have been damaged by the disease from which they suffer? Rather, the drug shall (in that case) weaken their strength and cause damage to their organs, due to the fact that the purgatives contain (an amount of) poison. However, (if) purgation causes damage to the retentive power of the bodily mixtures [temperaments], then one should (rather) refrain from it (completely). Therefore, purgative drugs should only be administered in an adjusted form with their impact broken, and in appropriate measures which, in only a few days, are able to redress the damage which the purgative drugs have left behind in the body, so that one can (start) purging (once again) with lubricants. Purging by means of lubricants stands very close to (employing) the natural condition of foodstuff such as for instance the black prune, the tamarind and (various) mucilaginous [= slimy] decoctions (such as different types of honey). However, the dryness which (likewise) occurs should neutralize the strong fever in the stomach, the intestines and the places which border these organs, so when it happens that these organs are not dry, these (lubricants) can (also) cause harm therein [i.e. to the organs].

One has already praised the merits of barley-water, but is also cautious of it. Barley-water is an outstanding and useful nutrient, but it is nevertheless very harmful when it is not properly administered. One has already enumerated its harm in chronic and acute diseases, when a dose of fourteen was (for instance) increased to a dose of twenty.[244]

(73r) Whenever we warn healthy persons, who are in possession of their full strength, of the harm of the purgative, it is even more appropriate that we should warn ill persons, whose strength has been weakened, of the harm of the purgative. It is desirable thus, to very seriously warn them; especially those persons who suffer from acute fevers and (are treated) with warm(ing) purgatives. Therefore, the physicians already put it into practice to purge with lubricants which are cool(ing) and moist(ening). From (all) this it has become clear that the risk of blood-letting is less than the risk of drinking poisonous drugs. For blood-letting by no means diminishes the functioning of the bodily mixtures (temperaments). It leaves the

[244] For the treatment with barley-water and barley-gruel, see: Kahl, *Ya'qūb ibn Isḥāq al-Isrā'īlī's "Treatise...*, 22-24, 45-47.

body in full strength and does not damage its principal organs. Blood-letting can replenish perfectly good blood in a (relatively) short period, but purgation merely weakens the internal organs. As a consequence, purgation can only replace blood (and fluids) after a (very) long time. Purgation can weaken the drugs which are given to (cure) the organs. The damage which purgation brings to them [these organs] delays the replacement (of blood and fluids), because it is exactly these organs which contribute to the replacement of blood (and fluids). Consequently, if these organs become damaged, their functioning will diminish with the exact quantity of damage that healthy people will receive. Then, nourishment and replacement becomes impossible for them. And if they accept nourishment, then in an amount which is not enough to bring back the dead [i.e. in an amount which is not enough to save the organs].

We have already discussed in a separate treatise (bearing the title) *On the man who started the medical art* [*Maqāla fī al-bādi' bi-ṣinā'at al-ṭibb*][245] that this art arose when mankind felt the need for it. Whenever the medical art declined in the course of time, God, may he be praised and exalted, sent someone to breathe new life into its practices and traditions and to restore its obliterated outlines and demolished cornerstones, just as it happened in the time of Hippocrates that (the latter) restored the medical science of his great forebear Asclepiades, and then in the time of Galen that (the latter) restored Hippocrates' medical science. The last (physician) which I like to acknowledge in the Islamic period [lit.: within the religious community of Islam] is Abū Ja'far Aḥmad ibn Muḥammad ibn abī l-Ash'ath.[246]

(73v) Those who occupy themselves at this time with the art of medicine usually read a bit in the *Generalities* of the *Canon* [i.e. the first part of the *K. al-Qānūn* (*fī al-ṭibb*) (by Ibn Sīnā) dealing with general principles [*kullīyāt*].[247] Then they learn by heart the definition of medicine, the definition of the element, the definition of the temperament, and the like. They carry on a dispute about them, repeat them on top of their voices during social gatherings, and in bazaars and markets. Afterwards, they proceed to treat (patients) in the (false) opinion that this (alone, i.e. basic book learning) is beneficial and suffices, and that he who knows the definition of medicine correctly is able to cure (patients) of fevers and other (diseases), and know their different kinds. I admonish those who take my advice, if they want to be physicians, not to abandon Galen's and Hippocrates' books. And if they regard my advice as insincere, they should start (preparing their studies) by (analyzing) a (small) area of the medical science. I would, for example, assign them the *Book on mixtures/On Temperaments* [*K. al-Mizāj*].[248] Consequently, they should read what has been written about the (same) concept in the *K. al-Qānūn* (*fī al-ṭibb*) (of Ibn

---

245 Cf. Ibn abī Uṣaybi'a, *K. 'Uyūn al-anbā' fī ṭabaqāt al-aṭibbā'*, ed. Imru'ulqais b. aṭ-Ṭaḥḥān (August Müller), Juz' 1-2 (Cairo-Königsberg 1299 H./1882 A.D.) [Reprint: F. Sezgin *et alii* (editor): *Islamic Medicine*, vol. 1-2, Frankfurt am Main 1995] vol. 2, at 211, ultimate line.

246 Cf. Kruk, *Ibn abī l-Ash'ath's Kitāb al-Ḥayawān*, 119-168.

247 Cf. Carl Brockelmann, *GAL*, S. I, 812-28.

248 Cf. Sezgin, *GAS*, III, 87-88, 146, 302.

Sīnā) and other works. If they find in what goes beyond Galen's discussion something which makes it [Galen's discussion] superfluous, then they should not accept other things which I said. Yet when they read Galen and find for themselves that they may be able to compose (works) just as them [Galen and Hippocrates], then they should rely on my words and continue their studies. They should do the same thing with *The small book on the pulse* [*K. an-Nabḍ aṣ-ṣaghīr*] by Galen[249] and the section on the pulse of the *K. al-Qānūn* (*fī al-ṭibb*). They should proceed in a similar fashion with all the other books of Galen as they have done with the *Book on mixtures/On Temperaments* [*K. al-Mizāj*], which Galen made into a kind of model, experience, and test [*ja'alahu (Jālīnūsu) ka-l-unmūdhaji wa-l-tajribati wa-l-imtiḥāni*]. Accordingly, they should do the same with *The large book on the pulse* [*K. an-Nabḍ al-kabīr*][250] and likewise with (all of) his [Galen's] (other) practical and theoretical books. If this should become too overbearing for them, they may prefer to restrict themselves to abridgements of these books[251] such as *The small book on the art of medicine* [*K. aṣ-Ṣinā'a aṣ-ṣaghīra*] which is an introduction (to medicine),[252] *The small book on the pulse* [*K. an-Nabḍ aṣ-ṣaghīr*], *The book to Glauco* [*K. (ilā) Ighlūqun*],[253] *The compendium of the* [Galen's] *book on the stratagem of healing* [*Ikhtiṣār Ḥīlat al-bur'*],[254] and *The two treatises on the restoration of health* [*al-Maqālatān al-Shāfīyatān*] by him.[255] If they want to read works by recent authors in order

(74r) to enjoy [*'alā l-tanazzuh*] the extant of the scholar's knowledge, their different abilities to understand, the quality of their abridgments and explanations, then so be it [i.e. then nothing can be said against it].[256] Those, however, who think that *The Royal Book* [*K. al-Malakī*] (by al-Majūsī),[257] *The Hundred Books on the*

---

249 That is the *K. an-(fī) Nabḍ aṣ-ṣaghīr ilā Ṭuthrūn wa-ilā sā'ir al-muta'allimīn*, cf. Sezgin, *GAS*, III, 70-71, 81-82, 213.

250 'Abd al-Laṭīf apparently got confused with the first example, for he again wrote *K. an-Nabḍ aṣ-ṣaghīr* here. Perhaps he meant to write *K. an-Nabḍ al-kabīr*, cf. Sezgin, *GAS*, III, 70, 91-94, 213.

251 An optional rendering of this sentence may be: 'If this takes too much time, they can limit themselves to abridgements [of these books] of which they are (usually) very fond'.

252 For the *K. aṣ-Ṣinā'a aṣ-ṣaghīra* or *K. aṣ-Ṣinā'a aṭ-ṭibbīya*, cf. Sezgin, *GAS*, III, 80-81, 146.

253 The *K. ilā Ighlūqun fī t-ta'attī li-shifā' al-amrāḍ* or *K. fī Mudāwāt al-amrāḍ ilā Ighlīqūn*, cf. Sezgin, *GAS*, III, 82-83, 146.

254 Cf. Sezgin, *GAS*, III, 115.

255 Or: 'The two medical treatises'. Perhaps 'Abd al-Laṭīf is referring here to the separate tractates which are registered under the collective name *K. al-'Ilal wa-l-a'rāḍ*, cf. Sezgin, *GAS*, III, 89-90.

256 An optional rendering of this sentence may be: 'If he wants to read works by recent authors to amuse himself with the extant of the knowledge of these scholars, their different abilities to understand, the quality of their abridgements and explanations, then so be it'.

257 The *K. al-Malakī* or *K. Kāmil aṣ-ṣinā'a aṭ-ṭibbīya* ('The complete book on the medical art'), cf. Sezgin, *GAS*, III, 320-22.

Medical Art [*al-Kutub al-Mi'ah fī al-ṣinā'a al-ṭibbīyah*] (by Abū Sahl al-Masīḥī),[258] or the *Canon* [*K. al-Qānūn* (*fī al-ṭibb*)] (by Ibn Sīnā) suffice and make Galen's works superfluous adhere to a false opinion, for the (former) works do not contain a selection of Galen's words, nor are their authors thoroughly acquainted with Galen's words. These works, however, contain imitations, falsehoods and lies. Only the words which are clearly better than the (other) words therein are excerpted from (the works of) Galen. The words of (these other authors) do not enter anyone's heart, are long-winded to anyone but themselves, do not give pleasure to anyone else besides themselves, and do not attract anyone else but themselves, nevertheless with the exception of *The Hundred Books on the Medical Art* [*al-Kutub al-Mi'ah fī al-ṣinā'a al-ṭibbīya*] (by Abū Sahl al-Masīḥī), which is an outstanding book (at heart). And where *The Small Compendium* [*al-Kunnāsh aṣ-ṣaghīr*] of [Yūḥannā] Ibn Serapion [Ibn Sarābiyūn] is concerned, this constitutes the basis of the majority of the medical handbooks.[259]

I have observed a group of people of whom one man had turned away from the words of Galen. He deceived himself into thinking that he was one of those who had already been given an insight into the secrets of the existence and had (already) received a deeper understanding of the mysteries of the world, by stating that the medicine of those (ancients) has become worthless by now, since nature has changed (considerably) and time has become different due to the movement of the fixed stars [i.e. the medical handbooks of the ancients cannot be applied as they are, since the ancient physicians wrote their books in a different period and in a different climate]. He considered it something of the past that the people of Baghdād received medical treatment by way of warm(ing) drugs, and stated that nowadays the physicians do not value (the application of) warm(ing) drugs at all, but rather eagerly devote themselves to (the application of) cool(ing) drugs. He has (also) said that the medicine of Hippocrates and Galen was appropriate for the country of the Greeks, but that the lands of Syria and Iraq do not allow for it [i.e. that the medicine of Greece is not appropriate for other regions]. Only someone who has not read the books of the ancients and has not tested their content at all could think this! Do you believe that when the stars circle (in the sky) they change the nature of people only, without changing the nature of the plants and all the other living beings? If this were the case, it would indeed be amazing. If they changed everything, however, then the opium will be hot, and the pepper cold;

(74v) the meat of fish hot and the meat of the lion cool; the lion will be cowardly and the hare brave. Thus their opinions change about the nature of drugs

---

[258] Cf. Sezgin, *GAS*, III, 326-27; There is an excellent Arabic edition of this work available: Floréal Sanagustin, *Le livre des cents questions en medicine d'Abū Sahl 'Isa b. Yaḥyā al-Masīḥī (m. ca 401h./1010 apr. J.-C.)*, 2 vols. (Damas 2000); For an overview of this interesting work, cf. Ghada Karmi 'A Mediaeval Compendium of Medicine: Abū Sahl al-Masīḥī's *Book of the Hundred*', in: *Journal for the History of Arabic Science* (Aleppo), 2 (1978), 270-90; cf. also Emilie Savage-Smith, 'New Evidence for the Frankish Study of Arabic Medical Texts in the Crusader Period', in: *Crusades* 5 (2006), 99-112.

[259] Cf. Sezgin, *GAS*, III, 240-42.

and foods-whether derived from plants, animals or minerals! Moreover, we find that Hippocrates agreed with those (living) long before him about the nature of things. He tested what people of old had said and found that in his day things had not changed; their [the ancients'] judgments still applied. Likewise, Galen tested all of Hippocrates' opinions and found them to agree (with what he thought); and between them there are six hundred years. People still test until today what Galen said and find it to agree (with what they observed); and Galen lived roughly one thousand two hundred years before![260] The *Book of (Nabataean) Agriculture* [*K. al-Filāḥa an-nabaṭīya*][261] which Ibn Waḥshīya translated from the language of the Nabataeans contains (some) tedious and long-winded discussions. The 'natures [i.e. the natural properties]' in it, however, are stable in one state. This is something very absurd to say.[262] Had it not been for the fact that it had been written in books, I would not have deemed it proper to refute and relate it. I have observed (people) who firmly believed in his [i.e. Ibn Waḥshīya's] words, who said and did strange and amazing things in order to keep his reputation alive, and who built a name on his knowledge [*lege*: the product of his thoughts]. I have observed others who had similar thoughts and who (also) uttered foolish words: (for example) that the medical science of Hippocrates and Galen was sufficient (only) for Greece; that they were not sure of the fact that the sayings of Galen and Hippocrates were universal matters which are not subject to change and which do not undergo alteration; that the only possibility to cure a person is by applying the opposite; that health can be preserved (only) through something similar; that fever can only be neutralized by applying a cool(ing) and moist(ening) substance; that a pure and unadulterated tertian fever requires cool(ing) and moist(ening) (only) and to a large extent, and that the latter is not the case with regard to phlegmatic [mucous] diseases and a quartan fever; that one cannot apply hot liquids to quotidian fever in its early stages in excess, but (rather in moderation) and with gentleness; and that accordingly one should apply (these) hot liquids by force when the substance [*mādda*][263] is well-cooked and matured. The (same) people have (also) warned for the application of hot liquids by force in the early stages of hemiplegia.

---

260 Cf. likewise Joosse and Pormann, *Decline and Decadence*, 12-15.

261 Cf. Sezgin, *GAS*, IV, 318-29. For a recent analysis of the religious, philosophical and folkloristic content of Ibn Waḥshīya's *Nabataean Agriculture*, cf. Jaakko Hämeen-Anttila, *The Last Pagans of Iraq. Ibn Waḥshiyya and his Nabatean Agriculture* (Leiden/Boston 2006) [= Islamic History and Civilization; 63]; cf. for background study: John F. Healey, *The Religion of the Nabataeans. A Conspectus* (Leiden/Boston/ Köln 2001).

262 That is, the previous statement that the nature of plants etc. changes according to time/climate. In other words, 'Abd al-Laṭīf al-Baghdādī proclaims that even the *Book of (Nabataean) Agriculture* agrees with this point, namely that plants have one nature. But he immediately follows this statement by boldly saying that Ibn Waḥshīya's point is fairly banal.

263 That is, the medicaments, the drugs.

(75r) Rather, progress should proceed step by step. Galen already reported about such-and-such a person (who) suffered from quartan fever: 'the doctors (at his bedside) advised him to take warm(ing) drugs (immediately), but I advised against it. I said: "If you do this [i.e. if you take the drugs] (now), the quartan fever shall recur as a fever composed of two quartan fevers [a double quartan fever]". So, when he obeyed the doctors, the quartan fever recurred as a fever composed of two quartan fevers [a double quartan fever]. When he gave in to (receive) medical treatment (from me), I stayed with him, treated him with gentleness and tolerance, and did not use force until the substance was well-cooked and matured. Thereupon, I personally administered him these warm(ing) drugs, whereupon the (fierce) quartan fever departed from him altogether'.[264] Thus, all that which is written in the books of the (different) peoples is not subject to change and alteration, but is rather one set of (well-defined and) universally established principles. Furthermore, these peoples filled their books with instructions (and directions) which took into account the age (of a person), the country (a person lived in), the habits (of a person), the climate (in which a person lived), the seasons, the present moment, and so on. They blamed those who disregarded to pay attention to all these (instructions and directions) and ascribed mistakes and errors to them. Their medicine was applicable to the Slavs and the Abyssinians and to those peoples who lived between these two extreme regions. The people of Baghdād did not fall beyond the center, let alone beyond the extreme boundaries [i.e. the people of Baghdād followed the golden mean and thus belonged to the abovementioned category]. Therefore, an end should be put to the story that phlegmatic [mucous] diseases [*amrāḍ al-balgham*] such as hemiplegia [*fālij*], facial paralysis [*laqwa*], apoplexy [*sakta*], epilepsy [*sarʿ*], dropsy [*istisqāʾ*] and others could not befall the inhabitants of Baghdād.[265] In the same way,

---

264 This fragment apparently refers to Galen's skills in prognostication. Most of the doctors whom Galen met when he first arrived in Rome did not prognosticate. It appears that ʿAbd al-Laṭīf wants to make the point that also the Arabic doctors of his time did not prognosticate, but merely guessed and computed by conjecture. The story in question deals with Galen and his former teacher Eudemus. When Eudemus felt ill, he summoned Galen to his sickbed. When Galen arrived, he told the patient that he had a quartan fever. Galen stayed with him, treated him with gentleness and tolerance, and made predictions about the outcome of the fever. Galen was proved correct and Eudemus recovered, cf. Roger French, *Medicine before Science. The Business of Medicine/The Rational and Learned Doctor from the Middle Ages to the Enlightenment* (Cambridge 2003), 42-45. According to French (*Medicine before Science*, 44), Galen 'was telling Eudemus the Good Story of the Rational and Learned Doctor: I am the doctor, I have specialist knowledge of what it is you are suffering from, I can predict the outcome because of my knowledge and medical first principles, and I can trace your very symptoms back to the axiomatic first principles of the natural world'.

265 The notion that certain diseases could not befall the citizens of Baghdād may ultimately refer to Ptolemy's *Tetrabiblos*, which includes a section on chorography or mundane astrology, being the study of the influence of the stars on cities or regions of the world. The people of Baghdād were said to live in the temperate zone, i.e. the place where the best people live: they are of medium coloring, of moderate stature, have an even temper,

an end should be put (to the story) that these diseases should be treated with cool(ing) substances due to the movement of the fixed stars.[266] Do you (actually) believe that quotidian, nocturnal and quartan fevers cannot befall them? An end should (also) be put (to the story) that the aforementioned diseases should be treated with blood-letting, cool(ing) and bringing relief by alleviating the suffering as in the case of sanguinary diseases or with cool(ing) and moist(ening) as in the case of choleric [bilious] diseases. Do you (truly) accept as right that they are protected against phlegmatic [mucous] colic [*qaulanj al-balghamī*]? I wish I knew which part of nature undergoes changes due to the movement of the fixed stars, or which medical treatment, which is characteristic of Greece only, cannot be employed in Iraq. Verily, this is (all) plain imbecility and foolish and stupid reasoning!

---

group together (in cities) and are civilized in their habits. The followers of the abovementioned theories therefore believed that the people of Baghdād were not exposed to the different diseases due to these traits. The *Tetrabiblos*, moreover, offers explanations of the physical appearance and customs of the peoples living in the different *climata*, which more or less correspond with the discussions of physiognomists such as Polemon of Laodicea on the influence of the climate on customs and behavior of man. The theories of physiognomists and (geographical) astrologers were used by the physician Galen in his discussion of the different blends of humors (the bodily fluids) in the various parts of the body, cf. Tamsyn S. Barton, *Ancient Astrology* (London/New York 1994), 179-207; *idem, Power and Knowledge: Astrology, Medicine and Physiognomics under the Roman Empire* (Ann Arbor/Michigan 1995); cf. also Joseph Schacht and Max Meyerhof, *The Medico-Philosophical Controversy between Ibn Butlan of Baghdad and Ibn Ridwan of Cairo* (Cairo 1937), 89-90 where it is among others stated that amid the inhabitants of Baghdād 'one rarely sees a mangy or scabby individual, or someone suffering from asthma or eczema'. There it has also been mentioned that Ibn al-Jawzī [d. 1200 A.D.] wrote a treatise called *Manāqib Baghdād* ('Outstanding features of Baghdād') of which the last chapter is entitled 'That Baghdād is superior to the other places'.

266 According to Vivian Nutton, *Ancient Medicine* (London/New York 2004), 267-68, 'Galen accepted the factual basis behind some of the theories of the astrologers' although he claimed 'that medical astrology was far too crude to allow for the inevitable variations in events or in individuals'. ‘Abd al-Laṭīf, on the other hand, vehemently rejected the whole concept of medical astrology or iatromathematics. It is remarkable that the famous Muslim thinker al-Ghazālī (d. 1111 A.D.) regarded astrology as a useless science and therefore a waste of time, but still stated that: "The conviction that the stars are causes that have effects that come about on earth in plants and in animals by the creation of God –Exalted– is not damaging to religion but it is the truth", cf. Frank Griffel, *Al-Ghazālī's Philosophical Theology* (Oxford 2009), 244. However, al-Ghazālī's statement may not have been self-contradictory. He may well have rejected what we call astrology in our modern sense, but accepted that, excepting miracles, customarily the celestial bodies affect climate, tides, and therefore, which plants or animals can live where, i.e., what is part of climatology and geography. He may have been very aware of the influence of the celestial bodies on climate and, therefore, the common ways of life of people in a certain area.

(75v) Although they [the Indians] are situated in the first clime, the Indian medicine has already been transmitted to us a long time ago and stuffed up our books. At the same time, its vast amount of salves and ointments found its way into (our) composite medicaments/pharmacopoeia [*aqrabādhīnāt*]. Greece is situated in the fourth and fifth clime, but Iraq is situated in the third and fourth clime, which is nearer to Greece than India. Moreover, the Egyptian and Syrian people often kept up (deep-rooted) friendships with the peoples with which they made contact. Galen had already traveled through Egypt and Syria and had expressed an opinion about the natural environment (of these countries). He witnessed the customs of the people of Alexandria, visited Baghdād, and reported about it in his books. Dioscorides originated from *'Ain Zarbā* [*Anazarbus* in Asia Minor]. Many of the Greek philosophers from Egypt, Syria and *Qūnyah*, [Konya, the ancient *Iconium* in Asia Minor] were originally from the country of the philosophers [i.e. Greece]. This is the same for (the philosophers) in (the city of) *Malaṭya* [Malatya]. In Malaṭya was an enormous library and a (teaching) academy for philosophers [*dār ta'līm lil-ḥikma*]. Malaṭya was, moreover, closely connected to (greater) Syria. The name Dioscorides can be explained as 'God's herbalist' [*'ashshāb allāh*], because Dioscorides occupied himself for thirty years with traveling through the regions of the earth in order to learn and find out about the essence of plants and their benefits. He learnt this by carrying out scientific experiments on the plants which he sampled. It has been said that he used to form a theory about them before he put them to practice [i.e. before he applied them to tests]. Therefore, his judgment has been accepted as correct. I shall tell you something (now) with which I like to conclude this section. Did you test the drugs of the ancients by attaching all kinds of (pre)conditions to them? (If you did), you were not very successful! For I shall tell you the truth: every one of you may reach ninety years of age and (still) treat the diseased, but you will (not be capable) of using any of those things which have been described in the books of the ancients. Hence, it shall not become known to you whether something is wrong or right. By the everlasting existence of God, I say unto you that the medicine of the ancients must be revealed

(76r) to you, because of your incapability to apply it and because of your (complete) ignorance about the (pre)conditions which are attached to it. For who among you is capable of bleeding someone with a fever until (such a person swoons) and becomes unconscious, and of causing him to recover on the spot, or who among you dares to give water chilled with ice to drink to a feverish person, so that the latter shall cool off and his fever shall abate at once, or who among you shall in case of pleurisy give (a patient) a burning substance to drink and lets (the patient) vomit black bile, or who (among you) knows the reason for the need of letting someone, who is affected by the disease called pleurisy, vomit black bile? And how can it be that this (black bile) is brought forth by the patient's body, since the base of his disease is sanguinary? Who (among you) is able to stabilize an inflamed wound in its initial stages by applying the most approved (and costly) sort of theriac, and can prevent the generation of pus in the wound, and the onset of phthisis [or: consumption]? And who among you is capable of treating an epileptic with the aid of the *dūlāb*?[267] The ancient sages were rather proud of (their ability) to stop diseases before they could spread and consolidate, for the methods of stopping them from spreading were few. Who among you has the audacity to give vinegar to drink in case of a purulent wound? Thus, if you do not practice the medicine of the ancient (wise men), then where does your notion come from that something is either right or wrong, or that something is suitable for such-and-such country and harmful for another country? Do you (actually) believe that the knowledge which can be found in the *Book on the pulse* [*K. al-Nabḍ*], in the *Book on urinary science* [*K. 'Ilm al-baul*],[268] in (all that) which is written in the *Book of Aphorisms* [*K. al-Fuṣūl*],[269] in the *Book of the forecasting of knowledge* [*K. Taqdimat al-ma'rifa*] or *Prognosticon*,[270] and in the *Book of airs and places* [*K. al-Ahwiya wa-l-buldān*][271] shall undergo an alteration caused by the movement of the fixed stars? And do you (really) believe that a medicament which contains asafetida resin [*ḥiltīt*] and an electuary which contains pepper [*ma'jūn al-falāfilī*] shall stop the impact of the disease, and that there shall be no disease which can do without these remedies?[272]

I have given you my advice and I have disclosed to you my well kept secret intention. Thus, if you accept it, then benefit from it, but if you sweep it away, then that is up to you! I gave you the same advice which I gave to myself when I was consulted about the case of a patient: do not to be (too) quick with a diagnosis, but

---

267 *Dūlāb*: wheel, tire, gearing, gears, wheels, mechanism, machine, machinery, closet, locker, cabinet, cupboard, artifices, tricks, attendants. It is also a machine in the walls of (...) hospitals, or lazarettos, into which people on the outside put victuals or other necessaries (...), and then, turning it upon its axis, leave them to be carried off by those within, cf. Franz Steingass, *A Comprehensive Persian-English Dictionary* (London 1892) [reprint: Beirut 1975], 546.

268 This is the *K. al-Baul* (*De Urinis*) by Hippocrates, cf. Sezgin, *GAS*, III, 46.

269 N. Peter Joosse and Peter E. Pormann, 'Commentaries on the Hippocratic *Aphorisms* in the Arabic Tradition: The Example of Melancholy', in: Peter E. Pormann (editor): *>Epidemics< in Context: Greek Commentaries on Hippocrates in the Arabic Tradition* (Berlin/Boston 2012) [= Scientia Graeco-Arabica Band 8], 211- 249. [Info on ALB on 231-33].

270 Cf. Sezgin, *GAS*, III, 32-33; N. Peter Joosse and Peter E. Pormann, ''Abd al-Laṭīf al-Baġdādī's *Commentary on Hippocrates' 'Prognostic'*: A Preliminary Exploration', in: Peter E. Pormann (editor): *>Epidemics< in Context: Greek Commentaries on Hippocrates in the Arabic Tradition* (Berlin/Boston 2012) [= Scientia Graeco-Arabica Band 8], 251-283.

271 This is the *K. al-Ahwiya wa-l-azmina wa-l-miyāh wa-l-buldān* by Hippocrates, cf. Sezgin, *GAS*, III, 36-37.

272 Compare Kahl, *Ya'qūb ibn Isḥāq al-Isrā'īlī's "Treatise...*, 37 and 56: "And dare nobody listen to my words and then speak to me like that physician who, when he heard me say: "The electuary of cumin and the peppered electuary are both applied to phlegmatic and black-bilious fevers", replied: "My dear friend! Leave it! This was done in Galen's time, but not in this day and age!" – and off he went, the simpleton, thinking that he had said something!"

seek clarification, consider (everything) carefully, examine (the case) well, discover and question,

(76v) and ponder your opinion thoroughly. If a patient consults you, you should imagine that you are the patient himself, and make a diagnosis as you would make it for yourself, if you had the disease. You should (also) be afraid of making a mistake with regard to the patient such as you would be afraid to make a mistake about yourself, even if he [the patient] is not a friend of yours [lit.: even if the patient is your foe]. I shall give you a new and wondrous piece of information (now), which reflects something that often happens to me, and that is, that when a disease befalls each one of the doctors, (or) his offspring and his loved ones, he will come to me and ask for my opinion. He shall not come into action himself, for confusion and dismay have taken the upper hand of him. But if a person who is unknown to him appears before him, he will react promptly, make a diagnosis, rush into the case with undue haste, proceed independently, and shall not ask for my opinion, as if he is a doctor who is proficient in the medicine for strangers, but not in the medicine for relatives! Thus, it is desirable for you that you should reflect on matters (first). Accordingly, you should (slightly) postpone your diagnosis, for man shall not be discarded from the rank of the learned and the virtuous when the correct decision [*lege*: diagnosis] comes with a (slight) delay. Where the person who is mistaken is concerned, he shall not come into possession of a (single) portion of the virtue, no matter whether he delays his decision or not! If he accustoms himself (to do) it like this [i.e. the right way], the power of his reasoning shall reply to him with less effort, and he shall reach a right decision far more quickly. But if he accustoms himself to do things in a careless and hasty manner without contemplating the truth, then a bad quality shall firmly take root in him. If he tries to get rid of this bad quality by putting something else in its place, he shall not be able to do so, and it shall not be possible for him to pick up his own mistakes, just like a person who lets his speech get accustomed to grammatical errors and his hand to bad penmanship. But if you practice the proper things from the start, and from the very outset urge yourself to do things in the right way, all this shall be easy for you, and a good quality, which can be practiced easily, shall firmly take root in you. Many of the things which induce (the doctors) to proceed with undue haste, like for instance the fact that they do not postpone their diagnosis, are their own choice, lest it shall not become obvious to the patients that they possess weaknesses and shortcomings. (They believe that) a (certain) hesitation in replying to the patient shall diminish the esteem which patients have for their doctor. Thus, they continue to make mistakes, and subsequently these mistakes become a trait of character and a nasty habit. If they want to get rid of this nasty habit and are capable of doing that, and if they delay their diagnosis, reflect (on the case), learn (to deal) with both defeat and success [i.e. learn (to deal) with it by trial and error],

(77r) and converse (with the patients) in a pleasant manner (or: have fine bedside manners), then the masses would put more trust in them, and might begin to believe that their doctors are virtuous men who possess an excessive compassion and care (for their patients), and take the utmost pains in forming a right judgment [i.e. in making the right diagnosis]. It is (truly) astonishing (to know) that Galen and his likes hesitated to make a diagnosis in many diseases. They postponed it to the second and the third day and (even) longer than this. Yet, among these spongers you do not find anyone at all for whom a disease is ever difficult (or represents the slightest problem). They (pretend to) know everything, and can diagnose anything right away (without any delay). You, however, who seek advice for yourself and love to acquire virtue, beware (of these things)! Beware (even more) of haste, because it is something which comes from the devil. You ought to proceed slowly, gently, and lovingly, and strive to obtain (your goal) through persistence. You should take pleasure in doing the right thing [i.e. making the right judgment], because when you do that, the hidden things shall become manifest to you, the solutions (for your problems) shall follow as a matter of course, the truth shall give you a (positive) answer in (all kinds of different) matters,[273] and the appropriate solutions (for your problems) shall become most obvious. The truth, at its onset, shall wear you out, but accordingly it shall put you at ease in all that you may come to face, like sound and solid pillars [i.e. foundations]. Where the untruth is concerned, it shall put you at ease at first, but accordingly it shall wear you out enduringly, like the house which is built on a feeble foundation is (always) in danger of collapsing. I have witnessed some of the physicians of Cairo and Baghdād and of (certain) places which lie in between these cities, and I took a close look at some of the matters which I (still) remember to have taught them and which they have taught me, but I can (truthfully) state that I have never experienced a doctor who was any worse than this damned North African [*maghribī*] devil who (nowadays) resides in Aleppo, and I have never seen a better doctor than (Raḍī al-Dawla Abū Naṣr) ibn Hibat Allāh (b.) Ṣā'id who is better known under the name of Ibn at-Tilmīdh. I do not mean the learned and venerable sheikh who composed (so many books), because I (of course) never caught up with him, but (I am referring to) his son! He has already passed the age of seventy, but I (hereby) testify that he possesses an unbelievable talent. He can diagnose the diseases as though he views them with his own eyes, as if the body is a transparent glass which displays all that which lies behind it. As one might say, he does not hesitate for one moment (when making his diagnosis), does not make mistakes, does not unnecessarily complicate prescriptions, and only sparingly employs the (prescription) of compound remedies. In most cases

(77v) he treats (the patients) only with simple remedies. When he uses compound medicines, they are but slightly compounded. He does not transfer from one treatment to another, because of his strong self-confidence. Rather, he sticks to (one remedy) until his assumption appears to him (to be true),[274] as Hippocrates

---

[273] The Arabic text reads the word *umam* ('nations', 'peoples', 'communities', 'generations') here, which does not make much sense in the specific context. Instead of the reading *umam*, which is in my view corrupt, we should perhaps adapt the more adequate reading *umūr* ('matters', 'affairs', 'things').

[274] 'Abd al-Laṭīf's portrait of his tutor and mentor Ibn Hibat Allāh b. Ṣā'id a.k.a. (the son of) Ibn at-Tilmīdh can be found in a slightly altered version in the biographical dictionary of

said: 'You have done all the necessary things, but have not seen what is necessary, therefore do not transfer from what is necessary, so long as what you first saw remains valid'. The trickery and falsehood (of these spongers) extends to lengthening prescriptions and multiplying ingredients without any regard to how their powers interact with each other, and without having any experience with their effect.

They do this either to make the common crowd stand in awe of themselves and the extent of their knowledge, or to achieve a tidy profit when people buy the necessary drugs from them or from an apothecary who is in cahoots with them.[275] One of (these spongers) may enter the patient's (sickroom) many times a day, each time prescribing some new drug. He thereby intends to leave a lasting impression behind when he enters, and to display each time some practical (skill, *'amal*). The most cunning [lit.: virtuous] (persons) among them employ changes (in the prescription) which resemble each another (but make little difference). Perhaps they use another physician's recipe, adding or reducing things which neither have any benefit, nor cause any damage. Their aim is thus to show that they are more erudite than other doctors, and to point out their (high) rank [i.e. their high status]. These and other men like them do not disgust me as much as (some of) the aforementioned men have disgusted me. For these men provide some benefit to (the patient) and do not cause harm to anyone. But how much does the one whom I despise profoundly damage people! May God provide refuge! Hence, be careful that you do not become one of those who trade their place in the hereafter for worldly and temporal matters

---

Ibn Khallikān (who was himself a pupil of 'Abd al-Laṭīf): *K. Wafayāt al-a'yān wa-anbā' abnā' al-zamān*, ed. I. 'Abbās, 8 vols. (Beirut 1968-72); tr. [E]: Baron W. McGuckin de Slane, *Ibn Khallikan's Biographical Dictionary*, 4 vols. (Paris-London 1842-1871) [also Paris 1842-43] [Reprint: Beirut 1970], III, 596-603, especially 602-03. The report on Ibn at-Tilmīdh in Ibn Khallikān's dictionary apparently refers to a different source than the passage from the *Book of the Two Pieces of Advice*, because in the latter version Ibn at-Tilmīdh was in his seventies and still alive, whereas in the former work it is mentioned that he had already passed away at the age of nearly eighty years. Ibn Khallikān's version runs as follows: ('Abd al-Latīf states): "I profited greatly under the tuition of this Amīn ad-Dawla's son. He lived nearly eighty years. His great experience and his profound acquaintance with the secrets of the human constitution were such that he could discern every malady as clearly as if he saw it through a pane of glass; and he had never the least hesitation in deciding on its nature and mode of treatment. He usually prescribed simple remedies or such as were but slightly compounded, and he thought no one worthy of practicing medicine but himself. He used to say 'A prudent man should wear such clothes as may not draw upon him the envy of the lower order or the contempt of the higher.' So he wore white clothes of a fine quality." - He ('Abd al-Latīf) then adds: "This (doctor) was strangled in the court of his house, in the first third of the night; he became a Muslim before his death. I have often regretted his loss."

275 For an exploration of the full spectrum of pharmacy in the medieval Arabic world, cf. Leigh Chipman, *The World of Pharmacy and Pharmacists in Mamlūk Cairo*, (Leiden/Boston 2010).

and concerns, and whose religion is influenced by carnal desire [*hawāhu*].[276] This is the last topic which I wish to discuss with you in this advice to the general public and to those who are devoted to the art of medicine in particular. There is no (further) need for me to tell you anything else, apart from the fact that you should not neglect to read the books of Galen. There is no harm and discomfort for you in reading them, but there is (also) no need for me to request from you to neglect the works of the later [i.e. contemporary] authors. But by

(78r) having read Galen's books, you may have disregarded (these) other (authors). Hence, your innermost feeling should have told you to work with books (by other authors) which are of similar purport. It shall bring you no harm to read these together with Galen's books.

Peace be upon you!

May God, the Lord of the Worlds, be praised. May God bless our Master Muḥammad, his Prophet, the members of his house [i.e. the family of the Prophet], the good and the pure-hearted.

---

[276] Cf. Joosse and Pormann, *Decline and Decadence*, 15-17.

The *Book of the Two Pieces of Advice* or *Kitāb al-Naṣīḥatayn* by ʻAbd al-Laṭīf ibn Yūsuf al-Baghdādī (1162-1231): Arabic Edition of the Medical Section on the basis of the unique Ms. Bursa (Turkey): Hüseyin Çelebi 823 (fol. 62r-78r)

(62r)

كتاب النصيحتين من عبد اللطيف بن يوسف إلي الناس كافةً.

(62v)

بسم الله الرحمن الرحيم. هذا كتاب من المتقرب إلى خالقه سبحانه وتقدس يبذل جهده متحوباً في المناصحة والإرشاد إلى خلصائه وأودّائه على تفرقهم في البلاد وتنقلهم في القرى وفي الأمصار. ثم إلى ملوك الأطراف والولاة والأمراء. ثم إلى السواد كافةً ممن يؤثر الخير لنفسه والسعادة لها ينزل الهوى والعصيبة والأنفة من التقليد والحمية وباستعمال النظر والتأمل والروية. فأول ما يبتدئ به حمد الله سبحانه الذي هو مفتاح كل خيرٍ واستيفاقه الذي هو قائد إلى كل مكرمةٍ والثناء عليه بما هو أهله. ثم الصلوة على نبي الرحمة ومرشد الأمة والمنقذ من كل ضلالةٍ وغمةٍ. فالدال على سبل النجاة والسعادة محمد النبي الأمي وعلى آله الطاهرين. وعلى الأولياء والشهداء والصديقين. ثم الشكر للحكماء العظماء الذين اقتدوا بالأنبياء على غاية الإمكان بأن أصلحوا نفوسهم أولاً ثم نحلوا العامة النصيحة ما وضعوا لهم من العلوم الفاضلة والصنائع النافعة. فجعلوا الحكمة غايتهم من حياتهم الداثرة وزادهم إلى الدار الآخرة وصرفوا وقتهم وقوتهم في اقتنائها وغنوا بها عن المقتنيات الفانية والأعراض البالية واقتصروا من ضرورة البدن على ما يوصلهم إلى المحل ولا يصدفهم عن المبتغي وعزفت نفوسهم

(63r)

عن كل ما سوى الحكمة ورأوا أن اقتنائها أفضل القرب إلى الحكيم الأزلي الواحد الفرد القديم الأبدي وصرفوا فضل حكمتهم إلى ما يعود على العامة بالمنفعة في نفوسهم وأبدانهم وبثوا فيهم من أصناف العلوم والصنائع النافعة في دنياهم وأخراهم مما أثاره مشكورة وأفعاله ظاهرة محمودة كالطب والنجوم والفلاحة والملاحة والحساب والهندسة والمساحة. وكل من جاء بعدهم وأم حزبهم وأخذ أخذهم وامتثل سمتهم كان معدوداً منهم ومحسوباً في زمرتهم وله أجر مثل أجرهم واستحق الحمد والشكر بقدر غنائه وصدق قصده. ومن أعان على ذلك من الملوك وأولي الأمر كان له الأجر أضعافاً والفضيلة أصلاً ومضافاً لان الملك يتبعه الناس ويتشبهون به ويتآمرون له ويستقيلونه وهذا لهم في أصل فطرهم ومعجون بجبلتهم كما ترى الصبي يحاكي شيم والديه ومؤدبه ثم لهم منه الرغبة والرهبة ومن خذل عن ذلك كان عليه من الوبال كفاء وكثرهم ما للأول من الثواب إذ الحسنات أضداد السيئات. وقصدي في هذا الكتاب إلى خلصائي أرشدهم الله وأحسن توفيقهم أن أنحلهم النصيحة وأوقظهم من رقدة الغفلة وسنة الإلف والعادة وأنبههم على بليةٍ انتشرت يعم ضررها النفوس والأبدان وأحذرهم من الوقوع فيها فمن كان عارفاً بصحة ما أقول ازداد تمسكاً به وثقةً ومن لم

(63v)

يكن عارفاً رجوت له أن يعرف ولو اهتدي بما أقول واحد من العالم احسبني أجره وكفاني فخره ونكاية هذه البلية في الملوك والعظماء إضعاف نكايتها في الرعاع والغثاء وأفتها أعظم من أفة عدم الحكمة فإن سألتَ وقلتَ أي أفة هي أعظم من عدم الحكمة فأقول اسمع مني وافهم عني واعلم أن اقتناء الحكمة المموهة أشد أفة وأعظم مضرة من عدم الحكمة الحقة فإن من عدم الحكمة رأساً شعر بالخلو عنها والفراغ منها والحاجة إليها فكان يتشوقها ويطلبها ويحرص مجتهداً في اقتنائها فأما من عنده حكمة مموهة فانه يظن انه غني وهو أفقر الفقراء ويوهل نفسه للتعليم والإصلاح وهو أحوج إلي التعلم والصلاح فمن لا دين له أسرع إجابةً ممن له دين فاسد ومن ينطوي على اعتقادٍ خطأ أعسر إجابةً ممن لا اعتقاد له لذلك كانت العوام أسرع تعلماً وأسلس قياداً ممن تمكنت فيه اعتقادات فاسدة. كم بين صحيفة بيضاء وأخرى مشغولةٍ بخطوط فاسدة وقد أشارت النبوة المقدسة إلى هذا المعنى بهذا القول كل مولودٍ يولد على الفطرة حتى يكون أبواه هما اللذان يهودانه وينصرانه ويمجسانه. وقال

فلاطن في كتاب السياسة أنّ الشر أشد مضادةً للخير من سلب الخير. وقال العلم صبغ النفس وليس يشرق صبغ الشئ حتى ينظف أدناسه. وهذه البلية

(64r)

العظمى والفادحة الكبرى التي قصدت الأجر في التنبيه عليها وقعت في الطب للموضوع لخلاص الأبدان من الأسقام وفي الحكمة للموضوعة لخلاص النفوس من آلام الجهل إلى سلامة المعرفة وصحة إدراك الحق ونحن نشرح أولاً البلية الواقعة من جهة الطب إذ كان شرها عاماً للجمهور ولكل احد فيها نصيب إذ كل احد يهمه خلاص بدنه من الآلام فليس كل احد يهمه خلاص نفسه من الجهل فنقول أولاً أن صناعة الطب خطيرة شريفة قد أقر بفضلها الجمهور وأصفقت الأمم مع تباينهم على حلالتها وعظم الحاجة إليها وفيها ما هو وحي والهام ورؤىً صادقة وهي منسوبة إلى الأنبياء عليهم السلام وإلى الحكماء الربانيين وجعلت في المنام من أعظم القرب إلى الله سبحانه وتقدس ولمن يعانيها مرتبه من الشرف لا يدفع ومدح من جميع الطوائف لا يجحد وذلك لما يظهر من فضلها ونفعها وأفعالها التي يشبه السحر. لكن هؤلاء المسترزقة بها أطفئوا نورها واخمدوا ذكرها ومحوا محاسنها وأساءوا سمعتها وأذلوا قدرها والحقوا بها العجز والقصور. وصناعة الطب إذا استوفيت شرائطها لا تخطي أبداً وإنما يخطي الطبيب الحاذق فيها مرةً ويصيب مائة مرةً كما قال جالينوس ولا يكون خطوه قطيعاً ولا كثيراً ولا بعيداً من الصواب فعاله الحاذق في الرماية فانه

(64v)

يصيب الغرض غالباً وإن اخطأ فلا يبعد عنه بعداً كثيراً وإنما يقع سهمه قريباً من الغرض سديداً وأما أن يقع في ضد الجهة وكلاً فهكذا يكون خطأ الطبيب وإنما قلنا أن الطب لا يخطي بل الطبيب الحاذق يخطي على الأقل ويصيب على الأكثر من قبل أن الصنائع التي شانها أن تعمل في المادة لها شروط كثيرة من جهة الصورة وشروط كثيرة من جهة المادة وكل ذلك من جهة الأمر الكلي ومن جهة الأمر الجزئي فأما الكلي فعليه يقع التعليم والتعلم وأما الجزئي اعني الأشخاص فلا يأتي عليه القول وإنما الملكة الحاصلة بالمزاولة هي التي تحدس عليه وتقارب فيه والمسامحة اليسيرة من شان الطبيعة لا يعبأ بها ويستدركها ولاسيما في الأمراض التي ليست في غاية الحدة والخطر وأنا اضرب لك مثلاً من مساحة الدائرة وجذر الأصم كالعشرة مثلاً فإن الحاذق في الصناعة يستخرج ذلك على اقرب ما يمكن ويسامح بأقل جزء مما لا يظهر له تفاوت في الحس ولا كثير اختلاف عند العقل فهذا الحكم

يعد صواباً وإن كان فيه تسامح حيث أخل بجزء لا يكاد يعتد به وكلما قل ذلك الجزء المتسامح به كان الحكم أصح وصاحبه أحذق فلحدس الصناعي في الطب بهذه المنزلة وما خالف ذلك وبعد عنه فهو ظاهر الخطأ وصاحبه لا يعد من أهل الصناعة كما أن من قال أن جذر العشرة مثلاً ثلاثة لم يعد حاسباً ولم يؤخذ

(65r)

بقوله وكذلك من كان بهذه المثابة ممن يدعى صناعة الطب لم يكن طبيباً وينبغي أن يردع عنها ويخرج من أهلها ويحذر أشد من حذر السباع الضارية والسموم الموجبة وجميع الآفات التي تأتي على النفوس لأنها أعداه كأشره قد استعد لها وحذر منها. وأما الطبيب الجاهل فانه عدو مبين في ثياب صديق وسم في صورة ترياق وهو يعطي أدويةً مشهورةً بالنفع فيقتل بها إذا لم يصادف موقعها فيكون لذلك سماً قاتلاً وإن شربة ماء في غير وقتها أو بغير شرطها قد تقتل فدع أدويةً مسهلةً سميةً كالسنا والبسفايج والتربد وشحم الحنظل والسقمونيا وأمثال ذلك مما هو سم أو سمي وكلما كان المرض أحد وأخطر كان الضرر في خطأ الطبيب أعظم حتى أن بعض المرضي يكون شفاؤه في شربة ماء إذا مُنعها هلك وآخر شفاؤه المنع منها إذا أعطيها هلك فلا يحقرن احد خطأ الطبيب فقليله كثير ويسيره له وقع عظيم. وقد قال بقراط إنه لما كان الطبيب يستعمل الأسماء التي يستعملها المتطبب لم يفرق العامة بين الطبيب والمتطبب وذلك أن الطبيب يصادف بها الوقت والمتطبب يخيطه وهذا المعنى لا تدركه العامة. وقد قال في مبتدئ كتاب الأمراض الحادة نحو هذا القول وله كتاب في أدب الطبيب وكتاب آخر في صفة الطبيب

(65v)

كيف ينبغي أن يكون ولجالينوس كتاب في امتحان الطبيب وهو كتاب فاضل حقيق ممن يحتاج أن يستطب أن يقف عليه ويتأدب بما فيه فمما قال فيه انه لما كان كثير من الرؤساء وأرباب الثراء لا يتسع وقتهم للاشتغال بصناعة الطب وكانوا يحتاجون إلى الأطباء عندما يقعون في الأمراض وكان الطبيب الحاذق ينحيهم من الآلام والجاهل يوقعهم فيما هو أشد منها وهو الهلاك وحب أن تكون عندهم علامات يفرقون بها بين الطب والمتطبب ويسبرون بها أحوالهما حتى يتوقوا هذا ويسلموا مهجهم إلى الآخر كما يحب على الإنسان أن يكون عنده معرفة بالفرق بين السم والغذاء فلا يلتبس عليه احدهما بالآخر. ثم قال فحب أن تأمل وتسبر من يدعي الطب في ماذا صرف صدر عمره وفي ماذا يصرفه في حالته الراهنة بعد

أن يعلم جودة فطرته وحسن استعداده وصحة عقله وفطنته التي وهبت له من أصل مولده ثم يسبر دينه وأمانته ومروءته وكتمانه للسر ويفقد ذلك كله في أفعاله لا من أقواله فإن كل احد يحسن في قوله ويتجمل فيما يظهر من فعله للناس وإنما يجب أن يتتبع حاله في خلواته وما يبدوا منه عند من يبسط إليه ثم يمتحن عفته في بطنه وفرجه ومقدار حرصه في تحصيل الدرهم فإن كان عبد ذلك فلا خير عنده فانه لا يؤمل أن يتبيع

(66r)

دنياه وآخرته بدرهمٍ واحدٍ أو بفسقةٍ واحدةٍ فإن كان غبياً بالفطرة ردي الطباع بالجبلة فلا ترج منه خيراً ولا يتوقع منه فضيلةً وايس من فلاحه ولا تطمع في صلاحه ولا يتربص به أن يصلحه الرياضة بالعلوم بل يوقع أن تزيده شراً وفساداً كما قال بعض الشعراء العلم للرجل اللبيب زيادة ونقيصة للأحمق الطياش مثل النهار يزيد أبصار الوري نوراً ويعشي أعين الخفاش وكان هذا مأخوذ من قول فلاطون العلم يزيد الشرير شراً لأنه يقوم له مقام الأنياب والمخالب للسباع. فإن كان فيه مع ذلك حسد وملق وجشع فقد اجتمعت فيه آلات الشر كلها ودواعيه فإن أضاف إلى ذلك الكذب وقلة التدين فالحذر منه كل الحذر. فإن كان مطبوعاً جيد الفهم والفطنة لكنه أذهب صدر عمره في البطالة والتجارة فلا ترج منه الحذق في الصناعة والبراعة ولا يئس منه كل اليأس فإن صرف وقته الراهن في اللذات فذلك بعيد من الفضيلة بقدر استغراقه في الرذيلة. وقد قال في هذا الكتاب يحب أن ينظر في ماذا يصرف الطبيب وقته ووكده فإن صرفهما بالليل في نيل اللذات وبالنهار في لقاء الرؤساء في الأهنية والأعزية فلا خير عنده ولا فضل لديه وإن كان يصرف ليلة وساعات فراغة

(66v)

في القراءة والتعلم والتفكر والتزيد ويصرف سائر وقته في مصالح الناس ومعالجه المرضى وبذل الجهد في نفعهم والحرص على تخليصهم من الآلام والإسقام على سبيل الفرح بذلك والابتهاج والتقرب به إلى خالق الكل والمطلع على خفيات القلوب فذلك طبيب فاضل يحب أن يوثق بعلمه ويستنام إلى تدبيره ورأيه ومن صفاته أن يكون مع ذلك فيه رأفة ورحمة وشفقة بعيداً عن القساوة والغلظة يكون فرحه بإصابته في حدسه أضعاف فرحه تحصيل الدرهم والدينار وكيف يحسن بعاقل أن يسلم مهجته إلى من يبيت سكران ويصبح مخموراً فمثل هذا مريض النفس والجسم فكيف يداوي صاحب مرضين صاحب مرض وحال المعاقر للشراب مضاد لحال العالم الحاذق فإن المعاقر مريض يتواتر الأبخرة المتضاغطة

الرطبة الضبابية المتزاحمة في بطون الدماغ فإنها تسد منافس البدن وتكدر الأرواح وتظلم منها الحواس وتطفئ نور الحياة وبهجة النفس وتتعطل موضع الفكر وتخرب بيت الرأي فهل يستوي هذا ممن بات ليلة مكباً على التعلم والتفكر والبحث والتبحر يصقل مرآه وعقله ويشحذ غرار فهمه ويرهف قواه ويستثير خواطره وسوانحه ويصبح وهمه إفادة الناس بعلمه وعمله وتجربة ما علمه وحدسه هل يستوي هذا ومن يصبح والدنيا غاية

(67r)

همه يسعى لغازية ودرهم يقتنيه أحب إليه. ولتغض الشعراء في ذم المعاقر للشراب ذر الخمر يسلم من عيوب كثيرة وإياك أن تزداد ما يورث الجهلاء فما عاقل يرضي بإنفاق عقله على الخمر أن الخمر يستلب العقلاء وما زال بقراط وجالينوس ومن سلك سبيلهما يشكون من جهل أطباء زمنتهم وقلة معرفتهم وكثرة تهجمهم ولقد تهكم بهم بقراط كثيراً في كتاب في الأمراض الحادة. وأما جالينوس فإنه يفتتح جل كتبه بمناقصتهم والتحذير منهم والإعلان نقصهم ومع هذا فإنه لم يشاهد زماننا ولم يرَ ما رأينا ولم يبل بما بلينا به فإن شكواه كانت من فرقة أصحاب الحيل وفرقة أصحاب التجربة وكل هؤلاء لهم مع تقصيرهم ضوابط ومع نقصهم فضائل يصلح أن نقتني ونتعلم ولسيما أصحاب التجربة فإن جالينوس ينقل عنهم كثيراً من أعمالهم في الميامر وفي قاطاجانس وأما أهل زماننا فليسوا من الفرق الثلاث الذي حددهم في كتاب الفرق وإنما هم من باب البخت والاتفاق مثل الأعمى يرمي ولا يدري في أي جهة هو الغرض فإن فرقتي الحيل والتجربة يعلمان جهة الغرض ولكن يرميانه مع عدم تحصيل موضعه الخاص وأما

(67v)

أرباب القياس فيعلمون الجهة ويحصلون موضع الغرض ويسددون نحوه السهم أكملَ تسديدٍ وأفضلَ تصويبٍ وأهل التجربة يحصلون عرضاً من أعراض الغرض كظله مثلاً فهم جدراء بالإصابة فأما أهل زماننا فلا يحصلون الغرض ولا جهة فلذلك صار العجب من صوابهم لا من خطئهم وأما أرباب القياس فالعجيب من خطئهم لا من صوابهم لأنهم يصيبون على الأكثر وبالذات ويخطئون على الأقل وبالعرض وأما هؤلاء المسترزقة فصوابهم على الأقل وبالعرض وخطؤهم على الأكثر وبالذات.

ونحن نزيد ذلك بياناً بمثال نضعه فأنزل رجلاً حُمّ فأتاه من كل فرقة طبيب أما صاحب الحيل فإنه يقصد لاستفراغه حيث كانت الحمى اختناقاً. وأما صاحب التجربة فيقول إني رصدت مرات كثيرة من به مثل هذه الحمى ففصدته وأخرجت له من الدم مقدار كذا أو كذا إلى أن غشي عليه فأفرق دفعة واحدة وأما صاحب القياس فإنه يجعل الحمى جنساً ويقسمها بفصول ذاتية إلى أنواعها الثلاث وينظر حمى هذا الرجل من أي هذه الثلاث هي فيجدها من الحمى ذات المادة ثم يقسم هذه الحمى إلى أنواعها بحسب المواد فيجدها دموية ويقسم الدموية إلى الخالصة والمشوبة فيجدها خالصة ويقسم هذه الخالصة إلى ما عفن وإلى ما أخذ في الغليان فيجدها مما أخذ في الغليان ثم يعتبر البلد والسن

(68r)

والوقت الحاضر والعادة وسالف التدبير وسائر ما شأنه أن تغير الحكم ثم يستخرج من مجموع ذلك كله صورة التدبير الواجب ثم يفصده حتى يعرض الغشي فمن ترى ليت شعري أقمن بالصواب وأبعد من الخطأ من هؤلاء الثلاثة الأطباء فلا عاقل ألا وهو يختار صاحب القياس ويحكم له بالحذق ويرجو له الظفر والفلاح. وأما الواحد من أطباء زماننا فإنه يقدم فيفصده أو يمنع من فصده كيف جاء واتفق لا عن معرفه بشيء من هذه القوانين المذكورة بل بحسب ما يظن ظناً غير صناعي ويحدس حدساً بحسب ما يقع في خياله لا عن قياسٍ وحجةٍ أو تجربةٍ ورصدٍ هذا هو الغالب فيهم ولا يحد من يعتبر بعض الشروط المذكورة إلا الواحد بعد الواحد. وأظن أن هذا الفساد كله راجع إلى إهمال الملوك والرؤساء امتحان الأطباء وربما قدموا الناقص ورفعوه على الكامل فانكسرت همته وهمه الشادي ورأوا أن الدنيا إنما تنال بالبخوت لا بالفضيلة فقصروا في طلبها. والعجب أن الملك ينظر من تولي طعامه وشرابه ويفتقد أحواله وينظر مثل ذلك لرعيته وخاصيته ويهمل جانب الطب وهو أشرف وأهم وأعلى وأنفس وأخطر وهو أحق بالنظر والرعاية والحياطة من جميع ما عددناه لأن التفريط في ذلك يخل بالألذ والأنفع والتفريط في حال الطب يخل بالمهج فحب ألا تكون للملك

(68v)

عناية بشي أكثر من عنايته بأمر الطب والأطباء والعجب من إنسانٍ يختار لحماره وفرسه أجود البياطرة وأحذقهم ثم يسلم مهجته إلى من لا يثق بحذقه ولا معرفته والعجب ممن يحتسب على السوقة في الطبيخ والشواء والخبز ويهمل جانب الأطباء ويتركهم يتلاعبون

بالمهج والعجب من إهمال الفقهاء هذا الباب واحتياطهم على باب الأموال فلا يثقون عليها إلا الأمين ولا يقبلون على الدرهم إلا بشهادة العدل ويقبلون قول الواحد من هؤلاء في مهج من غير اختبار دينه وأمانته وعلمه وفهمه والعجب من فقيهٍ قد بلغ درجة الاجتهاد أو كاد ويسلم مهجته إلى عامي لا يحفظ من الطب كراسةً واحدةً والعجب منهم كيف أهملوا ذلك ولم يعملوا بقول النبي صلى الله عليه وسلم من تطبب ولم يعلم منه طب فقتل فهو ضامن
والعجب أنه قد سبق في لسان الجمهور لمن أخطأ عليه الأطباء أن يقولوا مات بأجله فإن الله قضي عليه مع أنهم يعتقدون أن جميع أفعال العباد خلق الله سبحانه وتعالى ومع هذا فيقتلون القاتل ويقتصون من الجاني كان الله سبحانه إنما يتولى قتل من يخطئ عليه الأطباء دون من تذبح وتضرب عنقه ولم أسمع بقوم يحتاطون على صناعة الطب ويعتبرون الأطباء
ويأخذون على أيديهم كأهل قسطنطينية فإنهم لا يمكنون أحداً من مزاولة الطب دون أن يكون قد تدرج في أجزائه

(69r)

وتمرن في أعماله ومضى عليه سنون كثيرة وشهد له بذلك الشيوخ الأفاضل ثم يعقد مجلس ويمتحن في محفلٍ منهم بان يحضر له عدة مرضي مختلفي الأمراض ويديرهم بحضرة جميع الأفاضل فإذا رضوا أفعله بعد ما رضوا قوله أخذوا عليه عهداً بقراط الذي كان عهده إلى الغرباء حتى دخلوا به في زمره الأولاد والاقرباء وهذه كانت حالهم لما كان يملكهم الروم وفي هذه السنين انتقل الملك إلى الإفرنج وغيروا كثيراً من الأوضاع الحسنة ومحوا معظم الرسوم القديمة فلا أدري كيف حالهم اليوم. ورأيتُ لأهل بغداد بالأطباء بعض العناية وكذلك لأهل مصر لا يطلق المباشرة إلا من معه محضر فيه خطوط شيوخ الصناعة وعلى نحو هذا يجري حال الأطباء بدمشق ولم أرَ أشد إهمالاً من هذه الصناعة بمدينة حلب فلذلك كانت سيرتهم في غاية الرداءة وطرق أطبائها على حال من الفساد لا يكون أحط منها فلا سلطان يزعهم ولا دين يردعهم ولا علم يرشدهم ولا رئيس عليهم يرشدهم ويرهبهم ولهم أسلوب متشابه قلما يخالفونه وهو أن كل من شكا إليهم مرضاً عاجلوه بشربة مسهل ليتعجلوا ثمنها ويغتنموا فضيلتها ولا يعتبرون نضجاً ويهملون سائر الشرائط ويطلقون ذلك لمن سمعوا خبره من غير معاينته وليس همهم سوى اختلاس ثمن المسهل والتحيل عليه بكل وجه ولا يبالون

(69v)

كيف قتلوا بها ويبيعون مهجة إنسان بربع درهم وأظن أن الذي جراهم على هذه الأفعال القبيحة والشيم الرذيلة شيخ منهم مغربي كان مسلماً وارتد وعاد يهودياً في الظاهر وهم يعتقدون أنه مهمل لجانب دينهم متهاون بوظائف عباداتهم منحل في الشريعة أكذب ما يكون إذا حلف بالتوراة والعشر الكلمات وكان فقيراً يتركض في البلاد بخدمة التجار وعاني بصناعة الطب على الكبر وفيه من الحرص على الدنيا وشدة الكلب والجشع ما يحمله على الفتك بالمهج والإقدام على النفوس الضرغام على الفريسة وأجمعوا على أنه لا يخاف خالقاً ولا مخلوقاً وأهون بشيء عليه قتل ألف نفسٍ في ساعةٍ واحدةٍ قالوا وأنه يلتذ بذلك ويسر به. وقتل في سنة ثلاث عشرة وأربع عشرة وستمائة جماعةً من الملوك والأكابر شهدت بعضهم والباقي اتصل في خبرهم وممن قتل في سنة ثلاث عشرة سلطان المدينة الملك الظاهر غازي بن يوسف فإنه حم يوم السبت السادس والعشرين من جمادى الأولى من السنة المذكورة وكان عبلاً قد أرمى على الأربعين سنةً ويقدم له فكر وهموم في تعبية عساكر ومداوسة حروبٍ ونفقاتٍ فهجر لأجل ذلك الشراب وأقل الطعام وأكثر السهر وإعمال الفكر فأشار طبيب مسلم يفصده ووافقه على ذلك

(70r)

الأطباء فمنعهم هذا الملعون من الفصد وقال لهم في السر أن فصده هذا حظي عنده وتقدم عليكم فصدفوه عن الفصد فسقاه شربته المجربة في اليوم السادس من مرضه قبل النضج فمشاه أربعة والعشرين مجلساً سقطت قوته في المجلس الرابع وبرد جسمه وبطلت حركته نحو ثلثين ساعة ويئسوا منه وقعد الملعون يضحك ويعمل رأيه فيمن يكون بعده فقام منهم رجل ذو حمية ومعرفة لينظر قوته فنظروا به وقالوا أنتَ تريد أن تحيى الموتى قال فطمعتُ في حياته إذ كان سقوط قوته من قبل التدبير لا من قبل خبث المرض فسقاه شيئاً من أمراق الفراريج بعد أن فتح فاه بجهدٍ فتراجع نبضه وقوته وفتح عينه وتكلم ثم طلب الماء والغذاء ونهض على نفسه فعادوا إليه وكان هذا الملعون رأى أن سهمه لم ينفذ فأعطاه حقنةً بعد أخرى وفي أثنائهما فتائلاً كثيرة ورفقاؤه من الأطباء ينهونه ويردعونه وهو يكفهر في وجوههم ويسبهم ويستحمقهم ويقول إنما قصدي أن أغسل بدنه وبهذا وأمثاله كان يقنع خدمه وأهله إلى أن أوثقه وأسلمه إلى المنون فانحلت القوى الماسكة وانبثقت فأخذوا حينئذٍ في

المقبضات المفرطة يظنون أن الأدوية تعمل بأنفسها من غير أن تكون في البدن قوة تدبرها وتفعل بها وأنا أقول أن الأدوية لا تفعل بأنفسها إنما هي آلات

(70v)

لقوى البدن فإذا فسد ذو الآلة بطلت الآلة ولم تفعل ولذلك لا تحدي ولم يزل رحمة الله يسيل حتى مات في الرابع والعشرين من مرضه. واجتمع كل واحد من الأطباء الذين كانوا معه وصرحوا بأنه قتله ووصف كل واحد منهم صفاً من التدبير الردى الذي ارتكبه غير ما وصفه الأخر ومن دقيق مكره في هذه المرضة أنه وهم من يتولى أمره من الخدم أن كثرة الأطباء يضجره فاقتصروا على اثنين يشير إلى نفسه وإلى شيخ منهم صالح العلاج متلطف ولو قدر على العادة لفعل فاختلى بالسلطان والشيخ مغلوب معه فحكم فيه كيف شاء حتى أفاق السلطان وطلب أخر منهم كان يأنس به وهو رجل كهل حسن التدبير سديد الرأي فتسلمه ولكن بعد أن يقدم ذلك الملعون فأسلمه وكثيراً ما رأيت هذا الملعون يروم أن يحفظ الصحة بالضد ويزيل المرض بالشبيه فيسقي في الأمراض البلغمية بزر القثاء وماء الشعير وشراب الورد وفي الأمراض الصفراوية والدموية والمسلولين المعالي المفتحة المسخنة والمسهلات الحارة وقد ظن بعض العقلاء أن فعله هذا عن قصدٍ منه لإهلاك النفوس والتذاذٍ بإفساد الصور. ويحكي عن المبرد أنه مر بطرقي يلحن في هاذورة لحناً مفرطاً فقال لصاحبه أظن هذا يعرف طرفاً من العربية فقال له بماذا عرفتَ فقال رأيته يتوقي الصواب بوقى

(71r)

من يعرفه فوقف حتى يفرق الناس عنه وسأله هل تعرف من العربية شيئاً فقال نعم وإنما أعدل عنها لئلا يلحقني حرفه الأدب. ونعود فنقول ما قال بقراط ترك الطبيعة مع المرض خير من تسليمها إلى طبيب سوء. وقال الرازي من جمع أطباء أوشك أن يجمع خطأهم. وأما جالينوس فقد شحن كتبه بالتحذير منهم والتنبيه على أصناف خطيهم فمن ذلك قوله إن حال الفقراء في أمراضهم خير من أحوال الرؤساء والمياسير لان الفقير لا يقدر على طبيب فيبقي مع طبيعته والغني يجتمع إليه الأطباء ويصبون عليه أصناف الأدوية والأشربة وفنون العلاج الخطأ فيصدفون الطبيعة عن جهتها ويقهرونها ويحيرونها ثم قال فمقدار ما يخرج جنازة الغني يكون الفقير قد أبل وربما شيع جنازته وأنا أقول إن طب العجائز أفضل من طب هؤلاء لأن العجوز تعمل ما رأت نجحه وجربت نفعه فهي قريبة من فرقة التجارب

وأما هؤلاء فيقدمون بقياسٍ فاسدٍ وظن مختل ثم أن العجوز قلما تقدم على دواء قوي ومسهل خطر فإن أقدمت على شيء منه لم تلج فيه ولم تبالغ لكن إن رأت إما رأت النجح ثبتت وإلا أقلعت وهؤلاء المسترزقة يقدمون بتهور ويصفون أدويةً لا يعرفون صورها ولا جربوا قواها ولا شاهدوا أثارها وكثيراً ما أسأل الواحد منهم بعد الواحد عن مفردات أدويتهم فلا

(71v)

أحدهم يعرفون صورها فضلاً عن قواها وغاية الفاضل منهم إن يسند ذلك إلى كتابٍ ويحيله على نقل فلا يعرفون قوى الأدوية المفردة معرفة امتحان وتجربة ولا القوة الحاصلة للمركب عنها وليتهم اقتصروا على التركيب المذكور في الكتب وتركوا عنهم أن يركبوا من قبل أنفسهم ويتصرفون في الكيفيات والكميات مع جهلٍ بهما وبالأمراض التي يقصدون مقابلتها وهم يقصدون أن يداووا الضد بالضد مع جهلٍ بهما وبمقدار البعد بينهما وبما بينهما من التضاد النوعي فضلاً عن جهلهم بالتضاد الشخصي فإن الطبيب لا يكتفي في صواب العلاج بمعرفة التضاد النوعي دون الشخصي فإنه إنما يداوي الأشخاص لا الأنواع فكذلك الحال في حفظ الصحة بالشبيه يجب عليه أن يعرف الشبيه الشخصي فإنه إياه يحفظ ولا يقف في شيء من ذلك على معرفة النوع فإن هذا غير كافٍ فإن هذه المعرفة ليست مقصودة لذاتها بل لأجل الشخص ليتوصل بها إلى المعرفة الشخص. وأقول إن الغرباء الذين يبيعون الشربات على قوارع الطرقات أمثل من هؤلاء أما أولاً فلأن أكثر الناس وخواصهم يحذرونهم ولا يسلمون نفوسهم إليهم وأما ثانياً فإنهم يسقون اليتوعات والشبوش الذي هو ورق الحنظل للأصحاء وأمزجتهم تحتمل الخطأ أكثر مما يحتمله المرضى وأكثر ما يسقون

(72r)

أدويتهم الفلاحين وأرباب الكد وأمزجتهم تحتمل الأدوية القوية ثم أن الغرباء عندهم أدوية مجربة ممتحنة وأعشاب مجربة هم يجتنونها ويمتحنونها ويتناقلون العلم بها. ويجب على الطبيب الحاذق العاقل الشفوق أن يحذر من شرب الدواء المسهل أشد الحذر ولا يقدم عليه إلا عند تحقق الضرورة وتوفر الدواعي والموجبات ويكون حذره منه في المرضى أشد من حذره في الأصحاء ويكون من الإسهال أشد حذراً من الفصد وإنما حذرنا من المسهلات لأنها إنما تسهل بسمية فيها والطبيعة تستعين بما فيها من السمية على دفع سمية مادة المرض فإذا وافق غرضها سهل احتمالها سمية الدواء إذ تدفع به سميةً أعظم منه كما تدفع الشر بشرٍ والعدو بعدوٍ فلذلك إذا صادف الدواء وقته ومحله حق على الطبيعة وسهل احتماله وحصلت

الراحة والحق عقيبه وإذا لم يصادف محله تمخضت مضرته وتضاعفت بليته وقد قالت الحكماء إن الأدوية الترياقية إذا شربت وفي البدن سمٌ ظهر نفعها وإذا شربت والبدن نقي عادت سماً وقالوا إن الترياق طبيعة متوسطة بين طبيعة السم المحض والدواء المحض وقال بقراط في كتاب الفصول من كان بدنه صحيحاً فأسهل أو فني بدواء أسرع إليه الغشى وكذلك من كان يغتذي بأغذيةٍ رديئةٍ وجالينوس يحذر غاية الحذر

(72v)

من سقي المسهل لمن بدنه كثير الامتلاء وقد شرح ذلك في كتاب حيلة البرء وذكر خطأ الأطباء على من هذه حاله ثم ذكر الحيلة في استفراغه بالدلك الدائم المتناسب والمرخ والدهن وتكرير ذلك حتى يستفرغ بعض المادة وينضج الباقي فحينئذٍ يمكنه إسهاله إن احتاج إلى ذلك أو فصده. فإنما قلنا إن الحذر من المسهل في المرضى أشد منه في الأصحاء من قبل أن الأصحاء موفور القوة صحيح الأعضاء ومع هذا فهو يضعفهم وينكي فيهم إذا صادف محله فضلاً عن أن لا يصادف فما ظنك بالمرضى الذين ضعفت قواهم ونكي المرض أعضاءهم الرئيسية وإنما كان الدواء يضعف القوى وينكي الأعضاء من قبل أن المسهلات سموم وإنما تسهل بأن ينكي القوى الماسكة لأمشاج البدن فتخلي عنها ولذلك لا تعطى إلا مصلحةً ومكسورة السَورة ومقداراً قصداً ويستدرك مضارها التي تخلفها في البدن في عدة أيام حتى أن التي تسهل بالتزليق وهي قريبة من طبيعة الغذاء مثل الإجاص وتمر الهندي والألعبة فمن شأنها أن ترخي وتحل القوة الماسكة وإنما يقاوم اليبس الحادث عن الحمي في المعدة والأمعاء وما يلي هذه الأعضاء فإذا اتفق أن لم تكن يابسةً نكت فيها وقد حذروا من ماء الشعير مع فضله ومدحه وإنه غذاء فاضل صالح ومع هذا فإذا لم يصادف موضعه أضر وقد عددوا مضاره في الأمراض المزمنة وفي الحادة إذا تجاوزت الرابع عشر وأكثره إلى العشرين

(73r)

وإذا كنا نحذر مضار المسهل في الصحيح الموفور القوى فما أجدرنا بالحذر منه في المرضى المهزولي القوى فينبغي أن نحذره فيهم غاية الحذر ولاسيما في أصحاب الحميات الحادة مع أن المسهلات حارة ولهذا قد احتال لهم الأطباء بما يسهل بالتزليق وفيه تبريد وترتيب. ومن هذا يتبين أن الخطر في الفصد أقل منه في شرب الدواء لأن الفصد ينقص الأمشاج والقوى موفورة والأعضاء الرئيسية بحالها فيمكنها أن تعوض عن الدم الصالح في

أمدٍ قريبٍ وأما الإسهال فلا يقع إلا بأن يضعف الأعضاء الباطنة فيعجز عن العوض إلا في زمان طويل ويقدر إضعاف الدواء لها ونكايته فيها يتأخر العوض لأن هذه الأعضاء هي التي تفعل العوض فإذا حلت بها آفة نقص فعلها بمقدار الآفة هذا في الأصحاء فلا يمكنهم الاغتذاء والعوض وإن تناولوا غذاء فبمقدار ما لا يفي برد الفائت. وقد كنا حدثنا في مقالةٍ لنا مفردة في بادي بصناعة الطب وإنها ناشئة معه (مع الإنسان) حيث كانت حاجته إليها معه وإنها كلما أخلقت على طول الزمان قيض الله سبحانه وتعالى لها من يحيى أثارها ويجدد ما انمحي من رسومها وتهدم من أركانها كما جرى ذلك على عهد ابقراط فإنه أحيا طب جده الأكبر اسقلبياذس ثم على عهد جالينوس فإنه أحيا طب ابقراط وأخر من أعرفه في ملة الإسلام أبو جعفر أحمد بن محمد بن أبي الأشعث

(73v)

وأما المشتغلون في هذا الزمان بالطب فشأنهم أن يقرؤوا شيئاً من كليات كتاب القانون فيحفظون حد الطب وحد الأسطقس وحد المزاج وأمثال ذلك ويتجادلون فيه ويرفعون بذلك أصواتهم في المجالس والأسواق ثم يقدمون على العلاج ظناً منهم أن ذلك يجدي عليهم وأنه كافيهم وأن من حقق حد الطب قدر أن يبرئ من الحميات وغيرها ويعرف أصنافها. وأنا أشير على من يقبل نصيحتي إن شاء أن يكون طبيباً ألا يعدوا كتب جالينوس وبقراط وإن استغشني في نصيحتي فليفعل ذلك في جزء من أجزاء الطب وأفرضه كتاب المزاج مثلاً فيقرؤه ثم يقرأ ما في هذا المعنى من كلام القانون وغيره فإن وجد في شيء مما عدا كلام جالينوس معنىً عنه فلا يقبل مني سائر أقوالي وإن وجد في نفسه عند قراءة كلام جالينوس قوةً على عمل تصنيف مثل تصانيفهم فليثق بقولي وليمض قدماً ويفعل ذلك في كتاب النبض الصغير لجالينوس والنبض من كتاب القانون ويمتثل في جميع كتب جالينوس ما امتثله في كتاب المزاج الذي جعله كالأنموذج والتجربة والامتحان ثم في كتاب النبض الصغير (الكبير) وهكذا جميع كتبه العلمية والعملية وإن استطالها فليقتصر على ما أحب من مختصراتها مثل كتاب الصناعة الصغير التي هي مدخل ومثل النبض الصغير واغلوقن واختصاره لحيلة البرء والمقالتين الشافيتين له وإن شاء أن يقرأ كلام المتأخرين على جهة

(74r)

التنزه على مقادير العلماء في علمهم وتفاوتهم في فهمهم وحسن اختصارهم وبسطهم فذلك إليه ومن زعم أن في الملكي وفي القانون كفايةً عن كتب جالينوس فقد زعم بطلاً ولم يقل

ذلك عن اختيار ولا عن إطلاع على كلام جالينوس بل عن تقليدٍ وافتراء وما استخرج من كلام جالينوس شيء إلا وكلامه أفضل منه ولا دخل كلامه قلب أحدٍ فوسع كلام سواه ولا راق له غيره ولا أطباءه ما عداه على أن كتاب المائة كتاب فاضل وأما كناش ابن سربيون فهو مادة تصانيف أكثرهم ولا أعرف كناشاً أفضل منه.

وقد رأيت جماعة ممن أعرض عن كلام جالينوس وحدث نفسه إنه ممن قد أطلع على أسرار الوجود ووقف على غوامض العالم بقول أن طب أولئك قد بطل اليوم واختلف الزمان بحركة الكواكب الثابتة وانتقلت الطبائع ويؤرخ أن أهل بغداد كانوا يتعالجون بالأدوية الحارة. وأما اليوم فلا يقدرون عليها أصلاً وإنما يكبون على المبردات. وقد يقول من هؤلاء إن طب بقراط وجالينوس كان يحسب بلاد الشام والعراق ولا تحتمل ذلك وهذه حال من لم يقرأ كتب القدماء ولا جرب شيئاً مما فيها أترى الكواكب حيث دارت غيرت طبائع الناس فقط دون النبات وسائر الحيوان إن كان هكذا فإن ذلك لعجيب وإن غيرت الجميع فإنه سيصير الأفيون حاراً والفلفل بارداً

(74v)

ولحم السمك حاراً ولحم الأسد بارداً ويصير الأسد جباناً والأرنب شجاعاً ويتبدل حكمهم على طبائع الأدوية والأغذية من النبات والحيوان والمعادن ثم إنا نجد أبقراط يوافق من قبله بالأحقاب الطويلة على طبائع الأشياء وامتحن ما قالوه قديماً فوجده في زمانه على ما حكموا عليه لم يتبدل وكذلك امتحن جالينوس على بقراط جميع ما حكم به فوجده موافقاً وبينهما من الزمان ستمائة سنة وما زال الناس يمتحنون ما قال جالينوس إلى زماننا هذا فوجدوه موافقاً ولجالينوس نحو ألف ومائتي سنة. وهذا كتاب الفلاحة الذي نقله ابن وحشية من لغة النبط له مدد متطاولة والطبائع فيه ثابتة على حال واحدة وهذا القول سخيف جداً لولا إنه قد سُطِرَ في الكتب لَما حَسُنَ بي مناقضته وحكايته ورأيت من يعتقده ويغرب بذكره وينتج بمعرفته ومثله في السخافة قولهم إن طب بقراط وجالينوس كان يحسب بلاد اليونان أو ما علم أن أقوالهم أمور كلية لا يقبل التبدل ولا تغير فإن قولهم أن الضد شفاء الضد وإن الصحة يحفظ بالشبيه وإن الحمى يقاوم بالتبريد والترطيب وإن الغب الخالصة يحتاج من التبريد والترطيب إلى مقدار كثير وليس كذلك البلغمية والربع وإن النائبة لا يستعمل في أولها ما تسخين بإفراط بل برفق فإذا نضجت المادة أعطي ما تسخين بقوة وقد حذروا من استعمال ما تسخين بقوة في أول الفالج

(75r)

وإنما يتدرج فيه وقد حكى جالينوس أن فلاناً كان به ربع فأشار عليه الأطباء بأدوية حارة فنهيته عنها وقلت إن فعلت عادت ربعين فلما قبل منهم عادت ربعه ربعين فلما سلم إلى علاجه رفقت به حتى نضجت المادة ثم أعطيته تلك الأدوية الحارة بعينها فأقلعتا جميعاً عنه وهكذا جميع ما في كتب القوم ليس فيه ما يقبل التبدل والتغير وإنما هي قوانين كلية ثابتة على حالة واحدة ثم أن القوم قد ملئوا كتبهم بالوصية بأن تعبر السن والبلد والعادة والهواء وأوقات السنة والوقت الحاضر وغير ذلك وعابوا من أغفل النظر في ذلك ونسبوه إلى الغلط والخطاء فطبهم ينطبق على الصقالبة وعلى الحبشان جميعاً وما بين هذين الطرفين وأهل بغداد لا يخرجون عن الوسط فضلاً عن الأطراف. ثم إنزال بقول أن أهل بغداد لا يعرض لهم أمراض البلغم كالفالج واللقوة والسكتة والصرع والاستسقاء ونحو ذلك إنزال يعالج هؤلاء بالأشياء الباردة لأجل حركة الكواكب الثابتة أتراهم لا يعرض لهم حميات نائبة وليلية وربع إنزال تعالجها بما تعالج به الدموية من الفصد والتبريد والتخفيف والصفراوية من التبريد والترطيب أتراهم أمنوا القولنج البلغمية فليت شعري أي صنفٍ من الطبائع تغيرت بحركة الكواكب الثابتة أم أي علاج خاصٍ ببلاد اليونان لا يستعمل في العراق إن هذا لسخيف بين وعقل مأفون وهذا طب الهند

(75v)

فد نقل إلينا وشحنت به كتبنا ومعاجينهم الكبار مبثوثة في الأقراباذينات هذا مع إنهم من الإقليم الأول وبلاد يونان من الإقليم الرابع والخامس والعراق من الثالث والرابع فهو أقرب إلى بلاد اليونان من الهند ثم أن مصر والشام قد كانت داخلةً في كثير من الأوقات في ولاية القوم متصلةً بهم وجالينوس قد سلك مصر والشام وحكم على طبائعها وشاهد عادات أهل الإسكندرية وحكاها في كتبه وعرض بغداد. وأما ديسقوردس فمن عين زربي وكثير من حكماء اليونان من مصر والشام وقونية قد كانت من بلاد الحكماء وكذلك ملطية وقد كان بها خزانة كتب عظيمة وكان بها دار تعليم للحكمة وملطية مختلطة بالشام وهذا ديسقوردس تفسير اسمه عشاب الله لأنه أقام ثلثين سنة يسيح في أقطار الأرض لتعرف أعيان النبات ومنافعه ويأخذ ذلك عمن وقع إليه فيه تجربة وقيل إنه كان يحكم عليه ثم يخبره فيصدق حكمه. وأنا أقول قولاً أختم به هذا الفصل هل جربتم أدوية القدماء بشرائطها فلم ينجح وحقاً

أقول أن الواحد منكم ليبلغ من العمر تسعين سنة يعالج المرضى ولم يستعمل شيئاً مما في كتب القدماء ولا يعلم أصحيح هو أم باطل ولعمر الله أن طب القدماء منزول

(76r)

عندكم لعجزكم عن استعماله وجهلكم بشروطه فمن فيكم يقدر أن يفصد المحموم حتى يعرض له الغشى ويبرئ في الحال أومن فيكم يجسر أن يسقي الماء المبرد بالثلج حتى بحصر المحموم وتنطفئ حماه على المكان أم من فيكم يسقي في ذات الجنب الحريق ويستفرغه السوداء أو من يعلم العلة في الحاجة إلى استفراغ السوداء من المجنوب وكيف يتولد في بدنه مع أن مادة مرضه دموية ومن ذا الذي يقدر أن يلحم قرحة الرئة في مبدأها بالترياق الفاروق ويمنع من تولد المدة فيها والوقوع في السل ومن يقدر منكم أن يداوي صاحب الصرع بالدولاب والحكماء القدماء إنما يفخرون بحسم الأمراض قبل تمكنها فإنها إذا تمكنت قلت فيها الحيلة ومن فيكم من يقدم فيسقي الخل في قرحه الرئة فإذا كنتم لا يجربون طب القدماء فمن أين لكم إنه صواب أو خطأ أو إنه يوافق بلد كذا ويضر بلد كذا. أترى كتاب النبض وعلم البول وما في كتاب الفصول وتقدمة المعرفة وكتاب الأهوية وبلدان تغير علم ما فيها بحركات الكواكب الثابتة أترى دواء الحلتيت والمعجون الفلافلي بطل فعله ولا يوجد مرض لا يحتاج إليه. وقد نحلتك نصيحتي وأبحتك حمي دخلتي فإن قبلت فلك وإن أتيت فعليك. وأنا أوصيك بما أوصي به نفسي إذا استفتيت في أمر مريضٍ اتصل ألا تعجل بالحكم بل تتبين وتثبت وتكشف وتسأل

(76v)

وتجيل فكرك وتتوهم إنك أنت صاحب المرض فتحكم له ما تحكم به على نفسك لو حل بك وتخاف من الغلط عليه كما تخاف من الغلط على نفسك ولو كان عدوك وأنا أطرفك بعجيبةٍ كثيراً ما يقع لي وهو أن الواحد من الأطباء إذا حل به مرض وبولده وعزيز عليه يشاورني فيه وتوقف وتحير فإذا عرض عليه مريض غريب بادر وحكم وسارع واستبد ولم يشاور كأنه أحكم طب الأجانب دون الأقارب فحب عليك أن تتفكر ثم تحكم فإن الصواب مع تأخر الجواب لا يخرج الإنسان عن مرتبة العلماء وأما المخطئ فلا حظ له من الفضيلة أسرع أو أبطأ وإذا عود نفسه أعمال فكرته صارت تجيبه بأهون سعى فيصير يسرع ويصيب وإذا عودها الإهمال والتسرع من غير حقيقةٍ صارت لنفسه ملكة ردية لو أراد أن يزول عنها عند الحاجة إلى غيرها لم يقدر على ذلك ولم ينقد له مثل من يعود لسانه اللحن ويده كتابةً

رديئةً فإذا أخذت نفسك بالسداد والصواب هان عليك وصار ذلك ملكةً لك تعمل عنها بسهولةٍ وأكثر ما يحملهم على المسارعة في الجواب إيثارهم ألا يظهر للناس نقصهم كان التوقف في الجواب بحط قدرهم فلا يزالون يسرعون في الخطأ حتى يصير ذلك ملكةً وعاده سوء لو أرادوا الانتقال عنه لما قدروا ولو توقفوا وتفكروا وظهر عليهم بشر والظفر

(77r)

وهشاشة المعرفة لكانت الثقة بهم من العامة أكثر واعتقدوا فيهم الفضيلة والحرص والاجتهاد والعجب أن جالينوس ونظراوه يتوقفون في كثير من الأمراض عن الحكم إلى اليوم الثاني والثالث وأكثر من ذلك ولا تجد الواحد من هؤلاء المسترزقة يشكل عليه مرض أصلاً بل يعلم كل شيء ويحكم في كل شيء فأنت أيها الناصح لنفسه المحب لها اقتناء الفضيلة إياك ثم إياك والعجلة فإنها من الشيطان وعليك بالتأني والرفق ومحبة الحق والالتداد بالإصابة فإنك إذا كنت كذلك انكشف لك المستور وانقادت لك الأمور وأجابك الحق عن أمور ولباك الصواب من كثب فالحق يتعبك عند حصوله ثم يريحك في جميع المستقبل كالأساس المحكم الصحيح وأما الباطل فيريحك في الأول ويتعبك دائماً كالبيت المبني على أساسٍ واهٍ لا يزال ينهدم. وقد رأيت من أطباء مصر وبغداد وما بين ذلك ومن ورد إلي ممن قرأت عليه أو قرأ علي فلم أر أسوأ حالاً من هذا الملعون المغربي الذي بحلب ولا أحسن حالاً من ابن هبة الله صاعد المعروف بابن التلميذ لا الشيخ المصنف فإن ذلك لم أدركه بل ولده وكان قد تجاوز سبعين سنةً فشاهدت له ملكةً عجيبةً كان يحكم على الأمراض كأنه يعاينها وكأن البدن زجاج شفاف يصف ما وراءه وكان كما يقال لا يبطئ ولا يخطئ ولا يطيل الوصفات ولا يكبر التركيبات وغالب ما كان

(77v)

يعالج به المفردات فإن يركب فتركيباً يسيراً ولا ينتقل من علاج إلى علاج لقوة ثقته بل كان يثبت عليه حتى يظهر له ما كان يتوقعه كما قال بقراط إذا أنت فعلت جميع ما ينبغي ولم تر ما ينبغي فلا تنتقل عما ينبغي ما دام ما رأيته منذ أول الأمر ثابتاً. ومن مخرقتهم وتمويههم تطويل النسخ وتكثير المفردات عن غير موازنة بين قواها ولا تجربة لما يكون عنها ويفعلون ذلك إما لتعجب العامة منهم ومن سعة علمهم وإما ليحصل لهم ربح إذا اشتريت الحوائج منهم أو من عطار هو شريكهم وقد يدخل الواحد منهم على المريض في اليوم مرات يصف في كل دخلة علاجاً جديداً وقصده في ذلك أن يكون لدخوله أثر ويظهر له في كل مرة

عمل فالفاضل منهم يجعل التغييرات متشابهة وربما عرضت عليه نسخة طبيب آخر فيزيد وينقص ما لا ينفع ولا يضر وقصده بذلك أن يري لنفسه فضيلة على غيره وينبه على مكانه وهذا ونحوه فلا أكرهه كما أكره الأول لأن هذا ينفعه ولا يضر به أحداً وأما الذي أكرهه جداً فما يضر به الناس أعاذنا الله وإياك أن تكون ممن يبيع آخرته بدنياه ويؤثر على دينه هواه. فهذا آخر ما أريد أن أقوله في هذه النصيحة للناس كافةً وللمشتغل بصناعة الطب خاصةً وليس لي عندك حاجة سوى أن تقرأ كتب جالينوس وليس في هذا مشقة عليك ولا كلفة يلحقك ولا احتاج أن أشير عليك بترك كتب المتأخرين فأنت إذا

(78r)

قرأت كتب جالينوس تركت ما عداها وحدثتك نفسك بعمل مثلها وإن قرأتها مع قراءة كتب جالينوس فلا ضير عليك والسلم عليك. والحمد لله رب العالمين وصلى الله على سيدنا محمد نبيه وعلى أهل بيته الطيبين الطاهرين.

Bibliography

1. 'Abd al-Laṭīf al-Baghdādī: manuscripts consulted

ms(s).: manuscript(s) used; **ed(s)**.: edition(s) used; **tr(s)**.: modern translation(s) used (often with commentaries) - [A] Arabic; [D] Dutch; [Dan] Danish; [E] English; [F] French; [G] German; [Gr] Greek; [It] Italian; [L] Latin; [Syr] Syriac; [T] Turkish; ALB: 'Abd al-Laṭīf al-Baghdādī; IAU: Ibn abī Uṣaybi'a; [Aut.]: biography and autobiography.

a: Ms. Bursa (Turkey): Hüseyin Çelebi 823, consisting of 10 treatises by 'Abd al-Laṭīf al-Baghdādī, as well as one by Alexander of Aphrodisias (No. 9), cf. Stern (1962) and Dietrich (1964), 100-113.

1. fol. 1b-19b, 28a-34a: *Al-Aurāq allatī 'amiltuhā 'alā kitāb Muḥammad b. 'Umar al-ma'rūf bi-Ibn Khaṭīb ar-Raiyī alladhī 'amilahu 'alā ba'ḍ al-juz' al-awwal min Kitāb al-Qānūn wa-huwa al-mulaqqab bil-Kullīyāt*: cf. partial tr. [F] in: Gannagé (2011).
2. fol. 34a-38b, 20a-23b: *Qaul li 'Abd al-Laṭīf b. Yūsuf 'alā ḥāl Ibn Khaṭīb ar-Raiyī fī tafsīr sūrat al-ikhlāṣ.*
3. fol. 23b-27b, 39a-52a: *'An māhīyat al-makān bi-ḥasbi ra'yi Ibn al-Haytham*: cf. ed. [A], annotated tr. [F] Rashed (1993-2002); cf. also the study by El-Bizri (2007).
4. fol. 52b-62a: *Maqāla fī-l-mizāj.*
5. fol. 62a-100b: *Kitāb al-Naṣīḥatayn min 'Abd al-Laṭīf b. Yūsuf ilā-l-nās kāffatan*. [medical section: fol. 62a-78a; philosophical section: fol. 78b-100b]: cf. full ed. [A], tr. [E] of the medical section: Joosse (2013/ new ed. 2014 - that is the present study); cf. partial ed. [A], tr. [E] of the medical section: Joosse and Pormann (2010); partial tr. [E] Joosse and Pormann (2008); partial tr. [E] Joosse (2007b); partial tr. [E] and study of the philosophical section: Martini Bonadeo (2013, 144-196), cf. also Gutas (2011). Unpublished ed. [A] en study [T] of both sections of the *Kitāb al-Naṣīḥatayn* by Enes Tas (2011).
6. fol. 100b-123b: *Risāla fī Mujādalat al-ḥakīmayn al-kīmiyā'ī wa-l-naẓarī*: cf. handwritten ed. [A], tr. [G] Allemann (1988); partial tr. [E]: Joosse (2008).
7. fol. 124a-132a: *Risāla fī-l-Ma'ādin wa-ibṭāl al-kīmiyā'.*
8. fol. 132b-135b: *Fuṣūl muntaza'a min kalām al-ḥukamā'*: cf. ed. [A], tr. [F] M. Rashed (2004), 9-63.
9. fol. 136a-137b: Alexander of Aphrodisias, *Risāla lil-Iskandar fī-l-faṣl khāṣṣatan wa-mā huwa*: cf. ed. [A], tr. [G] Dietrich (1964); ed. [A] Ghalioungui and Abdou (1972), 39-42.
10. fol. 138a-140a: *Fuṣūl ṭibbīya intaza'ahā 'Abd al-Laṭīf b. Yūsuf*: cf. tr. [G] Dietrich (1967), 42-60.

11. fol. 140b-149a: *(Fī) l-maraḍ al-musammā diyābīṭā*: cf. facs. ed. [A], tr. [G] Thies (1971); ed. [A] Ghalioungui and Abdou (1972), 123-152; study [G]: Degen (1977).

b: Ms. Paris (Bibliothèque Nationale de France): 2870, item 2 [= Ancient fonds 1088, fols. 128a-172b]: *Kitāb fī Uṣūl mufradāt aṭ-ṭibb wa-kayfīyāt ṭabā'ī'ihā* (*On the Principles of Simple Medical Substances and their Natural Qualities*), cf. Ullmann (1970), 279; *GAS*, vol. 3, 30-31; *GAL*, S. I, 881.

c1: Ms. Oxford: Bodleian Library Pococke 230: *Kitāb al-Ifāda wa-l-i'tibār fī-l-umūr al-mushāhada wa-l-ḥawādith al-mu'āyana bi-arḍ Miṣr*, cf. section 3 *infra* under *Ifāda* and in many other places; tr. [E]: cf. Zand and Videan under section 3.

c2: Ms. Riyadh (Saudi Arabia): King Faisal Center, 1894: *Mukhtaṣar Akhbār Miṣr* [= most probably: 'Abd al-Laṭīf b. Yūsuf al-Baghdādī, *Kitāb al-Ifāda wa-l-i'tibār fī-l-umūr al-mushāhada wa-l-ḥawādith al-mu'āyana bi-arḍ Miṣr*], cf. the unpublished catalogue of Adam Gacek under # 2784.

d: Ms. Damascus (Syria): Maktabat al-Asad 3152T (Ṭibb) = formerly Ms. Damascus (Syria): Ẓāhirīya, ṭibb 27: *K. Taqdimat al-ma'rifa li-Buqrāṭ wa-tafsīruhu*, pp. 2-143, cf. *GAS*, vol. 3, 33; *GAL*, S. I, 881, cf. for this Ms. and other Mss. of ALB's *Commentary on the Hippocratic Prognostic*: Joosse and Pormann (2012b).

2. 'Abd al-Laṭīf al-Baghdādī: autobiographical and biographical information

a: Biography and first list of his complete oeuvre in: ed. [A]: Ibn abī Uṣaybi'a, *K. 'Uyūn al-anbā' fī ṭabaqāt al-aṭibbā'*, ed. Imru'ulqais b. aṭ-Ṭaḥḥān (August Müller), Juz' 1.2., Cairo-Königsberg 1299 H./1882 A.D. [Reprint: F. Sezgin *et alii* (editor): *Islamic Medicine*, vol. 1-2, Frankfurt am Main 1995], Juz' 2, 201-13; likewise ed. Nizār Riḍā, Beirut 1965, 683-96; ed. Qāsim Muḥammad Wahb, Damascus 1997; ed. Muḥammad Bāsil 'Uyūn al-Sūd, Beirut 1998, 634-48; ed. Al-Najjār, Cairo 1996-2004 [= Aut. Version 1]; incomplete and rather unsatisfactory [E] tr. by Lothar Kopf (1971), cf. chapter 3 *infra*: *'Abd al-Laṭīf al-Baghdādī: editions, studies & translations*. The earliest complete manuscript copy of Ibn abī Uṣaybi'a's work is found in Istanbul, Süleymaniye Kütüphanesi: Ms. Şehid Ali Paşa 1923 (copied 774/1372 – complete annotated copy).

b: Autobiography in: ed. [A]: Ms. Bursa (Turkey), Hüseyin Çelebi 823 (No. 5): *Kitāb al-Naṣīḥatayn min 'Abd al-Laṭīf b. Yūsuf ilā-l-nās kāffatan*, philosophical section, fol. 88b-100b. [= Aut. Version 2]

c: Biography in: ed. [A], tr. [L]: J. Mousley, *Abdollatiphi Bagdadensis vita auctore Ibn Abi Osaiba; de codicibus mss. Bodleianis descripsit, et Latine vertit*, Oxonii 1808. [= Aut. Version 1]

d: Biography in: tr. [F]: A.-I. Silvestre de Sacy, *Vie de Mowaffik-eddin Abd-Allatif, de Bagdad, extraite de l'Histoire des médecins d'Ebn-Abi-Osaïba* (with added notes), Paris 1810, 457-494. [= Aut. Version 1]; ed. [A]: idem, *Texte de la Vie d'Abd-Allatif, extraite de l'Histoire des Médecins d'Ebn-Abi-*

Osaïba, 534-548. [= Aut. Version 1] [Reprint in: F. Sezgin *et alii* (editor), *Islamic Geography*, Volume 10: Antoine-Isaac Silvestre de Sacy (1758-1838), *Relation de l'Égypte, par Abd-Allatif, médecin arabe de Bagdad [1162-1231 A.D.]*, Reprint of the Edition Paris 1810, Part 2 (pp. 455-753), followed by *Abdollatiphi Compendium Memorabilium Aegypti*, arabice edidit D. Joseph White, Reprint of the Ed. Tübingen 1789, Publications of the Institute for the History of Arabic-Islamic Science at the Johann Wolfgang Goethe University, Frankfurt am Main 1992].

e: Biography in: tr. [E]: H.A.R. Gibb, "Life of Muwaffiq Ad-Din Abd al-Latif of Baghdad by Ibn Abi Usaybiya [Translated from the Persian, and for the first time rendered into English]", in: R.H. Saunders (editor), *Healing through Spirit Agency by the Great Persian Physician Abduhl Latif ("The Man of Baghdad") and information concerning The Life Hereafter of the deepest interest to all enquirers and students of Psychic phenomena*, London 1927, 65-90. [= Aut. Version 1]

f: Full [E] tr. and study of the biography [Aut. Version 1] in : C. Martini Bonadeo: *'Abd al-Laṭīf al-Baġdādī's Philosophical Journey: From Aristotle's* Metaphysics *to the 'Metaphysical Science'*, Leiden/Boston 2013, 110-43.

g: tr. (fragments of the biography) in: [F]: "Extrait de l'Autobiographie d'Abd el-Latif". Texte et traduction de Baron W. MacGuckin de Slane, in: *Recueil des historiens des croisades: historiens orientaux*, Paris, tomus 3 (1884), 431-39. [= Aut. Version 1]

h: tr. (fragments of the biograpy) in: [E]: "Curriculum Vitae of 'Abd al-Latif al-Baghdadi (d. 629/1231)", in: G. Makdisi, *The Rise of Colleges. Institutions of learning in Islam and the West*, Edinburgh 1981, 84-91. [= Aut. Version 1]

i: tr. (fragments of the biography) in: [E]: S.M. Toorawa, "The Autobiography of 'Abd al-Laṭīf al-Baghdādī (1162-1231): Selections from the Autograph Notes of 'Abd al-Laṭīf al-Baghdādī", in: D.F. Reynolds (editor); coauthored by Kristen Brustad…[et al.]: *Interpreting the self: autobiography in the Arabic literary tradition*, Berkeley and Los Angeles 2001, 156-164. [= Aut. Version 1]

j: Historical fragments by ALB as preserved in Shams al-Dīn al-Dhahabī's *Ta'rīkh al-Islām*, cf. Somogyi (1937): ed. [A], tr. [G]; Cahen (1970): ed. [A]; and Cahen (1971): tr. [F] of the part on the Khwārizm Turks (= ed. [A] Cahen [1970], 116-124). [= Aut. Version 3]. Rosenthal (1937), Somogyi (1937), Cahen (1970 & 1971), Allemann (1988) as well as the present author strongly believe that these fragments were once part of [Aut. Version 4], cf. under m *infra*.

k: Biographical remarks [A] with regard to 'Abd al-Laṭīf's life in: Ṭāhir (b. Ṣāliḥ) al-Jazā'irī, *At-Tadhkira*, Ms. Damascus: Zāhirīya (without date and number), Book 83, fol. 9a, 11a and 12a, cf. Dietrich (1964), 102; cf. also Vicomte Philippe de Tarrāzī, *Khazā'in al-kutub al-'arabīya fī l-khāfiqayn*, Beirut 1947, vols. 1-4, 1, 280; However, the text as such has not been registered by Ṣalāḥ Muḥammad al-Khaymī and Muḥammad Muṭī' al-Ḥāfiẓ in their *al-Fihris al-*

'āmm li-makhṭūṭāt dār al-kutub al-zāhirīya, Damascus 1407/1987, 564-65. It appears that the Ms. has been lost, or perhaps has been incorporated into a collective volume of texts by al-Jazā'irī.

l: Dimitri Gutas (Yale University, U.S.A) produced an [A] edition, [E] translation and some commentary of the autobiographical section in: Ms. Bursa (Turkey), Hüseyin Çelebi 823 (No. 5): *Kitāb al-Naṣīḥatayn min 'Abd al-Laṭīf b. Yūsuf ilā-l-nās kāffatan*, fol. 88b-100b. [= Aut. Version 2]. Gutas has been using [Aut. Version 2] in his Arabic seminar to train graduate students. He is planning to publish it at some point, but mentioned that this project is not yet on his front burner. (Personal e-mail communication, Sunday, July 6, 2003); cf. also the material in Gutas (2011) *infra* with regard to the philosophical section of the *Kitāb al-Naṣīḥatayn*.

m: *Kitāb Ta'rīkh wa-huwa yataḍammanu sīratahu allafahu li-waladihi Sharaf al-Dīn Yūsuf* – mentioned in IAU, *K. 'Uyūn al-anbā' fī ṭabaqāt al-aṭibbā'*, cf. ed. August Müller, vol. II, 211, line 28, but the text thereof is lost. [= Aut. Version 4]

n: Historical fragment by ALB preserved in: Al-Maqrīzī, *K. al-Sulūk li-ma'rifat duwal al-mulūk*, ed. Muḥammad Muṣṭafā Ziyāda, 2 vols., al-Qāhira 1956, I, I: 94. (see also tr. [E]: R.J.C. Broadhurst, 1980, 82-3, under secondary sources).

o: A second list of ALB's oeuvre in: Ibn Shākir al-Kutubī, *Fawāt al-wafayāt*, ed. M. Muḥyī al-Dīn 'Abd al-Ḥamīd, 2 vols., al-Qāhira 1951; ed. I. 'Abbās, 4 vols., Beirut 1973, vol. II, 385.1 – 388. 2. This second and later list of ALB's works is partially different from the earlier one as given in: Ibn abī Uṣaybi'a, *K. 'Uyūn al-anbā' fī ṭabaqāt al-aṭibbā'*, cf. under [a] *supra*.

p: Biographical information about ALB in: Abū Ja'far al-Idrīsī, *Kitāb al-Anwār 'ulūw al-ajrām fī l-kashf 'an asrār al-ahrām* ('Light on the Voluminous Bodies to Reveal the Secrets of the Pyramids'), Facsimile edition [Series C, Volume 44], ed. Ursula Sezgin, Frankfurt am Main 1988. This work may contain short fragments taken from ALB's larger work on Egypt, that is, from a work different than the *Kitāb al-Ifāda wa-l-i'tibār fī-l-umūr al-mushāhada wa-l-ḥawādith al-mu'āyana bi-arḍ Miṣr*, cf. Joosse (2011).

q: Biographical information about ALB in: Ibn al-Qifṭī, *Inbāh al-ruwāt 'alā anbāh al-nuḥāt*, ed. Muḥammad Abū 'l-Faḍl Ibrāhīm, 4 vols., al-Qāhira 1369-1374/1950-55. [Reprint: Beirut 2004], especially vol. II, 193-96, cf. Joosse (2007b).

r: Scattered quotations from ALB's work in: Ibn Khallikān [Info on ALB in: [E] tr. vol. III, 420, 602-03; vol. IV, 376, 378], Ibn abī 'l-Ḥawāfir, Ibn al-Athīr, al-Damīrī, Yaḥyā al-Wāṭwāṭ al-Kutubī, al-Qalqashandī and Ḥājjī Khalīfa, that is mainly with regard to zoology, cf. Kruk (2008), 345-362. Ibn Khallikān's *Biographical Dictionary* moreover contains interesting biographical information on ALB.

s: Notes and Remarks. London, Royal College of Physicians: Ms. GREEW/264/149, 150, 152, and 153. [unpublished translations and notes made about 1810 by William A. Greenhill on the lives of 'Abd al-Laṭīf al-Baghdādī, and two other Arab physicians].

3. 'Abd al-Laṭīf al-Baghdādī and his milieu: editions, studies & translations

Abdou, S., see: Ghalioungui, P. and S. Abdou (1392/1972).

Allemann, F. (1988): *'Abdallaṭīf al-Baġdādī: Ris. fī Mudjādalat al-ḥakīmain al-kīmiyā'ī wan-naẓarī ("Das Streitgespräch zwischen dem Alchemisten und dem* theoretischen *Philosophen)". Eine textkritische Bearbeitung der Handschrift: Bursa, Hüseyin Çelebi 823, fol. 100-123 mit Übersetzung und Kommentar*, (PhD diss.) Bern.

Anawātī, G.C. (1964): "Ṭibb al-Baghdādī", in: *Dhikrā* (1964), 73-89.

Al-'Ashrī [Al-'Ushrī?], 'Abd as-Salām (1963): [Al-'adad thalātha min *qiṣaṣ al-raḥḥāla wa l-mustakshifīn*], al-Qāhira.

Avci, Necati (1993; in [T]): "Abdüllatif Bağdādi'nin Dinī Ilimlerde Eğitimi ve Öğretimi" (in: TOC)/"Muvaffakuddin Abdullatif el-Bağdadi'nin Dini Ilimlerde Eğitim ve Öğretimi" (in: Book)/"Abdüllātif Bağdādi's Instructions and Lectures in Theology" (English title), in: *Kongresi*, 37-48.

Avci, Necati, see also: Köker, Ahmet Hulūsi and Necati Avci (1993b).

Badawī, 'Abd al-Raḥmān (1964): "Muwaffaq al-Dīn 'Abd al-Laṭīf al-Baghdādī, ḥayātuhu wa-mu'allifātuhu wa-falsafatuhu", in: *Dhikrā* (1964),1-29.

Balkar [Balkir], Faruk, see: Utaş, Cengiz and Faruk Balkar [Balkir] (1993).

Berendji, R. (1969): *Medizinisches in ABD-UL-LATIFs "Denkwürdigkeiten Ägyptens"*, (PhD Diss.) Düsseldorf.

Butterworth, C. (1980, review): (review of) "A. Neuwirth, *'Abd al-Laṭīf al-Baġdādī's Bearbeitung von Buch Lambda der aristotelischen Metaphysik*, Wiesbaden 1976 [= Veröffentlichungen der Orientalischen Kommission; Bd. 27]", in: *JA* 268, 198-99.

Cahen, C. (1971, tr. [F] of the part on the Khwārizm Turks [= ed. [A] Cahen [1970], 116-124]): "'Abdallaṭīf al-Baghdādī et les Khwārizmiens", in: C.E. Bosworth (editor): *Iran and Islam in memory of the late Vladimir Minorsky*, Edinburgh, 149-166. [see also *supra*: ALB Aut. under (j)].

Cahen, C. (1970, ed. [A]): "'Abdallaṭīf al-Baghdādī, Portraitiste et Historien de son Temps. Extrait inédits de ses Mémoires", in: *BEO* XXIII, 101-128. [see also *supra*: ALB Aut. under (j)].

Dabdūb [Dubdūb?], Faiṣal (1970): "Maqāla al-ḥawass: makhṭūṭa nādira li-'Abd al-Laṭīf al-Baghdādī", in: *Majallat majma' al-lugha al-'arabīya bi-dimashq*, 45, 332-341 [= sābiqan: *Majallat al-majma' al-'ilmī al-'arabī*].

Degen, R. (1977): "Zum Diabetestraktat des 'Abd al-Laṭīf al-Baġdādī", in: *Annali Istituto Universitario Orientale di Napoli* 37 (N.S. 27), 455-462.

Dhikrā (1964) = Dawlat Ṣādiq (editor): 'Abd al-Laṭīf al-Baghdādī commemorative volume: *Fī al-dhikrā al-mi'awiyya al-thamina li-mīlādihi*: nadwa fī yawmay 29-30 min Yūniyū sanat 1963, bi-munāsabat murūr 800 sana 'alā mīlād Muwaffaq al-Dīn 'Abd al-Laṭīf al-Baghdādī, al-Qāhira 1384/1964.

Dietrich, A. (1967, tr. [G]): "Ein Arzneimittelverzeichnis des 'Abdallaṭīf Ibn Yūsuf al-Baġdādī", in: W. Hoenerbach (editor): *Der Orient in der Forschung. Festschrift für Otto Spies zum 5. April 1966*, Wiesbaden, 42-60.

Dietrich, A. (1966): *Medicinalia Arabica. Studien über arabische medizinische Handschriften in türkischen und syrischen Bibliotheken*, Göttingen. [= Abhandlungen der Akademie der Wissenschaften in Göttingen; Philologisch-historische Klasse 3. F., Nr. 66]. [Info on ALB on 217-236].

Dietrich, A. (1964, ed. [A], tr. [G]): *Die arabische Version einer unbekannten Schrift des Alexander von Aphrodisias über die Differentia specifica* (Nachrichten der Akademie der Wissenschaften in Göttingen: I. Philologisch-historische Klasse; Jahrgang 1964, Nr. 2, Göttingen), 85-148. [Info on ALB on 100-113].

Drossaart Lulofs, H.J. and E.L.J. Poortman (1989, ed./tr.): *Nicolaus Damascenus. De plantis: Five Translations* (Verhandelingen der Koninklijke Nederlandse Akademie van Wetenschappen, Afd. Letterkunde, Nieuwe Reeks, deel 139; ASL 4), Amsterdam/Oxford/New York. [Info on ALB on 4-8: *The Fragments of De plantis in 'Abd al-Laṭīf*].

El-Bizri, N. (2007): "In Defence of the Sovereignty of Philosophy: Al-Baghdādī's Critique of Ibn al-Haytham's Geometrisation of Place", in: *Arabic Sciences and Philosophy*. A historical journal 17: 1, 57-80.

El-Bizri, N. (forthcoming?): "The physical or the mathematical? Interrogating al-Baghdādī's critique of Ibn al-Haytham's geometrisation of place", in: Graziella Federici Vescovini (editor): *Les Actes du Colloque de la Société Internationale d'Histoire des Sciences et des Philosophies Arabes et Islamiques (Circulation des savoirs autour de la Méditerranée, IXe-XVIe siècles*, Florence.

Gannagé, E. (2011): "Médecine et philosophie à Damas à l'aube du XIIIème siècle: un tournant post-avicennien?", in: *Oriens* 39, 227-256.

Garrett, E.J. (1968): *Many Voices. The Autobiography of a Medium*, New York. [Info on ALB on 85-89].

Genequand, C. (1978, review): (review of) "A. Neuwirth, *'Abd al-Laṭīf al-Baġdādī's Bearbeitung von Buch Lambda der aristotelischen Metaphysik*, Wiesbaden 1976 [= Veröffentlichungen der Orientalischen Kommission; Bd. 27]", in: *Der Islam* 55 (2), 362-64.

Ghalioungui, P. (1985): *'Abd al-Laṭīf al-Baghdādī ṭabīb al-qarn al-sādis al-hijrī: shakhṣīyatuhu, injāzatuhu*, al-Qāhira. [= *A'lām al-'Arab*; No. 114, 232 pp.].

Ghalioungui, P. (1977): "The Legend of Abdullatif al-Baghdady's «Spirit»", in: *Annales Islamologiques* XIII, 257-267. [*Usṭūra rūḥ 'Abd al-Laṭīf al-Baghdādī* also in Ghaloungui (1985), 33-38 (shortened version; in Arabic)].

Ghalioungui, P. and S. Abdou (1392/1972, eds. with commentary [A]): *Maqālatān fī l-Ḥawāss wa- Masā'il Ṭabi'ya/Risāla li l-Iskandar fī l-Faṣl/Risāla fī l-maraḍ al-Musammā Diābīṭis by Abd Al-Latif Al-Baghdadi*, Kuwait. [= The Arab Heritage series/*Wizārat al-I'lām* No. 18].

Grotzfeld, S. (1970): art. "(Kitāb) al-Ifāda wal-i'tibār (Das Buch des Nutzens und der Belehrung)", in: *Kindlers Literatur Lexikon* (Einmalige zwölfbändige Sonderausgabe), Band V: Gib-Iz, Zürich, 4740b.

Gül, Ahmet and Ahmet Hulūsi Köker (1993; in [T]): "Hipokrat ve Galen'in Hekimlere ve Filozoflara Öğütleri" (in: TOC)/"Hekimlere Nasihat Abdüllatif Bağdādī (1161-1231)" (in: Book)/"Hippocrates and Galen's Advice to Doctors and Philosophers" (English title), in: *Kongresi*, 21-26.

Gutas, D. (2011): "Philosophy in the Twelfth Century: One View from Baghdad, or the Repudiation of al-Ghazālī", in: Peter Adamson (editor): *In the Age of Averroes: Arabic Philosophy in the Sixth/Twelfth Century*, London/Turin, 9-26.

Gutas, D. (1980, review): "Editing Arabic Philosophical Texts" = (review of) "Angelika Neuwirth, *'Abd al-Laṭīf al-Baġdādī's Bearbeitung von Buch Lambda der aristotelischen Metaphysik*, Wiesbaden 1976 [= Veröffentlichungen der orientalischen Kommission; Bd. 27]", in: *Orientalistische Literaturzeitung* 75/3 (1980), 213-222.

Ifāda = [A] editions of Muwaffaq al-Dīn 'Abd al-Laṭīf al-Baghdādī's *Kitāb al-Ifāda wa l-i'tibār fī l-umūr al-mushāhada wa l-ḥawādith al-mu'āyana bi-arḍ Miṣr*. [among others eds. al-Qāhira 1869, 1934, and Beirut 1983]. For mss., see: section 1c *supra*.

Joosse, N.P. and P.E. Pormann (2012a): "Commentaries on the Hippocratic *Aphorisms* in the Arabic Tradition: The Example of Melancholy", in: Peter E. Pormann (editor): *>Epidemics< in Context: Greek Commentaries on Hippocrates in the Arabic Tradition*, Berlin/Boston [= Scientia Graeco-Arabica Band 8], 211- 249. [Info on ALB on 231-33].

Joosse, N.P. and P.E. Pormann (2012b): "'Abd al-Laṭīf al-Baġdādī's *Commentary on Hippocrates' 'Prognostic'*: A Preliminary Exploration", in: Peter E. Pormann (editor): *>Epidemics< in Context: Greek Commentaries on Hippocrates in the Arabic Tradition*, Berlin/Boston [= Scientia Graeco-Arabica Band 8], 251-283.

Joosse, N.P. and P.E. Pormann (2010): "Decline and Decadence in Iraq and Syria after the Age of Avicenna? 'Abd al-Laṭīf al-Baghdādī (1162-1231) between Myth and History", in: *BHM* 84, 1-29.

Joosse, N.P. and P.E. Pormann (2008): "Archery, mathematics, and conceptualising inaccuracies in medicine in 13th century Iraq and Syria". Available from: www.jameslindlibrary.org (Sir Iain Chalmers and Jan P. Vandenbroucke (editors)). [Republished as: "Archery, mathematics, and conceptualizing inaccuracies in medicine in 13th century Iraq and Syria", in: *Journal of the Royal Society of Medicine* 101 (2008), 425-27].

Joosse, N.P. (2013): "A Newly-Discovered Commentary on the Hippocratic *Prognostic* by Barhebraeus: Its Contents and Its Place within the Arabic *Taqdimat al-ma'rifa* Tradition", in: *Oriens* 41.2-4, 499-523 [contains info on ALB].

Joosse, N.P. (2011): "'Abd al-Laṭīf al-Baghdādī as a Philosopher and a Physician: Myth or Reality, Topos or Truth?", in: Peter Adamson (editor): *In the Age of Averroes: Arabic Philosophy in the Sixth/Twelfth Century*, London/Turin [= Warburg Institute Colloquia 16], 27-43.

Joosse, N.P. (2010): "Expounding on a Theme: Structure and Sources of Bar Hebraeus' 'Practical Philosophy' in *The Cream of Wisdom*", in: Herman Teule & Carmen Fotescu Tauwinkl with Bas ter Haar Romeny & Jan van Ginkel (editors): *The Syriac Renaissance*, Leuven/Paris/Walpole, MA [= Eastern Christian Studies 9], 135-150. [Info on ALB on 135-38].

Joosse, N.P. (2008): "Unmasking the Craft'. 'Abd al-Laṭīf al-Baghdādī's Views on Alchemy and Alchemists", in: Anna Ayşe Akasoy and Wim Raven (editors): *Islamic Thought in the Middle Ages. Studies in Text, Transmission and Translation, in Honour of Hans Daiber*, Leiden/Boston, 301-17.

Joosse, N.P. (2007a, in [D]): "De Geest is uit de Fles'. De middeleeuwse Arabische arts 'Abd al-Laṭīf ibn Yūsuf al-Baghdādī: zijn medische werk en zijn bizarre affiliatie met het twintigste-eeuwse spiritisme"; [E] title: "The spirit has left the bottle': the medieval Arabic physician 'Abd al-Laṭīf ibn Yūsuf al-Baghdādī: his medical work and his bizarre affiliation with twentieth-century spiritualism", in: *Gewina* 30, nummer 4, 211-29.

Joosse, N.P. (2007b): "Pride and Prejudice, Praise and Blame'. 'Abd al-Laṭīf al-Baghdādī's Views on Good and Bad Medical Practitioners", in: Arnoud Vrolijk and Jan P. Hogendijk (editors): *O ye Gentlemen: Arabic Studies on Science and Literary Culture in Honour of Remke Kruk*, Leiden/Boston, 129-141. [= Hans Daiber (general editor): Islamic Philosophy, Theology and Science. Texts and Studies, Volume LXXIV].

Karabulut, Ali Riza (1993; in [T]): "Abdüllātif Bağdadi'nin Eserleri" (in: TOC)/"Abdullātif Bağdādi'nin Eserleri" (in: Book)/"Abdüllātif Bağdadī's Works" (English title), in: *Kongresi*, 79-108.

Karabulut, Ali Riza, see also: Köker, Ahmet Hulūsi and Ali Riza Karabulut (1993c).

Kaya, M. (n.d.; in [T]): art. "Abdüllatif el-Bağdadi" [or: "Abdullatif Bağdadī"], in: *Islam Ansiklopedisi*, 254-55.

Keleştimur, Fahrettin and Şaban Kuzgun (1993; in [T]): "Diyabetes Risalesi" (in: TOC)/"Diabetes Risalesi" (in: Book)/"Booklet of Diabet" (English title), in: *Kongresi*, 17-19.

Kirca, Celal (1993; in [T]): "Abdüllatif Bağdādi'nin Fahreddin Razi'yi Tenkidi" (in: TOC)/"Abdüllatif el-Bağdadi'nin Fahreddin er-Razi'yi Tenkidi" (in: Book)/"Abdüllatif Bağdādi's Critic for Fahreddin Razi" (English title), in: *Kongresi*, 49-55.

Köker, Ahmet Hulūsi (1993a; in [T]): "Abdüllātif Bağdādi'nin Hayati ve Tibbi Eserleri" (in: TOC or Içindekiler)/"Abdüllātif Bağdādi'nin Hayati ve Tibbi Eserleri (1162-1231)" (in: Book)/"Abdüllātif Bağdadi's Life and Medical Works" (English title), in: *Kongresi*, 1-10.

Köker, Ahmet Hulūsi and Necati Avci (1993b; in [T]): "Rey'li Hatiboğlu'nun, Kanun el fi't Tip Hakkindaki Fikirleri" (in: TOC and Book)/"Hatiboğlu of Rey's Views on Kanun el fi't Tip" (English title), in: *Kongresi*, 11-15.

Köker, Ahmet Hulūsi and Ali Riza Karabulut (1993c; in [T]): "Abdüllatif Bağdādi'nin Eserlerindeki Anatomi Bilgileri" (in: TOC)/"Anatomi Bilgileri" (in: Book)/"Anatomical Data in the Works of Abdüllatif Bağdadi" (English title), in: *Kongresi*, 31-35.

Köker, Ahmet Hulūsi, see also: Gül, Ahmet and Ahmet Hulūsi Köker (1993).

Kongresi = Ahmet Hulūsi Köker, (1993, editor; in [T]): *Abdüllātif Bağdādi*, Kayseri: Erciyes Üniversitesi Matbaasi, Turkey [Erciyes Üniversitesi Gevher Nesibe Tip Tarihi Enstitüsü; Yayin No: 14 – Gevher Nesibe Sultan Anisina Düzenlenen Abdüllātif Bağdādī Kongresi tebliğleri 14 Mart 1992 Kayseri]; language note: articles in Turkish, but with a Turkish and English TOC.

Kopf, L. (circa 1971; tr. [E] unpublished): *Ibn Abu Usaibi'ah: History of Physicians*. Translated from the Arabic by Dr. L. Kopf with partial annotations by Dr. M. Plessner. Institute of Asian and African Studies, the Hebrew University, Jerusalem, Israel. Translated for the National Library of Medicine, Bethesda, Maryland, under the Special Foreign Currency Program, carried out under a National Science Foundation Contract with the Israel Program for Scientific Translations, Jerusalem, Israel [tr. prepared before 1969; library accession 1971; placed online by Roger Pearse (2011)]. [contains ALB Aut. Version 1].

Kraus, P. (1940-41): "Plotin chez les Arabes. Remarques sur un nouveau fragment de la paraphrase arabe des *Ennéades*", in: *Bulletin de l'Institut d'Égypte* XXIII, 263-95. [Info on ALB on 277]. [Reprint in: Rémi Brague (editor), *Alchemie, Ketzerei, Apokryphen im frühen Islam. Gesammelte Aufsätze*, Hildesheim/Zürich/New York 1994, 313-345]. [Info on ALB on 327].

Kruk, R. (2008): "'Abd al-Laṭīf al-Baghdādī's *Kitāb al-Ḥayawān*: A Chimaera?", in: Anna Ayşe Akasoy and Wim Raven (editors): *Islamic Thought in the Middle Ages. Studies in Text, Transmission and Translation, in Honour of Hans Daiber*, Leiden/Boston, 345-362.

Kuzgun, Şaban, see: Keleştimur, Fahrettin and Şaban Kuzgun (1993).

Leclerc, L. (1876): *Histoire de la médecine arabe*, vols. 1-2, Paris. [Info on ALB in: vol. 2, 182-87]. [Reprint: F. Sezgin *et alii* (editor): *Islamic Medicine*, vol. 48-49, Frankfurt am Main 1996].

MacGuckin de Slane, W. (1884, tr. (fragments) [F]): "Extrait de l'Autobiographie d'Abd el-Latif". Texte et traduction de Baron W. MacGuckin de Slane, in: *Recueil des historiens des croisades: historiens orientaux*, Paris, tomus 3, 431-39.

Makdisi, G., (1981): *The Rise of Colleges. Institutions of learning in Islam and the West*, Edinburgh. [Info on ALB on 84-91, cf. Aut. under (h) *supra*].

Mālallāh, 'Alī Muḥsin 'Īsā (1984): "Al-Ifāda wa l-i'tibār fī l-umūr al-mushāhada wa l-ḥawādith al-mu'āyana bi-arḍ Miṣr li-'Abd al-Laṭīf al-Baghdādī", in: *Maurid* (Baghdād) 13 (1), 163-182; 13 (2), 137-152.

Martini Bonadeo, C. (2013): *'Abd al-Laṭīf al-Baġdādī's Philosophical Journey: From Aristotle's* Metaphysics *to the 'Metaphysical Science'*, Leiden/Boston.

Martini Bonadeo, C. (2011): art. "'Abdallāṭīf al-Baġdādī", in: Henrik Lagerlund (ed.): *Encyclopedia of Medieval Philosophy: Philosophy between 500 and 1500*, Berlin/Dordrecht/Heidelberg/New York, Part 1, 1-4.

Martini Bonadeo, C. (2010): "'Abd al-Laṭīf al-Baġdādī's Reception of Book Beta of Aristotle's Metaphysics against the background of the competing readings by Avicenna and Averroes", in: *Documenti e studi sulla tradizione filosofica medievale* 21 (2010), 411-31.

Martini Bonadeo, C. (2002): *Il Libro della scienza della metafisica di 'Abd al-Laṭīf al-Baġdādī*, tesi di dottorato (PhD thesis), Università di Padova, Italia.

Mousley, J. (1808, ed. [A], tr. [L]): *Abdollatiphi Bagdadensis vita auctore Ibn Abi Osaiba; de codicibus mss. Bodleianis descripsit, et Latine vertit*, Oxonii. [see also *supra*: ALB Aut. under (c)].

Mūsā, Salāma (1937): *'Abd al-Laṭīf al-Baghdādī fī Miṣr*, al-Qāhira.

Nājī, Hilāl (1401/1981, ed. [A]): *Sharḥ Bānat Su'ād: qaṣīdat al-ṣaḥābī Ka'b b. Zuhayr* (by Muwaffaq al-Dīn 'Abd al-Laṭīf al-Baghdādī), Kuwait.

Al-Na'sānī, Muḥammad Badr al-Dīn (1325/1907, ed. [A]): *Dhail al-Fasīḥ* (by Muwaffaq al-Dīn 'Abd al-Laṭīf al-Baghdādī), al-Qāhira. [This volume also contains texts by Abū Sahl Muḥammad al-Harawī and Ibrāhīm al-Zajjāj].

Neuwirth, A. (2006): "'Abd al-Latif Ibn Yusuf al-Baghdadi Muwaffaq al-Din Abu Muhammad (557/1162-623/1231)", in: Josef W. Meri (editor): *Medieval Islamic Civilization: An Encyclopedia*, Volume 1, A-K, index, New York/Oxford, 2-3.

Neuwirth, A. (1976, ed. [A], tr. [G]): *'Abd al-Laṭīf al-Baġdādī's Bearbeitung von Buch* Lambda *der aristotelischen Metaphysik*, Wiesbaden. [= Veröffentlichungen der Orientalischen Kommission; Bd. 27].

Pinkerton, J. (1814, editor, tr. (fragments) [E]): "Extract from the relation respecting Egypt – Translation of Silvestre de Sacy's French translation", in: *A general collection of the best and most interesting voyages and travels*, vol. 15, 802-839.

Pococke, E(dward) the Elder (1702?, ed. [A], tr. [L]): *Abdollatiphi Historiae Aegypti Compendium* [Latine et Arabice, interprete Eduardo Pocockio. Edidit Thomas Hyde] by Ibn al-Labbād; Hyde, Thomas, 1636-1703; Pococke, Edward the Elder, 1604-1691], 1v (8vo), Oxonii.

Pococke, E(dward) the Younger, see: White, J. (1800).

Poortman, E.L.J., see: Drossaart Lulofs, H.J. and E.L.J. Poortman (1989).

Pormann, P.E., see: Joosse, N.P. and P.E. Pormann (2008, 2010, 2012a & b).

Provençal, P. (1995): "Nouvel essai sur les observations zoologiques de 'Abd al-Laṭīf al-Baġdādī", in: *Arabica* 42, 315-333.

Provençal, P. (1992): Observations zoologiques de 'Abd al-Laṭīf al-Baġdādī", in: *Centaurus* 35, 28-45.

{Qal'ajī, 'Abd al-Mu'ṭī Amīn (1406/1986, ed. [A]): *Al-Ṭibb min al-kitāb wa l-sunna* (by Muwaffaq al-Dīn 'Abd al-Laṭīf al-Baghdādī), Beirut. [The authorship of this work on prophetic medicine has not been disputed without reason. It has now become generally accepted that it is not a composition by 'Abd al-Laṭīf al-Baghdādī, but that it represents the *al-Ṭibb al-nabawī* by Shams al-Dīn al-Dhahabī (d. 1348)]}.

Al-Rāḍī, Fāṭima Ḥamza (1979): "Min Kitāb al-Mujarrad li-lughat al-ḥadīth li-'Abd al-Laṭīf al-Baghdādī", in: *Maurid* (Baghdād) 8 (2), 121-136.

Al-Rāḍī, Fāṭima Ḥamza (1397/1977, ed. [A]): *Al-Mujarrad li-lughat al-ḥadīth* (by 'Abd al-Laṭīf b. Yūsuf al-Baghdādī); vol. 1, Baghdād.

Rashed, M. (2004): "Priorité de l' EIDOS ou du GENOS entre Andronicos et Alexandre: vestiges arabes et grecs inédits", in: *Arabic Sciences and Pilosophy* 14, 9-63.

Rashed, R. (1993-2002, ed. [A], annotated tr. [F]): "Fī al-Radd 'alā Ibn Haytham fī al-makān; La réfutation du lieu d'Ibn al-Haytham", in: Roshdi Rashed: *Les mathématiques infinitésimales du IXe au XIe siècle*, vols. 1-4, London, IV, 908-53. [= Al-Furqan Islamic Heritage Foundation, 18].

Rizqāna, Ibrāhīm Aḥmad (1964): "Al-Āthār al-miṣrīya 'inda Muwaffaq al-Dīn 'Abd al-Laṭīf al-Baghdādī", in: *Dhikrā* (1964), 63-72.

Rosenthal, F. (1975, tr. (fragments) [E]): *The Classical Heritage in Islam*, London, 156-161: "About eternal providence, of the *Metaphysics* of 'Abd al-Laṭīf al-Baghdādī, according to the Istanbul MS Carullah 1279, 173b-175a".

Rosenthal, F. (1966): "Life is short, The Art is Long": Arabic Commentaries on the First Hippocratic Aphorism", in: *BHM* 40, 226-245. [Important info on ALB on 230 and 237-40].

Ṣādiq, Dawlat (1964): "Jughrāfiyā Miṣr fī kutub Muwaffaq al-Dīn 'Abd al-Laṭīf al-Baghdādī", in: *Dhikrā* (1964), 31-45.

Şahin, Hasan (1993; in [T]): "Abdüllātif Bağdadi'nin Mekan Hakkindaki Görüşleri" (in: TOC)/"Abdullatif Bağdadi'nin Mekan Felsefesi" (in: Book)/"Abdüllātif Bağdadi's Views on Setting" (English title), in: *Kongresi*, 69-78.

Saunders, R.H. (1928, editor): *Health: its Recovery and Maintenance. (Twelve addresses) by Abduhl Latif ("The Man of Baghdad") The Great Persian Physician and Philosopher*, London. [acquisition British Museum Library: 8 March 1929].

Saunders, R.H. (1927, editor): *Healing through Spirit Agency by the Great Persian Physician Abduhl Latif ("The Man of Baghdad") and information concerning The Life Hereafter of the deepest interest to all enquirers and students of Psychic phenomena*, London. [see also *supra*: ALB Aut. under (e)].

Saunders, R.H. (1924, editor/collaborator): *The Return of George R. Sims*, London.

Sédillot, J.J.E. (1812?): *Notice de l'ouvrage intitulé, Rélation de l'Égypte par Abd-Allatif...le tout traduit et enrichi de notes...par Silvestre de Sacy*, Paris.

Sevim, Seyfeddin [or in Book: Seyfullah Sevim] (1993; in [T]): "Abdüllātif Bağdadi'nin Kimya-Simya Hakkindaki Görüşleri" (in: TOC)/"Islam Dünyasinda Kimya (Simya) Bilminin Gelişimi ve Bağdadi'nin Görüşleri" (in: Book)/"Abdüllātif Bağdādi's Views on Chemistry-Alchemy" (English title), in: *Kongresi*, 57-67.

Silvestre de Sacy, A. -I. (1811): *Discours prononcé en présentant au corps législatif l'ouvrage intitulé: Relation de l'Égypte, par Abd-Allatif*, Paris.

Silvestre de Sacy, A. -I. (1810, tr. [F]): *Relation de l'Égypte, par Abd-Allatif, médecin arabe de Bagdad [1162-1231 A.D.]...le tout traduit et enrichi de notes historiques et critiques*, Paris. [Reprint in: F. Sezgin *et alii* (editor), *Islamic Geography*, Volume 9 & 10: Publications of the Institute for the History of Arabic-Islamic Science at the Johann Wolfgang Goethe University, Frankfurt am Main 1992].

Silvestre de Sacy, A. -I. (1802/1803?): *Notice de l'ouvrage intitulé: "Abdollatiphi Historiae Aegypti compendium arabice et latine, partim ipse vertit, partim a Pocockio versum edendum curavit, notisque illustravit J. White", Oxonii 1800*, Paris. [extrait du "Magasin encyclopédique"].

Silvestre de Sacy, A. -I. (no date): "Abrégé de l'Histoire d'Égypte par Abd-Allatif", *Magasin encyclopédique*, t. vi, 289-324, 452-486, (Paris?).

Al-Ṣiyyād, Muḥammad Maḥmūd (1964): "Muwaffaq al-Dīn 'Abd al-Laṭīf al-Baghdādī wa-jughrāfiyā Miṣr al-iqtiṣādīya", in: *Dhikrā* (1964), 47-62.

Somogyi, J. von (1937, ed. [A], tr. [G]): "Ein arabischer Bericht über die Tataren im "*Ta'rīkh al-Islām*" von aḏ-Ḏahabī", in: *Der Islam* 24, 105-130. [see also *supra*: ALB Aut. under (j)].

Stern, S.M. (1962): "A Collection of Treatises by 'Abd al-Laṭīf al-Baghdādī", in: *Islamic Studies*, (Karachi), vol. 1, 53-70. [Reprint in: Samuel Miklos Stern, *Medieval Arabic and Hebrew Thought*, London 1983: Variorum Reprints CS 183 under No. XVIII].

Stern, S.M. (1960): art. "'Abd al-Laṭīf al-Baghdādī", in: *EI²*, vol. I, 74.

Stone, C. and P. Lunde (2003): [Info from *Saudi Aramco World*, May-June 2003, 15: "...Caroline Stone working with Paul Lunde on translations of the Arab sources about the Vikings and peoples of the North and of 'Abd al-Latif al-Baghdadi's description of Egypt"].

Suter, H. (1900): *Die Mathematiker und Astronomen der Araber und ihre Werke* (= Abhandlungen zur Geschichte der mathematischen Wissenschaften mit Einschluss ihrer Anwendungen. X. Heft, Leipzig). [Info on ALB on 138 under No. 348].

Tas, Enes (2011, unpublished masters degree study: ed. [A] and study [T]): Abdüllatif el-Bağdâdî'nin Kitabü'n-Nasihateyn adli eseri: *tahkikli neşir ve muhteva analizi*. MA diss. Uludağ Universitesi, Bursa, Turkey.

Taylor, R.C. (1984, tr. [E]): "'Abd al-Latif al-Bagdadi's *Epitome* of the *Kalam fi Mahd al-Khayr (Liber de Causis)*", in: Michael E. Marmura (editor): *Islamic*

Theology and Philosophy: Studies in Honor of George F. Hourani, Albany, 236-248, 318-323.

Thies, H. -J. (1971, facs. ed. [A], tr. [G]): *Der Diabetestraktat 'Abd al-Laṭīf al-Baġdādī's. Untersuchungen zur Geschichte des Krankheitsbildes in der arabischen Medizin*, (Diss.) Bonn. [= Bonner Orientalistische Studien, Neue Serie, hsgb. von Otto Spies, Bd. 21].

Toorawa, S.M. (forthcoming?): "A detailed chronology and itinerary of 'Abd al-Latif al-Baghdadi", in: [...].

Toorawa, S.M. (2004a): "Travel in the medieval Islamic world: the importance of patronage, as illustrated by 'Abd al-Latif al-Baghdadi (d. 629/1231) (and other littérateurs)", in: Rosamund Allen (editor): *Eastward Bound: Travel and travellers 1050-1550*, Manchester and New York, 53-70.

Toorawa, S.M. (2004b): "A Portrait of 'Abd al-Laṭīf al-Baghdādī's Education and Instruction", in: Joseph E. Lowry, Devin J. Stewart and Shawkat M. Toorawa (editors): *Law and Education in Medieval Islam. Studies in Memory of Professor George Makdisi*, Oxford [E.J.W. Gibb Memorial Trust Series], 91-109. [= a revised version of S.M. Toorawa (1996)].

Toorawa, S.M. (2001, tr. (fragments) [E]): "The Autobiography of 'Abd al-Laṭīf al-Baghdādī (1162-1231): Selections from the Autograph Notes of 'Abd al-Laṭīf al-Baghdādī", in: Dwight Fletcher Reynolds (editor); coauthored by Kristen Brustad...[et al.], *Interpreting the self: autobiography in the Arabic literary tradition*, Berkeley/Los Angeles/London, 156-164. [see also *supra*: ALB Aut. under (i)].

Toorawa, S.M. (1997): "Language and Male Homosocial Desire in the Autobiography of 'Abd al-Laṭīf al-Baghdādī (d. 629/1231)", in: *Edebiyāt* NS 7 (2), 251-265.

Toorawa, S.M. (1996): "The Educational Background of 'Abd al-Laṭīf al-Baghdādī", in: *Muslim Education Quarterly* 13, no. 3, 35-53.

Ullmann, M. (1972, review): (review of) "Hans-Jürgen Thies, *Der Diabetestraktat 'Abd al-Laṭīf al-Baġdādī's. Untersuchungen zur Geschichte des Krankheitsbildes in der arabischen Medizin*, (Diss.) Bonn 1971", in: *Der Islam* 48 (1972), 339-340.

Utaş, Cengiz and Faruk Balkar [or in TOC: Balkir] (1993; in [T]): "Kennaş fi't Tibb" (in: TOC)/"Kennaş fi't Tib" (in: Book)/"Kennaş in Medicine" (English title), in: *Kongresi*, 27-30.

Vajda, G. (1959): "Une liste d'autorités du calife al-Nāṣir li-Dīn Allāh", *Arabica* 6, 173-77. [Reprint in: Georges Vajda, *La transmission du savoir en Islam (viie-xviiie siècles)*, London 1983: Variorum Reprints CS 181 under No. vii].

Vajda, G. (1956): *Les certificates de lecture et de transmission dans les manuscripts arabes de la Bibliothèque Nationale de Paris* [= Centre National de la Recherche Scientifique. Publications de l'Institut de Recherche et d'Histoire des Textes, VI], Paris, 5, No. 1c and 7, note 27.

Videan, J.A. and I.E., see: Zand, Kamal Hafuth.

Wahl, S.F.G. (1790, tr. [G]): *Abdallatif's, eines arabischen Arztes, Denkwürdigkeiten Egyptens*, aus dem Arabischen übersetzt und erläutert von Samuel Friedrich Guenther Wahl. In Hinsicht auf Naturreich und physische Beschaffenheit des Landes und seiner Einwohner, Alterthumskunde, Baukunde und Oekonomie, mit vielen medicinischen Bemerkungen und Beobachtungen, historischen, topografischen und andern beiläufig eingestreuten Nachrichten auch vornehmlich einer merkwürdigen Annale der Jahre 1200 und 1201, Halle.

White, J. (1801, tr. [E]): *Aegyptica: or observations on certain antiquities of Egypt*, (1): The history of Pompey's pillar elucidated; (2): Abdollatif's account of the antiquities of Egypt, transl. into English and illustrated with notes, Oxford.

White, J. (1800, ed. [A], tr. [L]): *Abdollatiphi Historiae Aegypti Compendium*, Arabice et Latine/partim ipse vertit, partim a Pocockio versum edendum curavit, notisque illustravit J. White, S.T.P, Oxonii [with a Latin version by Edward Pococke the Younger (1648-1727): Tractatus primus cap. i through cap. iv + stray fragments – remark: p. 99 at the bottom of the page: "Versionis Pocockianae Finis"].

White, J. (1789, ed. [A]): *Abdollatiphi Compendium Memorabilium Aegypti*, Arabice e codice mso Bodleiano edidit D. Joseph White, praefatus est Henricus Eberh. Gottlob Paulus, Tubingae.

Wüstenfeld, F. (1840): *Geschichte der Arabischen Aerzte und Naturforscher*, Göttingen. [Info on ALB on 123-127 under No. 220]; [Reprint: Hildesheim/New York 1978].

Zand, Kamal Hafuth and John A. and Ivy E. Videan (1204/1964, facs. ed. [A], tr. [E]): The Eastern Key: *Kitāb al-Ifādah wa'l-i'tibār of 'Abd al-Laṭīf al-Baghdādi* (The Book of Instruction and Admonition…Translated into English by…), Cairo/London.

4. Primary sources

Abū Shāma, *K. al-Rawḍatayn fī akhbār al-dawlatayn al-nūrīya wa l-ṣalāḥīya*, ed. Būlāq, 2 vols., 1287-92/1871-75, and ed. Muḥammad Ḥ. M. Aḥmad and Muḥammad Muṣṭafā Ziyāda, al-Qāhira 1956-62.

Al-Azdī, Muḥammad b. Aḥmad Abū l-Muṭahhar, *Ḥikāyat Abī l-Qāsim al-Baghdādī/ Abulḳāsim: Ein bagdāder Sittenbild*, mit Anmerkungen hg. von Adam Mez, Heidelberg 1902; tr. [F]: *Vingt-Quatre Heures de la vie d'une canaille* by René R. Khawam, Paris 1998.

Al-Baghdādī, Muḥammad b. al-Ḥasan b. Muḥammad b. al-Karīm, (tr. [E]): *A Baghdad Cookery Book. The Book of Dishes* (*Kitāb al-Ṭabīkh*). Newly translated by Charles Perry, Totnes 2005. [= Petits Propos Culinaires 79].

Barhebraeus, *Gregorii Barhebraei Chronicon syriacum*, ed. [Syr]: P. Bedjan, Paris 1890; facs. ed. [Syr], tr. [E]: E.A. Wallis Budge, *The Chronography of Gregory Abū'l Faraj, the son of Aaron, the Hebrew physician, commonly known as Bar Hebraeus*, 2 vols.,Oxford/London 1932.

Barhebraeus, *Kitāb Mukhtaṣar al-duwal li-l 'allāma Ghrīghūriyūs al-malaṭī al-ma'rūf bi-Ibn al-'Ibrī*, ed. Anṭūn Ṣālḥānī, Beirut 1890; second edition: Beirut 1958.

Al-Bundārī, al-Fatḥ b. 'Alī, *Sanā al-barq al-shāmī*, ed. Ramazan Şeşen, Beirut 1971; ed. Fatḥīya al-Nabarāwī, al-Qāhira 1979.

Al-Dhahabī, *Siyar a'lām al-nubalā'*, ed. S. al-Arna'ūṭ *et alii*, 25 vols., Beirut 1981-88.

Al-Dhahabī, *Ta'rīkh al-Islām*, Ms. London, British Library Or. 1540.

Ḥājjī Khalīfa (= Kātib Çelebi), *K. Kashf al-ẓunūn 'an asāmī l-kutub wa l-funūn*, ed. G. Flügel, 7 vols., Leipzig/London 1835-1858; ed. Ş. Yaltkaya and K.R. Bilge, 2 vols., Istanbul 1941-43.

Ḥunayn b. Isḥāq, *Masā'il Ḥunayn b. Isḥāq fī l-ṭibb li l-muta'allimīn ma'a ziyādāt Ḥubaysh*, tr. [E]: *Questions on Medicine for Scholars by Ḥunayn Ibn Isḥāq*: translated into English, with a preface and historical note…from a critical edition by Galal M. Moussa, Ph.D., of the Ninth Century Arabic text, "Al-Masa'il fi al-Tibb lil muta'allimin", Cairo 1980.

Ibn 'Abd al-Ẓāhir, *al-Rawḍ al-zāhir fī sīrat al-Malik al-Ẓāhir*, Riyadh 1976.

Ibn abī Uṣaybi'a, *'Uyūn al-anbā' fī ṭabaqāt al-aṭibbā'*, ed. Imru'ulqais b. aṭ-Ṭaḥḥān (August Müller), Juz' 1.2., Cairo-Königsberg 1299 H./1882 A.D. [Reprint: F. Sezgin *et alii* (editor): *Islamic Medicine*, vol. 1-2, Frankfurt am Main 1995]; ed. Nizār Riḍā, Beirut 1965; ed. Qāsim Muḥammad Wahb, Damascus 1997; ed. Muḥammad Bāsil 'Uyūn al-Sūd, Beirut 1998; ed. Al-Najjār, Cairo 1996-2004.

Ibn al-Athīr, *Al-Kāmil fī l-ta'rīkh*, 13 vols., Beirut 1965-67 and ed. C.J. Tornberg, 14 vols., Leiden-Uppsala 1851-1876.

Ibn al-Bayṭār, *K. al-Jāmi' li-mufradāt al-adwiya wa-l-aghdhiya*, 4 vols., Būlāq 1291. [Reprint: F. Sezgin *et alii* (editor): *Islamic Medicine*, 2 vols., vol. 69-70, Frankfurt am Main 1996], tr. [F]: Lucien Leclerc: *Traité des Simples par Ibn el-Beïthar*, 3 vols., Paris 1877-1883. [Reprint: F. Sezgin *et alii* (editor): *Islamic Medicine*, 3 vols., vol. 71-73, Frankfurt am Main 1996].

Ibn Buṭlān, *K. Da'wat al-aṭibbā'*, eds. [A] Bishāra Zalzal, Alexandria 1901, and Felix Klein-Franke, Wiesbaden 1985, tr. [G]: Felix Klein-Franke, Stuttgart 1984.

Ibn al-Furāt, *Ta'rīkh al-duwal wa l-mulūk*, 7 vols., ed. C.K. Zurayk and N. Izzeddin, Beirut 1936-42.

Ibn Ḥajar al-'Asqalānī, *Al-Durar al-kāmina fī a'yān al-mi'a ath-thāmina*, ed. M.S.J. al-Ḥaqq, 5 vols., al-Qāhira, *sine anno*; ed. Beirut, 4 vols., *sine anno*; ed. al-Qāhira 1966-67.

Ibn Hindū, *Miftāḥ al-ṭibb wa-minhāj al-ṭullāb*, *The Key to Medicine and a Guide for Students*. Translated by Dr Aida Tibi. Reviewed by Professor Emilie Savage-Smith, Reading 2010.

Ibn Hubal al-Baghdādī, *K. al-Mukhtārāt fī al-ṭibb*, 4 vols., Hyderabad 1943-45. [Reprint: F. Sezgin *et alii* (editor): *Islamic Medicine*, vol. 64-67, Frankfurt am Main 1996].

Ibn Jubayr, *Riḥla: The Travels of Ibn Jubayr*. Translated from the original Arabic by Roland J.C. Broadhurst with an introduction and notes, London 1952.

Ibn Jumay' (or: Ibn Jamī'), *Al-Maqāla al-ṣalāḥīya fī iḥyā' al-ṣinā'a al-ṭibbīya*, ed. [A], tr. [E]: *Treatise to Ṣalāḥ ad-Dīn on the Revival of the Art of Medicine*. Edited and translated by Hartmut Fähndrich, Wiesbaden 1983. [= Abhandlungen für die Kunde des Morgenlandes XLVI, 3].

Ibn Khallikān, *K. Wafayāt al-a'yān wa-anbā' abnā' al-zamān*, ed. I. 'Abbās, 8 vols., Beirut 1968-72; tr. [E]: Baron W. McGuckin de Slane, *Ibn Khallikan's Biographical Dictionary*, 4 vols., Paris-London 1842-1871 (also Paris 1842-43). [Reprint: Beirut 1970]. [Info on ALB in: vol. III, 420, 602-03; vol. IV, 376, 378].

Ibn al-'Imād, *Shadharāt al-dhahab fī akhbār man dhahab*, 8 vols., al-Qāhira 1350/1931.

Ibn Kathīr, *Al-Bidāya wa l-nihāya fī al-ta'rīkh*, 14 vols., al-Qāhira 1932-39.

Ibn Mammātī, As'ad, *K. Qawānīn al-dawāwīn*, ed. 'A.S. 'Aṭiya, Cairo 1943.

Ibn al-Maṭrān (or: Muṭrān), Abū Naṣr ibn Ilyās, *Bustān al-aṭibbā' wa-rawḍat al-alibbā' by Abū Naṣr ibn Ilyās ibn Maṭrān (d. 587/1191)*. Facsimile Edition of the Manuscript held at Malik public Library with an Introduction by Dr. Mahdi Muhaghghigh, Tehran 1989. [= Encyclopaedia Islamica Foundation: Center for the Publication of Manuscripts No. 5].

Ibn Qaiyim al-Jawzīya, (tr. [E]): *Medicine of the Prophet* (*Ṭibb al-nabawī*). Translated by Penelope Johnstone, Cambridge 1998. [= part of Ibn Qaiyim's *Zād al-Ma'ād*; eds. of the *Ṭibb al-nabawī*: 'Abd al-Mu'ṭī Amīn Qal'ajī, al-Qāhira 1398/1978 and 'Abd al-Ghinā 'Abd al-Khāliq, al-Qāhira, *sine anno*].

Ibn al-Qalānisī, *Dhayl ta'rīkh Dimashq*, ed. H.F. Amedroz, Leiden 1908.

Ibn al-Qifṭī, *Ta'rīkh al-ḥukamā'*, ed. J. Lippert, Leipzig 1903. [Reprint: F. Sezgin *et alii* (editor): *Islamic Philosophy*, vol. 2, Frankfurt am Main 1999].

Ibn al-Qifṭī, *Inbāh al-ruwāt 'alā anbāh al-nuḥāt*, ed. M. Abū l-Faḍl Ibrāhīm, al-Qāhira 1369-1374/1950-55. [Reprint: Beirut 2004].

Ibn Riḍwān, 'Alī, *Maqālat 'Alī b. Riḍwān fī al-taṭarruq bi l-ṭibb ilā al-sa'āda*, ed. [A], tr. [G]: *'Über den Weg zur Glückseligkeit durch den ärztlichen Beruf'*, hrsg. von Albert Dietrich, Göttingen 1982. [Abhandlungen der Akademie der Wissenschaften in Göttingen, Philologisch-historische Klasse; Folge 3, Nr. 129].

Ibn Riḍwān, 'Alī, *Risāla fī daf' maḍārr al-abdān bi-arḍ Miṣr*, ed. [A], tr. [E]: *Medieval Islamic Medicine: Ibn Riḍwān's Treatise " On the Prevention of Bodily Ills in Egypt"*, Translated, with an Introduction by Michael W. Dols. Arabic Text edited by Adil S. Gamal, Berkeley/Los Angeles/London 1984, 75-149; Arabic Text 1-63.

Ibn aṣ-Ṣābūnī, *Takmilat ikmāl al-akmāl*, ed. Muṣṭafā Jawād, Baghdād 1957.

Ibn Shaddād, *Al-Nawādir al-sulṭānīya wa l-maḥāsin al-Yūsufīya*, ed. Jamāl al-Dīn al-Shayyāl, al-Qāhira 1964. (see also tr. [E]: D.S. Richards, 2002 under secondary sources).

Ibn Shākir al-Kutubī, *Fawāt al-wafayāt*, ed. M. Muḥyī al-Dīn 'Abd al-Ḥamīd, 2 vols., al-Qāhira 1951; ed. I. 'Abbās, 4 vols., Beirut 1973.

Ibn Sīnā, *K. al-Qānūn fī al-ṭibb*, 3 vols., Būlāq 1294/1877. [Reprint: Beirut *sine anno*].

Ibn Taghrībirdī, *Al-Nujūm al-ẓāhira fī mulūk Miṣr wa l-Qāhira*, vol. II, part 2, no. 1, ed. William Popper, Berkeley and Los Angeles 1909-23, and ed. al-Qāhira, vols. I-XVI, 1929-1972.

Ibn al-Ukhūwa, *Ma'ālim al-qurba fī aḥkām al-ḥisba*, ed. Reuben Levy, London 1938. [= E.J.W. Gibb Memorial Series N.S. 12].

Ibn Wāṣil, *Mufarrij al-kurūb fī akhbār Banī Ayyūb*, ed. Jamāl al-Dīn al-Shayyāl, vol. I-III; vol. IV-V: ed. Ḥ. Rabī' and S. 'Āshūr, al-Qāhira 1953-1977 (i.e. until the year 645 A.H.).

Al-Idrīsī, Abū Ja'far, *Kitāb al-Anwār 'ulūw al-ajrām fī l-kashf 'an asrār al-ahrām* ('Light on the Voluminous Bodies to Reveal the Secrets of the Pyramids'), Facsimile edition [Series C, Volume 44], ed. Ursula Sezgin, Frankfurt am Main 1988.

Al-'Irāqī, Abū l-Qāsim Muḥammad ibn Aḥmad, *Kitāb al-'Ilm al-muktasab fī zirā'at adh-dhahab. Book of Knowledge Acquired Concerning the Cultivation of Gold by Abu 'l-Qāsim Muḥammad ibn Aḥmad al-'Irāqī*, ed./tr. by Erik John Holmyard, Paris 1923. [cf. Ullmann (1972), 235-37; Toorawa (1996), 45; Holmyard (1926), 403-26].

Al-Iṣfahānī, 'Imād al-Dīn al-Kātib, *Al-Barq al-shāmī*, ed. vol. 3: Muṣṭafā al-Ḥayārī; ed. vol. 5: Fāliḥ Ḥusayn, 'Ammān 1987.

Al-Iṣfahānī, 'Imād al-Dīn al-Kātib, *Kharīdat al-qaṣr (al-Shām)*, 3 vols., Damascus 1955-1964.

Al-Isnāwī, *Ṭabaqāt al-shāfi'īyah*, I-II, Baghdād 1390/1980.

Al-Isrā'īlī, Isḥāq ibn Sulaymān, *Kitāb al-Ḥummayāt: al-maqāla al-thālitha: fī al-sill* [= Isaac Judaeus: *On Fevers: the third discourse: on consumption*, edited and translated with introduction and notes by J.D. Latham and H.D. Isaacs], Cambridge 1981. [= Arabic Technical and Scientific Texts: Volume 8].

Jālīnūs, *K. Jālīnūs ilā Ṭūthrun fī al-nabḍ (al-saghīr) lil-muta'allimīn*, *naql*: Ḥunayn ibn Isḥāq; *taḥqīq*: Muḥammad Salīm Sālim, al-Qāhira 1986. [= Muntakhabāt al-Iskandarānīyīn: 3].

Judah al-Ḥarizi, *Sefer Taḥkemoni*, ed. Y. Toporovsky, *Rabi yehudah alḥarizi: Taḥkemoni*, Tel Aviv 1952. (see also tr. [E]: David Simha Segal, 2001 under secondary sources).

Al-Khaṭīb al-Baghdādī, *Ta'rīkh Baghdād*, I-XIV, al-Qāhira 1349/1931.

Al-Masīḥī, Abū Sahl 'Īsa ibn Yaḥyā, Kitāb al-mi'a fī l-ṭibb [Le livre des cent questions *en médecine d'Abū Sahl 'Īsa ibn Yaḥyā al-Masīḥī (m. ca 401h./1010 apr. J.-C.)*. Présenté et édité par Floréal Sanagustin], Tome I et II, Damas 2000.

Al-Maqrīzī, *K. al-Sulūk li-ma'rifat duwal al-mulūk*, ed. Muḥammad Muṣṭafā Ziyāda, 2 vols., al-Qāhira 1956. (see also tr. [E]: R.J.C. Broadhurst, 1980 under secondary sources).

Al-Maqrīzī, *K. al-Mawā'iẓ wa l-i'tibār fī dhikr al-khiṭaṭ wa l-āthār*, ed. Muḥammad Riyādah, Būlāq 1270/1853-54.

Al-Maqrīzī, *K. Ighāthat al-umma bi-kashf al-ghumma*, ed. Muḥammad Muṣṭafā Ziyāda and Jamāl al-Dīn al-Shayyāl, al-Qāhira 1940. (see also tr. [F]: Gaston Wiet, 1962 and tr. [E] Adel Allouche, 1994 under secondary sources).

Al-Nu'aymī, *Al-Dāris fī ta'rīkh al-madāris*, ed. J. al-Ḥasanī, 2 vols., Damascus 1367-70/1948-51.

Qusṭā ibn Lūqā, *K. fī l-Adwiya al-mushila wa-l-'ilāj bi-l-ishāl*, ed. and [E] tr. Lena Ambjörn, Frankfurt am Main 2004. [= Fuat Sezgin (editor), Publications of the Institute for the History of Arabic-Islamic Science: *Islamic Medicine*: Volume 100].

Al-Rāzī, Abū Bakr Muḥammad ibn Zakarīyā', *K. al-Murshid aw al-fuṣūl ma'a nuṣūṣ ṭibbīya mukhtāra*; *taqdīm wa-taḥqīq*: A.Z. Iskandar, no place [al-Qāhira?], no date.

Al-Ṣafadī, *Al-Wāfī bi l-wafayāt*, ed. H. Ritter *et alii*, Wiesbaden and Istanbul 1931-. For ALB, cf. especially ed. R. al-Sayyid, Beirut 1993: *Das biografische Lexikon des Ṣalāḥaddīn Khalīl Ibn Aibak aṣ-Ṣafadī*, Teil 19, No. 99, 107-15.

Ṣā'id ibn al-Ḥasan, *K. at-Tashwīq aṭ-ṭibbī*: cf. ed. [A]: *Das Buch At-Tashwīq aṭ-ṭibbī des Ṣā'id Ibn al-Ḥasan. Ein Adab-Werk über die Bildung des Arztes*, hrsg. u. bearb. von Otto Spies (Bonner Orientalistische Studien. N.S. 16), Bonn 1968; cf. tr. [G]: Taschkandi (1969) under secondary sources *infra*.

Sibṭ Ibn al-Jawzī, *Mir'āt al-zamān fī ta'rīkh al-a'yān*, ed. Hyderabad, volume VIII (parts 1 & 2), 1951-52.

Al-Subkī, *Ṭabaqāt al-shāfi'īyah al-kubrā*, I-VI, al-Qāhira 1323/24-1905/06.

Al-Sulamī, *K. Imtiḥān al-alibbā' li-kāffat al-aṭibbā'*, cf. ed. [A], tr. [E] by Gary Leiser and Noury al-Khaledy: *Questions and Answers for Physicians. A Medieval Arabic Study Manual by 'Abd al-'Azīz (b. 'Abd al-Jabbār) as-Sulamī*, Leiden/Boston 2004. [= The Sir Henry Wellcome Asian Studies: Volume 3. Edited by Lawrence I. Conrad, Dominik Wujastyk and Paul U. Unschuld].

Al-Suyūṭī, *Bughyat al-wu'āt fī ṭabaqāt al-lughawīyīn wa l-nuḥāt*, ed. M. Abū l-Faḍl Ibrāhīm, 2 vols., al-Qāhira 1964-65.

Al-Ṭabarī, 'Alī b. Sahl Rabban, *Firdaus al-ḥikma fī ṭ-ṭibb*, ed. Muḥammad Zubair al-Ṣiddīqī: *Firdausu'l Ḥikmat or Paradise of Wisdom*, Berlin-Charlottenburg 1928 [Reprint: F. Sezgin *et alii* (editor): *Islamic Medicine*, vol. 29, Frankfurt am Main 1996]; cf. also Siggel (1953) under secondary sources *infra*.

Al-Tha'ālibī, *Laṭā'if al-ma'ārif*, tr. [E]: *The Book of Curious and Entertaining Information. The Laṭā'if al-ma'ārif of Tha'ālibī.* Translated with introduction and notes by Clifford Edmund Bosworth, Edinburgh 1968.

Usāma b. Munqidh, *K. al-I'tibār*, tr. [E]: Philip K. Hitti, *An Arab-Syrian Gentleman and Warrior in the Period of the Crusades, Memoirs of Usāmah Ibn-Munqidh*, New York 1929. [Reprint: Princeton 1987]; cf. tr. [D]: Jan Just

Witkam, Usama ibn Munqidh, *Wat anders dan vechten en jagen? Memoires van een Syrisch edelman*, Amsterdam 1986.

Yaḥyā b. Sa'īd al-Anṭākī, *Histoire de Yahya-Ibn-Sa'ïd d'Antioche continuateur de Sa'ïd-Ibn-Bitriq*, éditée et traduite en français par I. Kratchkovsky et A. Vasiliev, Paris 1957 [= R. Graffin et F. Nau: *Patrologia Orientalis* Tome XVIII. – Fascicule 5 (No. 90)].

Yāqūt al-Hamawī al-Rūmī al-Baghdādī, *Mu'jam al-buldān*, 5 vols., Beirut 1399/1979.

5. Secondary sources

Ahmad, Jamil and Hakim Ashhar Qadeer (1999): *Unani, the Science of Graeco-Arabic Medicine*, New Delhi. [tr. [D]: *Unani: Grieks-Arabische geneeskunst* by Marlou Wijsman, *sine loco, sine anno*].

Algera, M. (2000, in [D]): *Mens en Medicijn. Geschiedenis van het geneesmiddel*, Amsterdam.

Ali, Salah Salim (1996): "Arabic References to Plato's Lost Atlantis", in: *Hamdard Islamicus* XIX (No. 3), 43-64.

Allouche, A. (1994): *Mamluk Economics: A Study and Translation of al-Maqrīzī's Ighātha*, Salt Lake City.

Álvarez-Millán, C. (2004): "Medical Anecdotes in Ibn Juljul's Biographical Dictionary", in: *Suhayl* 4, 1-18.

Álvarez-Millán, C. (2000): "Practice versus Theory: Tenth-century Case Histories from the Islamic Middle East", in: Peregrine Horden and Emilie Savage-Smith (editors): *The Year 1000: Medical Practice at the End of the First Millennium = Social History of Medicine* 13 (2), 293-306.

Álvarez-Millán, C. (1999a): "Graeco-Roman Case Histories and their Influence on Medieval Islamic Clinical Accounts", in: *Social History of Medicine* 12, (1), 19-43.

Álvarez-Millán, C. (1999b): "Galen's Influence on Rāzī's Clinical Accounts", in: John A.C. Greppin, Emilie Savage-Smith and John L. Gueriguian (editors): *The Diffusion of Greco-Roman Medicine into the Middle East and the Caucasus*, Delmar/New York, 57-71.

Amar, Zohar and Yaron Serri (2003): "Ibn al-Suri, Physician and Botanist of al-Sham", in: *Palestine Exploration Quarterly* 135/2, 124-130.

Ambjörn, L. (2004, ed. [A], tr. [E]): *Qusṭā Ibn Lūqā (9th century A.D.) On Purgative Drugs And Purgation*, Frankfurt am Main. [= Fuat Sezgin (editor), Publications of the Institute for the History of Arabic-Islamic Science: *Islamic Medicine*: Volume 100].

Amitai, R. (1986): "The Rise and Fall of the Mamluk Institution: A Summary of David Ayalon's Works", in: Moshe Sharon (editor): *Studies in Islamic History and Civilization in Honour of Professor David Ayalon*, Jerusalem/Leiden, 19-30.

Amundsen, D.W. (1996): *Medicine, Society, and Faith in the Ancient and Medieval Worlds*, Baltimore and London.

Anawātī, G.C. (1965): art. "Fakhr al-Dīn al-Rāzī, Abū 'Abd Allāh Muḥammad b. 'Umar b. al-Ḥusayn", in: *EI²*, vol. II, 751b-755b.

Arikha, N. (2007): *Passions and Tempers. A History of the Humours*, New York.

Arkomani, A.-A. (2005): "The Best Drink a Girl Can Get: *Skírnismál* 35, 6 and A Remedy for Epilepsy", in: Daisy L. Neijmann (editor): *Perkensian Rambles: A Collection of Essays in Honour of Richard Perkins*, London, 23-32.

Artelt, W. (1955): "Ossa mandibulae inferioris duo", in: *Sudhoffs Archiv* 39, 193-215.

Ashtor, E. (1969): *Histoire des prix et des salaires dans l'Orient médiéval*, Paris.

Ashtor, E. (1961): "Le coût de la vie dans la Syrie médiévale", in: *Arabica* 8, 59-73.

Azar, H. (2008): *The Sage of Seville. Ibn Zuhr, His Time, and His Medical Legacy*, Cairo and New York.

Baader, G. (1979): "Gesellschaft, Wirtschaft und ärztlicher Stand im frühen und hohen Mittelalter", in: *Medizinhistorisches Journal* 14, 176-185.

Bachmann, P. (1969): "Arzt und Krankheit in einigen Gedichten des arabischen Lyrikers al-Mutanabbī. Literar- und medizinhistorische Anmerkungen", in: *Medizinhistorisches Journal* 4, 99-120.

Bachmann, P. (1968): "Zum Medizin-Kapitel des Buches "al-Baraka" von al-Ḥabašī – Herrn Prof. Dr. Karl Deichgräber zum 65. Geburtstag", in: *Medizinhistorisches Journal* 3, 28-39.

Bachmann, P. (1965, ed. [A], tr. [G]): "Galens Abhandlung darüber, dass der vorzügliche Arzt Philosoph sein muss", in: *Nachrichten der Akademie der Wissenschaften in Göttingen aus dem Jahre 1965*; Philologisch-historische Klasse, 1/1965, 1-67.

Badawī, 'Abd al-Raḥmān (1947): *Arisṭū 'inda l-'Arab, Dirāsa wa-nuṣūṣ ghayr manshūra*, vol. 1 [= Dirāsāt islāmīya 5], al-Qāhira.

Baldwin, B. (1984a): "Beyond the House Call: Doctors in Early Byzantine History and Politics", in: John Scarborough (editor): *Symposium on Byzantine Medicine (1983: Dumbarton Oaks)*, [= Dumbarton Oaks Papers 38], 15-19.

Baldwin, B. (1984b, tr. [E]): *Timarion*. Translated with Introduction and Commentary by…, Detroit [= Byzantine Texts in Translation].

Balog, P. (1980): *The Coinage of the Ayyūbids*, London. [Royal Numismatic Society Special Publication Number 12].

Barton, T.S. (1995): *Power and Knowledge: Astrology, Medicine and Physiognomics under the Roman Empire*, Ann Arbor (Michigan).

Barton, T.S. (1994): *Ancient Astrology*, London and New York.

Basham, A.L. (1976): "The Practice of Medicine in Ancient and Medieval India", in: Charles Leslie (editor): *Asian Medical Systems: A Comparative Study*, Berkeley/Los Angeles/London, 18-43.

Beckwith, C.I. (2012): *Warriors of the Cloisters. The Central Asian Origins of Science in the Medieval World*, Princeton (New Haven) and Oxford.

Beeston, A.F.L. (1971): *Arabic Nomenclature. A summary guide for beginners*, Oxford.

Behrens-Abouseif, D. (1989): *Islamic architecture in Cairo: an introduction*, Leiden/New York/København/Köln.

BEO = *Bulletin d'études orientales*.

Berkey, J.P. (1992): *The Transmission of Knowledge in Medieval Cairo. A Social History of Islamic Education*, Princeton.

Berthelot, M. (1893): *La Chimie au Moyen Âge, Tome III: L'Alchimie arabe*, Paris. [Reprint: F. Sezgin *et alii* (editor): *Natural Sciences in Islam*, vol. 64, Frankfurt am Main 2002].

BHM = *Bulletin of the History of Medicine*.

Biesterfeldt, H.H. (2007): "Palladius on the Hippocratic Aphorisms", in: Cristina D'Ancona (editor): *The Libraries of the Neoplatonists*, Leiden/Boston, 385-398. [= Philosophia Antiqua 107]. [Brief info on ALB on 388].

Biesterfeldt, H.H. (1984): "Some Opinions on the Physician's Remuneration in Medieval Islam", in: *BHM* 58, 16-27.

Blair, A. (1999): "The *Problemata* as a Natural Philosophical Genre", in: Anthony Grafton and Nancy Siraisi (editors): *Natural Particulars. Nature and the Disciplines in Renaissance Europe*, Cambridge/Mass. and London, 171-204.

BMD = *Black's Medical Dictionary*, 39th edition, edited by Gordon Macpherson, Lanham/New York/Oxford 1999.

Bos, G. and M.R. McVaugh (2009): Maimonides, *On Poisons and the Protection against Lethal Drugs*. A New Parallel Arabic-English Translation by Gerrit Bos with Critical Editions of Medieval Hebrew Translations by Gerrit Bos and Medieval Latin Translations by Michael R. McVaugh, Provo (Utah).

Brain, P. (1986): *Galen on Bloodletting. A Study of the Origins, Development and Validity of his Opinions, with a Translation of the Three Works*, Cambridge.

Brandenburg, D. (1975): *Medizin und Magie: Heilkunde und Geheimlehre des islamischen Zeitalters*, Berlin.

Brandenburg, D. (1973): *Medizinisches in Tausendundeiner Nacht*, Stuttgart.

Broadhurst, R.J.C. (1980, tr. [E]): *A History of the Ayyūbid Sultans of Egypt*. Translated from the Arabic of al-Maqrīzī with Introduction and Notes by…, Boston. [= [E] tr. of [A]: al-Maqrīzī, *K. al-Sulūk li-ma'rifat duwal al-mulūk*].

Brock, S.P. (1995): "The Scribe Reaches Harbour", in: S. Efthymiadis (editor): *Bosporus: essays in honour of Cyril Mango* (ByF 21), Amsterdam, 195-202. [Reprint in: Sebastian P. Brock: *From Ephrem to Romanos. Interactions between Syriac and Greek in Late Antiquity*, Aldershot-Brookfield (VT) 1999 under no. XVI].

Brockelmann, C. (1937-49, editor): *GAL = Geschichte der arabischen Literatur*, vol. 1: Weimar 1898; vol. 2: Berlin 1902; 2nd edition: vol. 1: Leiden 1943; vol. 2: Leiden 1949; Suppl. (3 vols.): Leiden 1937, 1938, 1942. [Reprint: Leiden/New York/Köln 1996].

Browne, E.G. (1921): *Arabian Medicine*; being the Fitzpatrick lectures delivered at the college of physicians in November 1919 and November 1920, Cambridge.

Buckley, R.P. (1992): "The *Muḥtasib*", in: *Arabica* 39, 59-117.

Bürgel, J.C. (1991): *Allmacht und Mächtigkeit. Religion und Welt im Islam*, München.

Bürgel, J.C. (1988): *The Feather of Simurgh: The "Licit Magic" of the Arts in Medieval Islam*, New York/London.

Bürgel, J.C. (1986): "Pathology in Arabic Medicine: A View on its Ideological and Anthropological Setting", in: Teizo Ogawa (editor): *History of Pathology. Proceedings of the 8th International Symposium on the Comparative History of Medicine – East and West, September 18-24, 1983 Susono-shi, Shizuoka, Japan*, Tokio, 5-35.

Bürgel, J.C. (1976): "Secular and Religious Features of Medieval Arabic Medicine", in: Charles Leslie (editor): *Asian Medical Systems: A Comparative Study*, Berkeley/Los Angeles/London, 44-62.

Bürgel, J.C. (1975): "Der Mufarriḥ an-nafs des Ibn Qāḍī Ba'albakk, ein Lehrbuch der Psychohygiene aus dem 7. Jahrhundert der Hiğra", in: Frithiof Rundgren (editor): *Proceedings of the VIth Congress of Arabic and Islamic Studies, Visby 13-16 August, Stockholm 17-19 August 1972* [= Filologisk-filosofiska serien 15 Kungl. Vitterhets Historie och Antikvitets Akademien], Uppsala, 201-212.

Bürgel, J.C. (1973): "Psychosomatic methods of cures in the Islamic Middle Ages", in: *Humaniora Islamica* 1, 157-172.

Bürgel, J.C. (1972): "Dogmatismus und Autonomie im wissenschaftlichen Denken des islamischen Mittelalters – Albert Dietrich in Göttingen zum 60. Geburtstag", in: *Saeculum* 23, 30-46.

Bürgel, J.C. (1968a, ed. [A], tr. [G]): "Averroes «contra Galenum». Das Kapitel von der Atmung im Colliget des Averroes als ein Zeugnis mittelalterlich-islamischer Kritik an Galen", in: *Nachrichten der Akademie der Wissenschaften in Göttingen; I. Philologisch-historische Klasse*; Jahrgang 1967, Nr. 9, 263-340.

Bürgel, J.C. (1968b, review): "Martin Levey, *Medical Ethics of Medieval Islam with special reference to al-Ruhāwī's "Practical Ethics of the Physician "*, (= Transactions of the American Philosophical Society, N.S. 57/3), Philadelphia 1967", in: *Göttingische Gelehrte Anzeigen* 220, 215-227.

Bürgel, J.C. (1967a): "*Adab* und *i'tidāl* in ar-Ruhāwī's *Adab aṭ-Ṭabīb*. Studie zur Bedeutungsgeschichte zweier Begriffe", in: *ZDMG* 117, 90-102.

Bürgel, J.C. (1967b): "Die wissenschaftliche Medizin im Kräftefeld der islamischen Kultur", in: *Bustan* (Wien) 8 Jg., 9-19.

Bürgel, J.C. (1966): "Die Bildung des Arztes. Eine arabische Schrift zum 'ärztlichen Leben' aus dem 9. Jahrhundert", in: *Sudhoffs Archiv* 50, 337-360.

Burnett, C. (2005): "Arabic into Latin: the reception of Arabic philosophy into Western Europe", in: Peter Adamson and Richard C. Taylor (editors): *The Cambridge Companion to Arabic Philosophy*, Cambridge, 370-404.

Bylebyl, J. (1993): "The manifest and the hidden in the Renaissance clinic", in: William F. Bynum and Roy Porter (editors): *Medicine and the Five Senses*. Based on a Symposium on Medicine and the Five Senses, held at the Wellcome Institute for the History of Medicine on 11-12 June 1987, Cambridge 1993, 40-60.

Bynum, W.F. and R. Porter (1993, editors): *Medicine and the Five Senses*, Cambridge.

Cadden, J. (1993): *Meanings of sex difference in the Middle Ages: Medicine, science, and culture*, Cambridge. [= Cambridge History of Medicine].

Cahen, C. (2001): *The Formation of Turkey: The Seljukid Sultanate of Rum: Eleventh to Fourteenth Century*, Harlow, Essex.

Cahen, C. (1968): *Pre-Ottoman Turkey: A General Survey of the Material and Spiritual Culture and History c. 1071-1330*, New York.

Cameron, M.L. (1993): *Anglo-Saxon Medicine*, Cambridge. [Cambridge Studies in Anglo-Saxon England 7].

Cardano, G. (2000, tr. [D]): *Mijn Leven* (*De propria vita*), Amsterdam.

Carmona González, A. (1995): "El marco jurídico del ejercicio de la medicina en el mundo islámico medieval", in: Concepción Vázquez de Benito and Miguel Ángel Manzano Rodríguez (editors): *Actas XVI Congreso UEAI* [Union Européenne d'Arabisants et d'Islamisants, celebrado en Salamanca durante los días 27 de agosto a 2 de septiembre de 1992], Salamanca, 117-124.

Chamberlain, M. (1994): *Knowledge and social practice in medieval Damascus, 1190-1350*, Cambridge. [= Cambridge Studies in Islamic Civilization].

Chipman, L. (2010): *The World of Pharmacy and Pharmacists in Mamlūk Cairo*, Leiden/Boston.

Cloarec, F. (1998): *Bīmāristāns, lieux de folie et de sagesse. La folie et ses traitements dans les hôpitaux médiévaux au Moyen-Orient*, Paris.

Cohen, M.R. (1994): *Under Crescent & Cross. The Jews in the Middle Ages*, Princeton.

Conrad, L.I. (2001): "Ibn Buṭlān in *Bilād al-Shām*: the Career of a Travelling Christian Physician", in: David Thomas (editor): *Syrian Christians under Islam: The First Thousand Years*, Leiden/Boston/Köln, 131-157.

Conrad, L.I. (1999): "Usāma ibn Munqidh and Other Witnesses to Frankish and Islamic Medicine in the Era of the Crusades", in: Zohar Amar, Efraim Lev and Joseph Schwartz (editors): *Ha-Refu'ah bi-Yerushalayim le-doroteha* ('Medicine in Jerusalem Throughout the Ages'), Tel-Aviv, xxvii-lii.

Conrad, L.I. (1995): "Scholarship and social context: a medical case from the eleventh-century Near East", in: Don(ald) George Bates (editor): *Knowledge and the scholarly medical traditions*, Cambridge, 84-100.

Cooperson, M. (1997): "The Purported Autobiography of Ḥunayn ibn Isḥāq", in: *Edebiyāt* NS 7 (2), 235-249.

Corbin, H. (1960): *Avicenna and the Visionary Recital* [= Bollingen Series LXVI], Princeton. [= [E] tr. of [F]: *Avicenne et le recit visionnaire*, Paris 1954].

Coudert, A. (1980): *Alchemy: the philosopher's stone*, Boulder (Colorado).

Crone, P. (2004): *God's Rule: government and Islam. Six centuries of medieval Islamic political thought*, New York.

Culpeper, N. (1652): *Galens Art of Physick*, London (Peter Cole).

Daiber, H. (1999): *Bibliography of Islamic philosophy*, 2 Volumes: [i: Alphabetical list of publications; ii: Index of names, terms and topics], (Handbuch der Orientalistik: Abt. 1. Der Nahe und Mittlere Osten; Bd. 43), Leiden/ Boston/Köln.

Daiber, H. (1994): "The reception of Islamic philosophy at Oxford in the 17th century: The Pococks' (father and son) contribution to the understanding of Islamic philosophy in Europe", in: Charles E. Butterworth and Blake Andrée Kessel (editors): *The Introduction of Arabic Philosophy into Europe*, Leiden/New York/Köln, Ch. V, 65-82.

Daiber, H. (1989): art. "Masā'il wa-Adjwiba", in: *EI²*, vol. VI, 636a-639b.

Dallal, A. (2010): *Islam, Science, and the Challenge of History*, New Haven & London.

David, J.-C., see: Degeorge G. and J.-C. David (2002).

Davidson, H.A. (2005): *Moses Maimonides. The Man and His Works*, Oxford.

Degeorge, G. (2004): *Damas: Perle et Reine d'Orient*, Paris. [tr. [E]: *Damascus*, Paris 2004].

Degeorge, G. and J.-C. David (2002): *Alep*, Paris.

Deichgräber, K. (1970): *Medicus Gratiosus: Untersuchungen zu einem griechischen Arztbild*, Mainz. [= Akademie der Wissenschaften und der Literatur: Abhandlungen der Geistes- und sozialwissenschaftlichen Klasse, Jahrgang 1970 - Nr.3].

Demaitre, L.E. (2013): *Medieval Medicine: The Art of Healing, from Head to Toe*, Santa Barbara/Denver/Oxford. [= Praeger Series on the Middle Ages].

Dessing, N.M. (2001): *Rituals of Birth, Circumcision, Marriage, and Death among Muslims in the Netherlands*, Leuven. [= New Religious Identities in the Western World 2].

Dietrich, A. (1967, tr. [G]): "Ein Arzneimittelverzeichnis des 'Abdallaṭīf Ibn Yūsuf al-Baġdādī", in: W. Hoenerbach (editor): *Der Orient in der Forschung. Festschrift für Otto Spies zum 5. April 1966*, Wiesbaden, 42-60.

Dietrich, A. (1966): *Medicinalia Arabica. Studien über arabische medizinische Handschriften in türkischen und syrischen Bibliotheken*, Göttingen. [= Abhandlungen der Akademie der Wissenschaften in Göttingen; Philologisch-historische Klasse 3. F., Nr. 66].

Dietrich, A. (1964, tr. [G], ed. [A]): *Die arabische Version einer unbekannten Schrift des Alexander von Aphrodisias über die Differentia specifica* (Nachrichten der Akademie der Wissenschaften in Göttingen: I. Philologisch-historische Klasse; Jahrgang 1964, Nr. 2, Göttingen), 85-148. [Info on ALB on 100-113].

Dols, M.W. (1984a, tr. [E], ed. [A]): *Medieval Islamic Medicine: Ibn Riḍwān's Treatise "On the Prevention of Bodily Ills in Egypt"*, Berkeley/Los Angeles /London.

Dols, M.W. (1984b): "Insanity in Byzantine and Islamic Medicine", in: John Scarborough (editor): *Symposium on Byzantine Medicine (1983: Dumbarton Oaks)*, [= Dumbarton Oaks Papers 38], 135-148.

Dols, M.W. (1983): "The Leper in Medieval Islamic Society", in: *Speculum* 58, 891-916.

Dols, M.W. (1979): "Leprosy in medieval Arabic medicine", in: *JHMAS* 34, 314-33.

Dormandy, T. (2006): *The Worst of Evils: The Fight against Pain*, New Haven and London.

Dozy, R. (1881): *Supplément aux Dictionnaires Arabes*, 2 vols., Leiden. [Reprint: Beirut 1981].

Dubler, C.E. (1959): "Die "Materia Medica" unter den Muslimen des Mittelalters", in: *Sudhoffs Archiv* 43, 329-350.

Duffy, J. (1984): "Byzantine Medicine in the Sixth and Seventh Centuries: Aspects of Teaching and Practice", in: John Scarborough (editor): *Symposium on Byzantine Medicine (1983: Dumbarton Oaks)*. [= Dumbarton Oaks Papers 38], 21-27.

Ebrahimnejad, H. (2011): "Medicine in Islam and Islamic Medicine", in: Mark Jackson (ed.): *The Oxford Handbook of The History of Medicine*, Oxford, 169-89.

Eddé, A.-M. (2011): *Saladin* [Translated by Jane Marie Todd], Cambridge, Mass. and London.

Eddé, A.-M. (1999): *La principauté Ayyoubide d'Alep (597/1183 – 658/1260)*, Stuttgart. [= Freiburger Islamstudien; Bd. 21].

Eddé, A.-M. (1995a): "Hérésie et pouvoir politique en Syrie du Nord au XIIe siècle: l'exécution d'al-Suhrawardī en 1191", in: André Vauchez (editor): *La religion civique à l'époque médiévale et moderne (chrétienté et islam)*. Actes du colloque organisé par le Centre de recherche «Histoire sociale et culturelle de l'Occident. XIIe-XVIIIe siècle» de l'Université de Paris X-Nanterre et l'Institut universitaire de France (Nanterre, 21-23 juin 1993), [Collection de l'École Française de Rome-Palais Farnèse, 213], Rome, 235-44.

Eddé, A.-M. (1995b): "Les médecins dans la société syrienne du VIIe/XIIIe siècle", in: *Annales Islamologiques* XXIX, 91-109.

Eddé, A.-M. (1993): "Notes sur la fiscalité de l'État ayyoubide d'Alep au XIIIe siècle", in: Ph. Contamine, Th. Dutour and B. Schnerb (editors): *Commerce, finances et société (XIe-XVIe siècles). Hommage à M. le Professeur Henri Dubois*, Paris, 247-262.

Eijk, Ph.J. van der (1997): "Galen's use of the concept of 'qualified experience' in his dietetic and pharmacological works", in: A. Debru (editor): *Galen on*

Pharmacology. Philosophy, History and Medicine [= Studies in Ancient Medicine 15], Leiden, 35-57. [Reprint in: Philip J. van der Eijk, *Medicine and Philosophy in Classical Antiquity. Doctors and Philosophers on Nature, Soul, Health and Disease*, Cambridge 2005, 279-298].

El-Cheikh, N.M. (2004): *Byzantium Viewed by the Arabs*, Cambridge/Mass. and London. [= Harvard Middle Eastern Monographs XXXVI].

El-Daly, O. (2003): "Ancient Egypt in Medieval Arabic Writings", in: Peter Ucko and Timothy Champion (editors): *The Wisdom of Egypt: changing visions through the ages*, London, 39-63 [contains info on ALB].

El-Eswed, B.I. (2002): "Lead and Tin in Arabic Alchemy", in: *Arabic sciences and philosophy* 12 (1), 139-153.

Elgood, C. (1962, tr. [E]): "Tibb-ul-Nabbi or Medicine of the Prophet being a translation of two works of the same name", in: *Osiris* 14, 33-192.

Elias, J.J. (2012): *Aisha's Cushion. Religious Art, Perception and Practice in Islam*, Cambridge, MA.

Endress, G. (1982): *Einführung in die islamische Geschichte*, München.

Ephrat, D. (2000): *A Learned Society in a Period of Transition: The Sunnī 'Ulamā' of Eleventh-Century Baghdad*, Albany (NY).

Fahd, T. (1971): art. "Ibn Waḥshiyya", in: *EI*[2], vol. III, 963b-965b.

Fancy, N. (2013): *Science and Religion in Mamluk Egypt: Ibn al-Nafīs, Pulmonary Transit and Bodily Resurrection*, Abingdon (Ox)/New York.

Faris, Nabih Amin (1985): "Arab Culture in the Twelfth Century", in: Norman P. Zacour and Harry W. Hazard (editors): *A History of the Crusades* (general editor: Kenneth Meyer Setton), Volume V: *The Impact of the Crusades on the Near East*, Madison (Wisconsin), Chapter I, 3-32.

Filius, L.S. (1999, ed.): *The Problemata Physica attributed to Aristotle. The Arabic Version of Ḥunain ibn Isḥāq and the Hebrew Version of Moses ibn Tibbon*, Leiden/Boston/Köln. [= Aristoteles Semitico-Latinus; Vol. 11].

Flashar, H. (1962, tr. [G]): *Aristoteles, Problemata Physica* [= Ernst Grumach (editor): Aristoteles Werke in deutscher Übersetzung, Bd. 19], Darmstadt.

Fonahn, A.M. (1922): *Arabic and Latin anatomical terminology chiefly from the Middle Ages*, Kristiania.

Freeman-Grenville, G.S.P. (1995): *The Islamic and Christian Calendars AD 622-2222 (AH 1-1650). A complete guide for converting Christian and Islamic dates and dates of festivals*, Reading.

Freimark, P. (1967): *Das Vorwort als literarische Form in der arabischen Literatur*, (diss.) Münster.

Freind, J. (1725-26): *The History of Physick From the Time of Galen, to the beginning of the Sixteenth Century. Chiefly with Regard to Practice*, 2 vols., London. [Reprint from the London 1744-50 edition: New York 1973].

French, R. (2003): *Medicine before Science. The Business of Medicine/The Rational and Learned Doctor from the Middle Ages to the Enlightenment*, Cambridge.

French, R. (1999): *Dissection and Vivisection in the European Renaissance*, Aldershot/Brookfield/Singapore/Sydney. [= The History of Medicine in Context].

Freytag, G.W. (1830-37): *Lexicon Arabico-Latinum praesertim ex Djeuharii Firuzabadiique et aliorum arabum operibus adhibitis Golii quoque et aliorum libris confectum*, Bd. I-IV, Halle. [Reprint: Beirut 1975].

Fuess, A. and J.-P. Hartung (2010, eds.): *Court Cultures in the Muslim World: Seventh to Nineteenth Centuries*, [SOAS/Routledge Studies on the Middle East], Abingdon (Ox)/ New York.

Gacek, A. (2001): *The Arabic Manuscript Tradition. A Glossary of Technical Terms & Bibliography*, Leiden/Boston/Köln. [= Handbuch der Orientalistik. Section one: the Near and Middle East, vol. 58].

GAL = *Geschichte der arabischen Literatur*, see: Brockelmann, C.

Gambaccini, P. (2004): *Mountebanks and Medicasters. A History of Italian Charlatans from the Middle Ages to the Present*, Jefferson/North Carolina and London. [originally published in [It] as: *I Mercanti della Salute: le segrete virtù dell' imbroglio in medicina*, Firenze 2002].

García-Ballester, L. (1995): "*Artifex factivus sanitatis*: health and medical care in medieval Latin Galenism", in: Don(ald) George Bates (editor): *Knowledge and the scholarly medical traditions*, Cambridge, 127-150.

García-Ballester, L., see also: Kottek, S.S. and L. García-Ballester (1996).

GAS = *Geschichte des arabischen Schrifttums*, see: Sezgin, F.

Getz, F. (1998): *Medicine in the English Middle Ages*, Princeton.

Getz, F. (1997): "Roger Bacon and Medicine: The Paradox of the Forbidden Fruit and the Secrets of Long Life", in: Jeremiah Hackett (editor): *Roger Bacon and the Sciences. Commemorative Essays*, Leiden/New York/Köln, 337-364. [= Jan A. Aertsen *et alii* (editors): Studien und Texte zur Geistesgeschichte des Mittelalters, Bd. LVII].

Getz, F. (1992): "To Prolong Life and Promote Health: Baconian Alchemy and Pharmacy in the English Learned Tradition", in: Sheila Campbell, Bert Hall, David Klausner (editors) [Centre for Medieval Studies, University of Toronto]: *Health, Disease and Healing in Medieval Culture*, Basingstoke and London, 141-151.

Getz, F. (1991): *Healing & Society in Medieval England. A Middle English Translation of the Pharmaceutical Writings of Gilbertus Anglicus*. Edited with an Introduction and Notes by..., Madison (Wisconsin). [= Wisconsin Publications in the History of Science and Medicine Number 8].

Ghalioungui, P. (1980, tr. [E]): *Questions on Medicine for Scholars by Ḥunayn Ibn Isḥāq*: translated into English, with a preface and historical note...from a critical edition by Galal M. Moussa, Ph.D., of the Ninth Century Arabic text, "Al-Masa'il fi al-Tibb lil muta'allimin", Cairo.

Gibb, H.A.R. (1962): "The Aiyūbids", in: Robert Lee Wolff and Harry W. Hazard (editors): *A History of the Crusades* (general editor: Kenneth Meyer

Setton), Volume II: *The Later Crusades 1189-1311*, Philadelphia (Pennsylvania), Ch. XX, 693-714.

Gibb, H.A.R. (1953): "Al-Barq al-Shāmī: The History of Saladin by the Kātib 'Imād ad-Dīn al-Iṣfahānī", in: *Wiener Zeitschrift zur Kunde des Morgenlandes* 52, 93-115.

Gibb, H.A.R. (1950): "The Arabic Sources for the Life of Saladin", in: *Speculum* XXV, 58-72.

Gohlman, W.E. (1974, ed. [A]; tr. [E]): *The Life of Ibn Sīnā. A Critical Edition and Annotated Translation*, Albany/New York.

Goitein, S.D. (1967-1988): *A Mediterranean Society. The Jewish Communities of the Arab World as portrayed in the Documents of the Cairo Geniza*, Vols. I-V, Berkeley/Los Angeles/London. [Especially Vol. I: *Economic Foundations*, *passim*; Vol. II: *The Community*, 240-72 and 419f.]. [Volume VI: *Cumulative Indices* by S.D. Goitein and Paula Sanders, Berkeley/Los Angeles/London 1993].

Goitein, S.D. (1986): "The Moses Maimonides – Ibn Ṣanā' al-Mulk Circle (A Deathbed Declaration from March 1182)", in: Moshe Sharon (editor): *Studies in Islamic History and Civilization in Honour of Professor David Ayalon*, Jerusalem/Leiden, 399-405.

Goitein, S.D. (1961): "The mentality of the middle class in mediaeval Islam", in: *Actes du Colloque sur la sociologie musulmane, 11-14 Septembre 1961* [= Correspondance d'Orient, 5], Bruxelles, 249-63.

Goldziher, I. (1966): *A Short History of Classical Arabic Literature*, Translated, revised, and enlarged by Joseph DeSomogyi, Hildesheim.

Good, B.J. (1994): *Medicine, rationality, and experience. An anthropological perspective*, Cambridge. [The Lewis Henry Morgan Lectures: 1990].

Goodman, L.E. (1995): art. "al-Rāzī, Abū Bakr Muḥammad b. Zakariyyā'", in: *EI²*, vol. VIII, 474a-477b.

Grape-Albers, H. (1977): *Spätantike Bilder aus der Welt des Arztes. Medizinische Bilderhandschriften der Spätantike und ihre mittelalterliche Überlieferung*. Wiesbaden.

Graziani, J. (1976): "The Contributions of Arabic Medicine to the Health Profession during the Eleventh Century", in: *Episteme: Rivista Critica di Storia delle Scienze Mediche e Biologiche* (Milano), 10, 126-143.

Green, M. (1989): "Women's Medical Practice and Health Care in Medieval Europe", in: *Signs*. Journal of Women in Culture and Society (Chicago) 14/2, 434-473.

Griffel, F. (2009): *Al-Ghazālī's Philosophical Theology*, Oxford.

Grmek, M.D. *et alii* (1998, eds.): *Western Medical Thought from Antiquity to the Middle Ages*, Cambridge (Mass.)/London.

Grmek, M.D. (1989): *Diseases in the Ancient Greek World*, Baltimore and London. [= [E] tr. by Mireille and Leonard Muellner of [F]: *Les Maladies à l'aube de la civilisation occidentale*, Paris 1983].

Gutas, D. (1998): *Greek Thought, Arabic Culture. The Graeco-Arabic Translation Movement in Baghdad and Early 'Abbāsid Society (2nd 4th/8th-10th centuries)*, London/New York.

Hall, T.S. (1971): "Life, death and the radical moisture: a study of thematic pattern in medieval medical theory", in: *Clio Medica* 6 (1), 3-23.

Halm, H. (1997): *The Fatimids and their Traditions of Learning*, London/New York. [= Farhad Daftary (general ed.): The Institute of Ismaili Studies: Ismaili Heritage Studies, 2].

Hamarneh, S.K. (1983): HSEI = *Health Sciences in Early Islam. Collected Papers by Sami K. Hamarneh*. Edited by Munawar A. Anees, Volume 1, Blanco (Texas) 1403/1983. [= A Noor Health Foundation and Zahra Publications Monograph].

Hamarneh, S.K. (1979): "Medical Sciences under the Fatimiyyah Dynasty", in: *Hamdard Medicus* (Special Issue on Pharmacy and Medicine through the Ages) 22 (7-12), Karachi, 33-69. [Reprint in: *HSEI*, 61-93].

Hamarneh, S.K. (1978): "The Life Sciences", in: John R. Hayes (editor): *The Genius of Arab Civilization – Source of Renaissance*, Cambridge (Mass.), 143-172. [Reprint in: *HSEI*, 47-60].

Hamarneh, S.K. (1977): "Arab Manuscripts of the National Library of Medicine Washington, D.C.", in: *Journal for the History of Arabic Science* (Aleppo, Syria), 1 (1), 72-108. [Reprint in: *HSEI*, 331-358].

Hamarneh, S.K. (1976): "A Brief Survey of Islamic Medicine during the Middle Ages", in: *Journal of the Islamic Medical Association of the United States and Canada* 7 (1), 21-25. [Reprint in: *HSEI*, 39-46].

Hamarneh, S.K. (1973): "Some Aspects of Medical Practice and Institutions in Medieval Islam", in: *Episteme*: Rivista Critica di Storia delle Scienze Mediche e Biologiche (Milano), 7 (1), 15-31. [Reprint in: *HSEI*, 199-208].

Hamarneh, S.K. (1972): "Physicians and Practitioners during the Arabic Golden Age", in: *The Alexandria Medical Journal*, Alexandria, Egypt, 18 (4), 1-12. [Reprint in: *HSEI*, 191-198].

Hamarneh, S.K. (1971a): "Islamic Medicine and its Impact on Teaching and Practice of the Healing Arts in the West", in: *Convegno Internazionale, 9-15 Aprile 1969, Tema: Oriente e Occidente nel medioevo: Filosofia e Scienze (Accademia Nazionale dei Lincei, Fondazione Alessandro Volta, Ist. dalla Societa Edison di Milano, Atti dei Convegni, Vol. 13)*, 395-425. [Reprint in: *HSEI*, 169-190].

Hamarneh, S.K. (1971b): "The Physician and the Health Professions in Medieval Islam", in: *Bulletin of the New York Academy of Medicine* 47 (9), 1088-1110. [Reprint in: *HSEI*, 155-167 under the title "The Physician and the Health Professions in Early Islam"].

Hamarneh, S.K. (1970): "Medical Education and Practice in Medieval Islam", in: Charles D. O'Malley (editor): *The History of Medical Education*, Berkeley/Los Angeles, 39-71. [Reprint in: *HSEI*, 127-153].

Hamarneh, S.K. (1964): "Origin and Functions of the *Hisbah* System in Islam and its Impact on the Health Professions", in: *Sudhoffs Archiv* 48 (2), 157-173. [Reprint in: *HSEI*, 113-125].

Hamarneh, S.K. (1962): "Development of Hospitals in Islam", in: *JHMAS* 17 (2), 366-84. [Reprint in: *HSEI*, 97-111].

Hämeen-Anttila, J. (2006): *The Last Pagans of Iraq. Ibn Waḥshiyya and his Nabatean Agriculture*, Leiden/Boston [= Islamic History and Civilization; 63].

Hamilton, B. (2000): *The Leper King and His Heirs. Baldwin IV and the Crusader Kingdom of Jerusalem*, Cambridge.

Hau, F.R. (1983): "Die medizinische Geschichtsschreibung im islamischen Mittelalter", in: *Clio Medica* 18, 69-80.

Hau, F.R. (1979): "Gondeschapur – eine Medizinschule aus dem 6. Jahrhundert n. Chr.", in: *Gesnerus* 36 (1-2), 98-115.

Hau, F.R. (1978-79): "Die Bildung des Arztes im Islamischen Mittelalter", in: *Clio Medica* 13 (1978), No. 2, 95-124; 13 (1978), No. 3/4, 175-200; 14 (1979), No. 1, 7-25.

Hava, J.G. (1982, 5th edition): *Al-Faraid Arabic-English Dictionary*, Beirut.

Healey, J.F. (2001): *The Religion of the Nabataeans. A Conspectus*, Leiden/Boston/ Köln.

Heffening, W. (1927): "Die griechische Ephraem-Paraenesis gegen das Lachen in arabischer Übersetzung. Ein Beitrag zum Problem der arabischen Ephraemübersetzungen und ihrer Bedeutung für eine kritische Ausgabe des griechischen Ephraem", in: *OC* 3rd series 2 (1927) = whole series 24 (1927), 94-119.

Heijer, J. den (1993): "Muḥammad b. As'ad al-Ǧawwānī and his report on cannibalism. A study in source criticism", in: Frederik de Jong (editor): *Miscellanea Arabica et Islamica. Dissertationes in Academia Ultrajectina prolatae anno MCMXC*, Leuven, 255-266. [= Orientalia Lovaniensia Analecta 52].

Hein, C. (1985): *Definition und Einteilung der Philosophie. Von der spätantiken Einleitungsliteratur zur arabischen Enzyklopädie*, Frankfurt am Main/Bern/New York. [= Europäische Hochschulschriften Reihe XX: Philosophie; Band 177].

Helgadóttir, G.P. (1987): *Hrafns saga Sveinbjarnarsonar*, Oxford. [contains important info on medieval Icelandic medical knowledge: xci-cviii].

Hillenbrand, C. (1999; reprinted with corrections, 2006): *The Crusades: Islamic Perspectives*, Edinburgh.

Hirschler, K. (2012): *The Written Word in the Medieval Arabic Lands: A Social and Cultural History of Reading Practices*, Edinburgh.

Hirschler, K. (2011): "Reading certificates (*samā'āt*) as a prosopographical source: Cultural and social practices of an elite family in Zangid and Ayyubid Damascus", in: Andreas Görke and Konrad Hirschler (editors): *Manuscript*

Notes as Documentary Sources, Beirut, 73-92. [= Beiruter Texte und Studien 129].

Hitti, Yūsuf K. and Aḥmad Shafīq al-Khatīb (1989): *Hitti's New Medical Dictionary (English-Arabic with an Arabic-English Glossary)*, Beirut.

Hoffer, C. (2000, in [D]): *Volksgeloof en religieuze geneeswijzen onder moslims in Nederland. Een historisch-sociologische analyse van religieus-medisch denken en handelen*, Amsterdam.

Hoffer, C. (1997, in [D]): "Islamitisch volksgeloof en gezondheidszorg", in: Dik Pranger (editor): *Islam en gezondheidszorg* [= Annalen van het Thijmgenootschap jaargang 84 (1996), aflevering 3], Baarn, 50-71.

Holmyard, E.J. (1957): *Alchemy*. The story of the fascination of gold and the attempts of chemists, mystics, and charlatans to find the Philosophers' Stone, Harmondsworth (Middlesex). [Chapter 5 (58-101) deals with Islamic alchemy].

Holmyard, E.J. and D.C. Mandeville (1955): "L'Alchimie en Islam medieval", in: *Endeavour* 14, 117-125.

Holmyard, E.J. (1926): "Abu 'l-Qāsim al-'Irāqī", in: *Isis* VIII, 403-26.

Holmyard, E.J. (1923, ed. [A], tr. [E]): *Kitāb al-'Ilm al-muktasab fī zirā'at adh-dhahab. Book of Knowledge Acquired Concerning the Cultivation of Gold by Abu 'l-Qāsim Muḥammad ibn Aḥmad al-'Irāqī*, Paris.

Horstmanshoff, M. {= H.F.J.} (1999, in [D]): "Hoe ging Galenus met zijn patiënten om?", in: *Hermeneus* 71 (2), 131-139.

Horstmanshoff, H.F.J. (1990): "The Ancient Physician: Craftsman or Scientist?", in: *JHMAS*, 45, 176-197. [= (E) tr. of (D): "De antieke arts: ambachtsman of man van wetenschap?", in: *Lampas* 20 (1987), 340-55].

HSEI = *Health Sciences in Early Islam. Collected Papers by Sami K. Hamarneh.* Edited by Munawar A. Anees, Volume 1, Blanco (Texas) 1403/1983. [= A Noor Health Foundation and Zahra Publications Monograph].

Huizenga, E. (2003, in [D]): *Tussen autoriteit en empirie. De middelnederlandse chirurgieën in de veertiende en vijftiende eeuw en hun maatschappelijke context*, Hilversum.

Humphreys, R.S. (1977): *From Saladin to the Mongols. The Ayyubids of Damascus, 1193-1260*, Albany (New York).

Igarashi, H. (1986): "Traditional Greco-Islamic Pathology: A Search for Causes of Disease", in: Teizo Ogawa (editor): *History of Pathology. Proceedings of the 8th International Symposium on the Comparative History of Medicine – East and West, September 18-24, 1983 Susono-shi, Shizuoka, Japan*, Tokio, 37-52.

Inayatullah, Sh. (1944): "Contribution to the historical study of hospitals in mediaeval Islam", in: *Islamic Culture* (Hyderabad) 18, 1-14.

Irwin, R. (1986): *The Middle East in the Middle Ages: The Early Mamluk Sultanate 1250-1382*, Carbondale and Edwardsville (Illinois).

Isaacs, H.D. (1991): "A Medieval Arab Medical Certificate", in: *Medical History* 35, 250-57.

Iskandar, A.Z. (1985): "Development of Medical Education among the Arabic-Speaking Peoples", in: J.D. North and J.J. Roche (editors): *The Light of Nature. Essays in the History and Philosophy of Science presented to Alistair Cameron Crombie*, Dordrecht/Boston/Lancaster, 7-20. [= Archives Internationales d'Histoire des Idées 110].

Iskandar, A.Z. (1977): "An autograph of Ibn al-Tilmīdh's marginal commentary on Ibn Sīnā's Canon of medicine", in: *Le Muséon* 90, 177-236.

Iskandar, A.Z. (1976): "An Attempted Reconstruction of the Late Alexandrian Medical Curriculum", in: *Medical History* 20 (3), 235-258.

Iskandar, A.Z. (1962a): "Galen and Rhazes on Examining Physicians", in: *BHM* 36, 362-365.

Iskandar, A.Z. (1962b): "Al-Rāzī: al-ṭabīb al-iklīnīkī", in: *Al-Machriq* (Beirut) 56, 217-282.

Iskandar, A.Z. (1960): "Al-Rāzī wa-miḥnat al-ṭabīb", in: *Al-Machriq* (Beirut) 54, 471-522.

Issa Bey, A. (1928): *Histoire des Bimaristans (Hôpitaux) à l'époque islamique*, Le Caire. [Arabic title: *Ta'rīkh al-bīmāristānāt fī-l islām*, Damascus 1939 (Reprint: Beirut 1981)].

JA = *Journal Asiatique*.

Jacquart, D. and F. Micheau (1996): *La médecine arabe et l'Occident médiéval*, Paris.

Jacquart, D. (1992): "The Introduction of Arabic Medicine into the West: The Question of Etiology", in: Sheila Campbell, Bert Hall, David Klausner (editors) [Centre for Medieval Studies, University of Toronto]: *Health, Disease and Healing in Medieval Culture*, Basingstoke and London, 186-195.

Jadon, S. (1970a): "A Comparison of the Wealth, Prestige, and Medical Works of the Physicians of Ṣalāḥ al-Dīn in Egypt and Syria", in: *BHM* 44, 64-75.

Jadon, S. (1970b): "The Physicians of Syria during the Reign of Ṣalāḥ al-Dīn 570-589 A.H. 1174-1193 A.D.", in: *JHMAS* 25, 323-340.

Janssens, J. (2003): "Bahmanyār Ibn Marzubān: A Faithful Disciple of Ibn Sīnā?", in: David C. Reisman (ed.): *Before and After Avicenna. Proceedings of the First Conference of the Avicenna Study Group*, Leiden and Boston 2003, 177-197.

JHMAS = *Journal of the History of Medicine and Allied Sciences*.

Joosse, N.P. (2004): *A Syriac Encyclopaedia of Aristotelian Philosophy*. Barhebraeus (13th c.), *Butyrum sapientiae*, Books of Ethics, Economy and Politics. A Critical Edition, with Introduction, Translation, Commentary and Glossaries, Leiden/Boston. [= Hans Daiber and Remke Kruk (general editors): Aristoteles Semitico-Latinus Volume 16].

Joosse, N.P. (1993): "An example of medieval Arabic pseudo-hermetism: the tale of Salāmān and Absāl", in: *JSS* 38: 2, 279-293.

Jouanna, J. (1999): *Hippocrates*, Baltimore and London. [= [E] tr. of [F] *Hippocrate*, Paris 1992].

JRAS = *Journal of the Royal Asiatic Society*.
JSS = *Journal of Semitic Studies*.
Kaḥḥāla, 'Umar Riḍā (1376/1957-1381/1961): *Mu'jam al-mu'allifīn*. Tarājim muṣannifī l-kutub al-'arabīya, 15 vols., Damascus.
Kahl, O. (2007): *The Dispensatory of Ibn at-Tilmīḏ. Arabic Text, English Translation, Study and Glossaries*, Leiden/Boston. [= Hans Daiber (general editor): Islamic Philosophy, Theology and Science: Texts and Studies, Volume LXX].
Kahl, O. (2000): *Ya'qūb ibn Isḥāq al-Isrā'īlī's "Treatise on the Errors of the Physicians in Damascus"*. A critical edition of the Arabic text together with an annotated English translation, Oxford. [= *JSS* Suppl. 10].
Karamustafa, A.T. (1994): *God's Unruly Friends. Dervish Groups in the Islamic Later Middle Period 1200-1550*, Salt Lake City. [Reprint: Oxford 2006].
Karbstein, A. (2002): *Die Namen der Heilmittel nach Buchstaben. Edition eines arabisch-romanischen Glossars aus dem frühen 17. Jahrhundert*, Genève. [= Kölner Romanistische Arbeiten, Neue Folge – Heft 81].
Karmi, G. (1981): "State control of the physicians in the Middle Ages: an Islamic model", in: Andrew W. Russell (editor): *The Town and State Physician in Europe from the Middle Ages to the Enlightenment*, Wolfenbüttel, 63-84. [= Wolfenbütteler Forschungen Bd. 17].
Karmi, G. (1978): "A Mediaeval Compendium of Medicine: Abū Sahl al-Masīḥī's *Book of the Hundred*", in: *Journal for the History of Arabic Science* (Aleppo), 2 (1978), 270-90.
Kazhdan, A.P. and A. Wharton Epstein (1985): *Change in Byzantine Culture in the Eleventh and Twelfth Centuries*, Berkeley/Los Angeles/London.
Kazimirski, A. de Biberstein (1860): *Dictionnaire Arabe-Français*, 2 vols., Paris. [Reprint: Beirut *sine anno*].
Kedar, B.Z., see: Kohlberg, E. and B.Z. Kedar (1988).
Kenny, A. (2004): *Ancient Philosophy*, Oxford. [= A New History of Western Philosophy: Volume 1].
Khairallah, Amin A. (1946): *Outline of Arabic Contributions to Medicine*, Beirut.
Khan, M.S. (1986): *Islamic Medicine*, London.
Kholeif, F. (1966, tr. [E]): *A Study on Fakhr al-Dīn Rāzī and his Controversies in Transoxania*, Beirut.
Klein-Franke, F. (1986): "What was the Fatal Disease of al-Malik al-Ṣāliḥ Najm al-Dīn Ayyūb?", in: Moshe Sharon (editor): *Studies in Islamic History and Civilization in Honour of Professor David Ayalon*, Jerusalem/Leiden, 153-57.
Klein-Franke, F. (1984, tr. [G]): *Ibn Buṭlān: Das Ärztebankett*. Aus arabischen Handschriften übersetzt und mit einer Einleitung sowie Anmerkungen versehen von…, Stuttgart.
Klein-Franke, F. (1982): *Vorlesungen über die Medizin im Islam*, Wiesbaden. [= Sudhoffs Archiv, Beiheft 23].

Klemm, V. (1989): *Die Mission des fāṭimidischen Agenten al-Mu'ayyad fī d-dīn in Šīrāz*, Frankfurt am Main.

Kohlberg, E. and B.Z. Kedar (1988): "A Melkite Physician in Frankish Jerusalem and Ayyubid Damascus: Muwaffaq al-Dīn Ya'qūb b. Siqlāb", *Asian and African Studies* 22, 113-126. [The Gustav Heinemann Institute of M.E.S., Haifa, Israel].

Köhler, B. (1994): *Die Wissenschaft unter den ägyptischen Fatimiden* [= Arabistische Texte und Studien Bd. 6], Hildesheim/Zürich/New York. [Medical information especially on 65-67 & 111-133].

Kottek, S.S. and L. García-Ballester (1996, editors): *Medicine and Medical Ethics in Medieval and Early Modern Spain. An Intercultural Approach*, Jerusalem.

Krawulsky, D. (2011): *The Mongol Īlkhāns and their Vizier Rashīd al-Dīn*, Frankfurt am Main/Berlin/Bern.

Kraemer, J.L. (2008): *Maimonides: The Life and World of One of Civilization's Greatest Minds*, New York/London etc.

Kraus, P. (1942-43): *Jābir Ibn Ḥayyān. Contribution à l'histoire des idées scientifiques dans l'Islam*: Volume I: *Le corpus des écrits jabiriens*, Le Caire 1943; Volume II: *Jābir et la science grecque*, Le Caire 1942. [Reprint (both volumes): Hildesheim/Zürich/New York 1989].

Kraus, P. (1937): "Les "Controverses" de Fakhr al-Dīn Rāzī", in: *Bulletin de l'Institut d'Égypte* XIX, 187-214. [Reprint in: Rémi Brague (editor): *Alchemie, Ketzerei, Apokryphen im frühen Islam. Gesammelte Aufsätze*, Hildesheim/Zürich/New York 1994, 191-218].

Kraus, P. (1935): "Raziana I: La conduite du philosophe", in: *Orientalia* N.S. IV, 300-334. [Reprint in: Rémi Brague (editor): *Alchemie, Ketzerei, Apokryphen im frühen Islam. Gesammelte Aufsätze*, Hildesheim/Zürich/New York 1994, 221-255].

Kruk, R. (2001): "Ibn abī l-Ash'ath's *Kitāb al-Ḥayawān*: a Scientific Approach to Anthropology, Dietetics and Zoological Systematics", in: *ZGAIW*, 14, 119-168.

Kruk, R. (1999, in [D]): "De goede arts. Ideaalbeeld en werkelijkheid in de middeleeuws-Arabische wereld", in: *Hermeneus* 71, nr. 2, 140-148.

Kruk, R. (1998, in [D]): "Het artsenberoep in het middeleeuwse Arabische discours", in: *Gewina* 21, nr. 3, 94-107.

Kruk, R. (1976): "Pseudo-Aristotle: An Arabic Version of *Problemata physica X*", in: *Isis*, 67, 251-56.

Kudlien, F. (1979): "Die Unschätzbarkeit ärztlicher Leistung und das Honorar problem", in: *Medizinhistorisches Journal* 14, 3-16.

Kudlien, F. (1976): "Medicine as a 'Liberal Art' and the Question of the Physician's Income", in: *JHMAS*, 31, 448-459.

Kudlien, F. (1973): "''Schwärzliche'' Organe im frühgriechischen Denken", in: *Medizinhistorisches Journal* 8, 53-58.

Kudlien, F. (1969): "Antike Anatomie und menschlicher Leichnam", in: *Hermes* 97, 78-94.
Kudlien, F. (1968): "Der Arzt des Körpers und der Arzt der Seele", in: *Clio Medica* 3, 1-20.
Kuhne Brabant, R. (1993): "Al-Rāzī on when and how to eat fruit", in: Frederik de Jong (editor): *Miscellanea Arabica et Islamica. Dissertationes in Academia Ultrajectina prolatae anno MCMXC*, Leuven, 164-174. [= Orientalia Lovaniensia Analecta 52].
Lane, E.W. (1863-74, 1877-93): *Maddu-l Kamoos, an Arabic-English Lexicon derived from the best and the most copious Eastern sources*..., Parts 1-5: London 1863-1874, Parts 6-8: edited by Stanley Lane Poole: London 1877-1893. [Reprint: 2 vols., Cambridge 1984].
Langermann, Y. Tzvi (2007): "Ibn Kammūna at Aleppo", in: *JRAS* 17: 1, 1-19.
Lauer, H.H. (1984): "Ethik und Ärztliches Denken im arabischen Mittelalter", in: Eduard Seidler and Heinz Schott (editors): *Bausteine zur Medizingeschichte. Heinrich Schipperges zum 65. Geburtstag* (Sudhoffs Archiv Beiheft 24), Stuttgart, 72-86.
Le Coz, R. (2004): *Les médecins nestoriens au moyen âge: Les maîtres des Arabes*, Paris.
Le Goff, J. and Nicolas Truong (2004): *De geschiedenis van het lichaam in de Middeleeuwen*, Amsterdam. [= (D) tr. by T. Buckinx of (F): *Une histoire du corps au Moyen Âge*, Paris 2003].
Leezenberg, M. (2002, in [D]): *Islamitische Filosofie. Een Geschiedenis*, Amsterdam.
Leiser, G. (1983): "Medical Education in Islamic Lands from the Seventh to the Fourteenth Century", in: *JHMAS* 38, 48-75.
Leiser, G. and Noury al-Khaledy, cf., Al-Sulamī, *K. Imtiḥān al-alibbā' li-kāffat al-aṭibbā'* (see: under primary sources).
Lev, E. (2002): "Reconstructed *materia medica* of the Medieval and Ottoman al-Sham", in: *Journal of Ethnopharmacology* 80, 167-179.
Levey, M. (1967, tr. [E]): *Medical Ethics of Medieval Islam with special reference to al-Ruhāwī's "Practical Ethics of the Physician"* [= Transactions of the American Philosophical Society, N.S. 57/3], Philadelphia.
Levey, M. (1965): "Some Eleventh Century Medical Questions posed by Ibn Buṭlān and later answered by Ibn Ithirdī", in: *BHM* 39, 495-507.
Levey, M. (1963): "Fourteenth Century Muslim Medicine and the *Ḥisba*", in: *Medical History*, VII, 176-182.
Lieber, E. (1979): "Galen: Physician as Philosopher, Maimonides: Philosopher as Physician", in: *BHM* 53, 268-285.
Lindeboom, G.A. (1993, in [D]): *Inleiding tot de geschiedenis der geneeskunde*. Zevende, geheel opnieuw bewerkte uitgave door Prof. dr. M.J. van Lieburg, Rotterdam.
Lindemann, M. (1999): *Medicine and Society in Early Modern Europe*, Cambridge. [= New Approaches to European History 16].

Loots, G.M.P. (2007, in [D]): *Epilepsie in de zestiende eeuw. De Observationes van Pieter van Foreest*, Rotterdam.

Lory, P. (2004): *La science des lettres en islam*, Paris.

Lyons, M.C. (1961): "The *Kitāb al-Nāfi'* of 'Alī Ibn Riḍwān", in: *The Islamic Quarterly* 6 (1-2), 65-71.

MacKinney, L.C. (1937): *Early Medieval Medicine with Special Reference to France and Chartres. The Hideyo Noguchi Lectures*, Baltimore. [Reprint: New York 1979].

MacLean, I. (2002): *Logic, Signs and Nature in the Renaissance: The Case of Learned Medicine*, Cambridge. [= Ideas in context: 62].

Mandeville, D.C., see: Holmyard E.J. and D.C. Mandeville (1955).

Marcinkowski, Muḥammad Ismail (2003): *Measures and Weights in the Islamic World*. An English translation of Walther Hinz's handbook *Islamische Maße und Gewichte*, Kuala Lumpur.

Marenbon, J. (2007): *Medieval Philosophy: an historical and philosophical introduction*, London and New York.

Martini Bonadeo, C. (2005): "Avicenna: seguaci e critici", in: Cristina D'Ancona (editor): *Storia della filosofia nell'Islam medievale*, Torino, II, 627-668. [= Piccola Biblioteca Einaudi: Filosofia, 286].

Ma'ṣūmī, M. Ṣaghīr Ḥasan (1967): "Imām Fakhr al-Dīn al-Rāzī and his Critics", in: *Islamic Studies* 6 (1), 355-74.

Mattock, J.N. (1995): "The Medical Muse", in: Concepción Vázquez de Benito and Miguel Ángel Manzano Rodríguez (editors): *Actas XVI Congreso UEAI* [Union Européenne d'Arabisants et d'Islamisants, celebrado en Salamanca durante los días 27 de agosto a 2 de septiembre de 1992], Salamanca, 337-343.

Maxwell-Stuart, P.G. (2005, ed./tr. [E]): *The Occult in Mediaeval Europe, 500-1500. A Documentary History*, London/New York.

McDougall, I. (1992): "The Third Instrument of Medicine: Some Accounts of Surgery in Medieval Iceland", in: Sheila Campbell, Bert Hall, David Klausner (editors) [Centre for Medieval Studies, University of Toronto]: *Health, Disease and Healing in Medieval Culture*, Basingstoke and London, 57-83.

McVaugh, M.R., see: Bos, G. and M.R. McVaugh (2009).

McVaugh, M.R. (1997): "Bedside Manners in the Middle Ages" – The Fielding H. Garrison Lecture, in: *BHM* 71, 201-223.

McVaugh, M.R. (1993): *Medicine before the plague. Practitioners and their patients in the Crown of Aragon, 1285-1345*, Cambridge. [= Cambridge History of Medicine].

McVaugh, M.R. (1974): "The 'Humidum Radicale' in Thirteenth-Century Medicine", in: *Traditio* XXX, 259-283.

Mecit, S. (2014): *The Rum Seljuqs: Evolution of a Dynasty*, Abingdon (Ox)/ New York.

Meri, J.W. (2002): *The Cult of the Saints among Muslims and Jews in Medieval Syria*, Oxford.

Meyerhof, M. (1971): art. "Ibn al-Tilmīdh, Abu' l-Ḥasan Hibat Allāh b. Abi' l-'Alā' Ṣā'id b. Ibrāhīm", in: *EI*², vol. III, 956b-957a.

Meyerhof, M. (1945): "Sultan Saladin's Physician on the Transmission of Greek Medicine to the Arabs", in: *BHM* 18, 169-178. [Reprint in: Penelope Johnstone (editor): M. Meyerhof, *Studies in Medieval Arabic Medicine: Theory and Practice* (Variorum Reprints), London 1984 under No. III].

Meyerhof, M. (1944): "La surveillance des professions médicales et para-médicales chez les arabes", in: *Bulletin de l'Institut d'Égypte* 26, 119-134. [Reprint in: Penelope Johnstone (editor): M. Meyerhof, *Studies in Medieval Arabic Medicine: Theory and Practice* (Variorum Reprints), London 1984 under No. XI].

Meyerhof, M. (1940, ed. [A], tr. [F]: *Šarḥ asmā' al-'uqqār (L'explication des noms des drogues). Un glossaire de matière médicale composé par Maïmonide* [texte publié pour la première fois d'après le manuscript unique avec traduction, commentaries et index], Cairo. [Reprint: F. Sezgin *et alii* (editor): *Islamic Medicine*, vol. 63, Frankfurt am Main 1996].

Meyerhof, M. (1938): "Mediaeval Jewish Physicians in the Near East, from Arabic Sources", in: *Isis* XXVIII, 432-460. [Reprint in: Penelope Johnstone (editor): M. Meyerhof, *Studies in Medieval Arabic Medicine: Theory and Practice* (Variorum Reprints), London 1984 under No. VII].

Meyerhof, M. and J. Schacht (1937, tr. [E]): *The Medico-Philosophical Controversy between Ibn Butlan of Baghdad and Ibn Ridwan of Cairo. A Contribution to the History of Greek Learning among the Arabs* (= The Egyptian University – The Faculty of Arts publication No. 13), Cairo.

Meyerhof, M. (1935a): "Thirty-three clinical observations by Rhazes", in: *Isis* XXIII, 321-356 + 14 pages Arabic text. [Reprint in: Penelope Johnstone (editor): M. Meyerhof, *Studies in Medieval Arabic Medicine: Theory and Practice* (Variorum Reprints), London 1984 under No. V].

Meyerhof, M. (1935b): "Ibn An-Nafīs (XIIIth cent.) and his theory of the lesser circulation", in: *Isis* XXIII, 100-120. [Reprint in: Penelope Johnstone (editor): M. Meyerhof, *Studies in Medieval Arabic Medicine: Theory and Practice* (Variorum Reprints), London 1984 under No. VI; Reprinted also in: F. Sezgin *et alii* (editor): *Islamic Medicine*, Volume 79: 'Ali ibn Abi l-Ḥazm al-Qarshī Ibn al-Nafīs. Texts and studies: collected and reprinted, Frankfurt am Main 1997, 26-46].

Meyerhof, M. and G.P. Sobhy Bey (1932-1940, ed. [A], tr. [E]): *The Abridged Version of "The Book of Simple Drugs" of Ahmad Ibn Muhammad al-Ghāfiqī by Gregorius Abu'l Farag (Barhebraeus)* [Edited from the only two known Manuscripts with an English Translation, Commentary and Indices], vol. 1, Fasc. 1-4, Cairo. [Reprint: F. Sezgin *et alii* (editor): *Islamic Medicine*, vol. 51-52, Frankfurt am Main 1996].

Meyerhof, M. and J. Schacht (1931, ed. [A], tr. [G]): *Galen, Über die medizinischen Namen.* [Arabisch und Deutsch herausgegeben von] (Abhandlungen der Preussischen Akademie der Wissenschaften, Jahrgang 1931. Philosophisch-historische Klasse. Nr. 3), Berlin.

Meyerhof, M. (1930): "Von Alexandrien nach Bagdad. Ein Beitrag zur Geschichte des philosophischen und medizinischen Unterrichts bei den Arabern", in: *Sitzungsberichten der Preussischen Akademie der Wissenschaften, Phil.-hist. Klasse XXIII*, 1-43 [389-429].

Meyerhof, M. (1929a): "Autobiographische Bruchstücke Galens aus arabischen Quellen", in: *Sudhoffs Archiv* 22, 72-86.

Meyerhof, M. (1929b): "L'oeuvre médicale de Maimonide", in: *Archeion* (Rome) 11, 136-155. [Reprint in: Penelope Johnstone (editor): M. Meyerhof, *Studies in Medieval Arabic Medicine: Theory and Practice* (Variorum Reprints), London 1984 under No. VIII].

Meyerhof, M. and C. Prüfer (1913): "Die Lehre vom Sehen bei Ḥunain b. Isḥāq", in: *Archiv für Geschichte der Medizin* (= presently *Sudhoffs Archiv*) 6, 21-33.

Mez, A. (1922): *Die Renaissance des Islams*, Heidelberg. [Reprint: Hildesheim 1968].

Micheau, F. (1992): "Great Figures in Arabic Medicine, According to Ibn al-Qifṭī", in: Sheila Campbell, Bert Hall, David Klausner (editors) [Centre for Medieval Studies, University of Toronto]: *Health, Disease and Healing in Medieval Culture*, Basingstoke and London, 169-185.

Micheau, F., see also: Jacquart, D. and F. Micheau (1996).

Miller, T.S. (1985, revised ed. 1997): *The Birth of the Hospital in the Byzantine Empire*, Baltimore and London.

Minnaar, A. (2003): "Legislative and legal challenges to combatting witch purging and *muti* murder in South Africa", in: John Hund (editor): *Witchcraft Violence and the Law in South Africa*, Pretoria, 73-92.

Mitchell, P.D. (2004a): *Medicine in the Crusades. Warfare, Wounds and the Medieval Surgeon*, Cambridge.

Mitchell, P.D. (2004b): "Evidence for Elective Surgery in the Frankish States of the Near East in the Crusader Period (12th-13th Centuries)", in: Florian Steger and Kay Peter Jankrift (editors): *Gesundheit-Krankheit. Kulturtransfer medizinischen Wissens von der Spätantike bis in die Frühe Neuzeit*, Köln/Weimar/Wien, 121-138. [= Beihefte zum Archiv für Kulturgeschichte; Heft 55].

Mobayyed, Amer Rachid (2006): *Bimarestans of Aleppo. The distinction of the Islamic architecture*, Aleppo.

Moerman, D. (2002): *Meaning, Medicine and the 'Placebo Effect'*, Cambridge.

Montford, A. (2004): *Health, Sickness, Medicine and the Friars in the Thirteenth and Fourteenth Centuries* [= The History of Medicine in Context], Aldershot and Burlington.

Morray, D. (1994): *An Ayyubid Notable and his World. Ibn al-'Adīm and Aleppo as Portrayed in his Biographical Dictionary of People Associated with the City*, Leiden/New York/Köln. [Islamic History and Civilization; Vol. 5].
Müller-Bütow, H., see: Spies, O.
Munk, S. (1842): "Notice sur Joseph ben-Iehouda ou Aboul'hadjādj Yousouf ben-Ya'hya al-Sabti al-Maghrebi, disciple de Maïmonide", in: *JA* Série 3; Tome XIV, 5-70.
Musallam, B. (1990): "The human embryo in Arabic scientific and religious thought", in: Gordon Reginald Dunstan (editor): *The Human Embryo. Aristotle and the Arabic and European Traditions*, Exeter, 32-46.
Nasr, S.H. (1993): *An Introduction to Islamic Cosmological Doctrines. Conceptions of nature and methods used for its study by the Ikhwān al-Ṣafā', al-Bīrūnī, and Ibn Sīnā*, Albany.
Newman, W.R. (1997): "An Overview of Roger Bacon's Alchemy", in: Jeremiah Hackett (editor): *Roger Bacon and the Sciences. Commemorative Essays*, Leiden/New York/Köln, 317-336. [= Jan A. Aertsen *et alii* (editors): Studien und Texte zur Geistesgeschichte des Mittelalters, Bd. LVII].
Niebyl, P.H. (1971): "Old Age, Fever, and the Lamp Metaphor", in: *JHMAS* XXVI, 351-368.
Nisbet, H. (1888, editor): *Hermes, a disciple of Jesus: his life and mission work, also the evangelistic travels of Anah and Zitah, two Persian evangelists sent out by Hafed…*, Glasgow.
Nisbet, H. (1876; 6th ed. 1923, editor): *Hafed, Prince of Persia: his experiences in earth-life and spirit-life, being spirit communications received through Mr. David Duguid, the Glasgow trance-painting medium.* With an appendix, containing communications from the spirit artists, Ruisdal and Steen, London/Glasgow.
Noble, L. (2011): *Medicinal Cannibalism in Early Modern English Literature and Culture*, Basingstoke/New York.
Northrup, L. (2013): "Al-Bīmāristān al-Manṣūrī Explorations: The Interface Between Medicine, Politics and Culture in Early Mamluk Egypt", in: *Annemarie Schimmel Kolleg Working Paper* 12 [History & Society during the Mamluk Era (1250-1517)], Bonn, 1-37.
Nutton, V. (2004): *Ancient Medicine*, London and New York.
Nutton, V. (2001): "God, Galen and the Depaganization of Ancient Medicine", in: Peter Biller and Joseph Ziegler (editors): *Religion and Medicine in the Middle Ages*, York/Woodbridge/Rochester, 17-32. [York Studies in Medieval Theology III].
Nutton, V. (1997): "Hippocratic Morality and Modern Medicine", in: H. Flashar and J. Jouanna (editors): *Médecine et morale dans l'antiquité*. Dix exposés suivis de discussions. [= Entretiens sur l'antiquité classique publiés sous la direction de François Paschoud par Bernard Grange et Charlotte Buchwalder, Tome XLIII], Vandœvres-Genève 19-23 août 1996, Genève, 31-56.

Nutton, V. (1993): "Galen at the bedside: the methods of a medical detective", in: William F. Bynum and Roy Porter (editors): *Medicine and the Five Senses*. Based on a Symposium on Medicine and the Five Senses, held at the Wellcome Institute for the History of Medicine on 11-12 June 1987, Cambridge, 7-16.

Nutton, V. (1984): "From Galen to Alexander, Aspects of Medicine and Medical Practice in Late Antiquity", in: John Scarborough (editor): *Symposium on Byzantine Medicine (1983: Dumbarton Oaks)*, [= Dumbarton Oaks Papers 38], 1-14.

OC = *Oriens Christianus*.

O'Neill, Y.V. (1979): "Ossa mandibulae inferioris duo. A Recapitulation", in: *Clio Medica* 14 (2), 97-104.

Pahlitzsch, J. (2004): "Ärzte ohne Grenzen. Melkitische, jüdische und samaritanische Ärzte in Ägypten und Syrien zur Zeit der Kreuzzüge", in: Florian Steger and Kay Peter Jankrift (editors): *Gesundheit-Krankheit. Kulturtransfer medizinischen Wissens von der Spätantike bis in die Frühe Neuzeit*, Köln/Weimar/Wien, 101-119. [= Beihefte zum Archiv für Kulturgeschichte; Heft 55].

Paulus, H.E.G. (1792-1803): *Sammlung der merkwürdigsten Reisen in den Orient* [in: Übersetzungen und Auszügen mit ausgewählten Kupfern und Charten, auch mit den nothigen Einleitungen, Anmerkungen und kollectiven Registern herausgegeben von…], T. 1-T. 7, Jena.

Pavord, A. (2005): *The Naming of Names. The Search for Order in the World of Plants*, New York. [particularly chapter VII: The Arab Influence AD 600-1200].

Pedersen, J. (1984): *The Arabic Book*, Princeton. [= (E) tr. by G. French of (Dan): *Den Arabiske Bog*, København(?) 1946].

Perho, I. (1995): *The Prophet's Medicine: A Creation of the Muslim Traditionalist Scholars*, Helsinki. [= Finnish Oriental Society: Studia Orientalia 74].

Peters, F.E. (1968): *Aristotle and the Arabs: The Aristotelian Tradition in Islam*, New York/London. [= New York University Studies in Near Eastern Civilization Number 1].

Petry, C.F. (1981): *The Civilian Elite of Cairo in the Later Middle Ages*, Princeton.

Pormann, P.E. and E. Savage-Smith (2007): *Medieval Islamic Medicine*, Edinburgh.

Pormann, P.E. (2014, forthcoming): *Medicine in Abbasid Baghdad: Doctors and Diseases During the Golden Age*, Abingdon (Ox)/New York [Culture and Civilization in the Middle East].

Pormann, P.E. (2005): "The Physician and the Other: Images of the Charlatan in Medieval Islam", in: *BHM* 79, 189-227.

Pormann, P.E. (2004): *The Oriental Tradition of Paul of Aegina's ''Pragmateia,''* Leiden. [= Studies in Ancient Medicine, 29].

Porter, R. (2000): *Quacks, Fakers & Charlatans in English Medicine*, Stroud (Gloucestershire)/Charleston (South Carolina).

Porter, R. and G.S. Rousseau (1998): *Gout. The Patrician Malady*, New Haven and London.

Porter, R. (1993, editor), see: Bynum, W.F. and R. Porter.

Pouzet, L. (1995): "Médicine populaire et guérisons curieuses en Orient arabe au Moyen-Age", in: Concepción Vázquez de Benito and Miguel Ángel Manzano Rodríguez (editors): *Actas XVI Congreso UEAI* [Union Européenne d'Arabisants et d'Islamisants, celebrado en Salamanca durante los días 27 de agosto a 2 de septiembre de 1992], Salamanca, 409-416.

Pouzet, L. (1988): *Damas au VIIe/XIIIe siècle. Vie et structures religieuses dans une métropole islamique*, Beyrouth. [= Recherches: Nouvelle Série A: Langue arabe et pensée islamique 15].

Pouzet, L. (1975): "Maghrébins à Damas au VIIe-XIIIe siècle", in: *BEO* XXVIII, 167-199.

Prawer, J. (1985): "Social Classes in the Crusader States: the "Minorities", in: Norman P. Zacour and Harry W. Hazard (editors): *A History of the Crusades* (general editor: Kenneth Meyer Setton), Volume V: *The Impact of the Crusades on the Near East*, Madison (Wisconsin), Chapter III, 59-115.

Principe, L.M. (2013): *The Secrets of Alchemy*, Chicago/London.

Prüfer, C., see: Meyerhof, M. and C. Prüfer (1913).

Qadeer, Hakim Ashhar, see: Ahmad, Jamil and Hakim Ashhar Qadeer (1999).

Al-Qāḍī, W. (1995): "Biographical Dictionaries: Inner Structure and Cultural Significance", in: George Nicholas Atiyeh (editor): *The Book in the Islamic World. The Written Word and Communication in the Middle East*, Albany, 93-122.

Rabbat, N. (1997): "My Life with Ṣalāḥ al-Dīn: The Memoirs of 'Imād al-Dīn al-Kātib al-Iṣfahānī", in: *Edebiyāt* NS 7 (2), 267-287.

Rahman, F. (1987): *Health and Medicine in the Islamic Tradition: Change and Identity*, New York.

Rawcliffe, C. (1988): "The Profits of Practice: the Wealth and Status of Medical Men in Later Medieval England", in: *Social History of Medicine* 1, 61-78.

Reddig, W.F. (2000): *Bader, Medicus und Weise Frau. Wege und Erfolge der mittelalterlichen Heilkunst*, München.

Reynolds, D.F. (2001, editor); coauthored by Kristen Brustad...[*et alii*]: *Interpreting the self: autobiography in the Arabic literary tradition*, Berkeley and Los Angeles.

Richards, D.S. (2002, tr. [E]): *The Rare and Excellent History of Saladin or al-Nawādir al-Sulṭāniyya wa'l-Maḥāsin al-Yūsufiyya by Bahā' al-Dīn Ibn Shaddād translated by...*, Aldershot/Burlington. [= Crusade Texts in Translation 7].

Richards, D.S. (2000): "More on the death of the Ayyubid Sultan Al-Ṣāliḥ Najm al-Dīn Ayyūb", in: Çiğdem Balim-Harding and Colin Imber (editors): *The*

Balance of Truth. Essays in Honour of Professor Geoffrey Lewis, Istanbul, 269-274.

Richards, D.S. (1993): "'Imād al-Dīn al-Isfahānī: Administrator, Littérateur and Historian", in: Maya Shatzmiller (editor): *Crusaders & Muslims in Twelfth-Century Syria*, Leiden/New York/Köln, 133-146. [= The Medieval Mediterranean. Peoples, Economies and Cultures, 400-1453, Volume 1].

Richards, D.S. (1992): "A Doctor's Petition for a Salaried Post in Saladin's Hospital", in: *Social History of Medicine* 5, 297-306.

Richards, P. (1977): *The Medieval Leper and his northern heirs*, Cambridge. [Reprint: Woodbridge/Rochester 2000].

Richardson, K.L. (2012): *Difference and Disability in the Medieval Islamic World: Blighted Bodies*, Edinburgh.

Riddle, J.M. (1999): "Fees and Feces: Laxatives in Ancient Medicine With Particular Emphasis on Pseudo-Mesue", in: John A.C. Greppin, Emilie Savage-Smith and John L. Gueriguian (editors): *The Diffusion of Greco-Roman Medicine into the Middle East and the Caucasus*, Delmar/New York, 7-26.

Ringrose, K.M. (2003): *The Perfect Servant. Eunuchs and the Social Construction of Gender in Byzantium*, Chicago and London.

Robinson, C.F. (2003): *Islamic Historiography*, Cambridge.

Rosa Anglica (1929) = *Rosa Anglica Sev Rosa Medicinæ Johannis Anglici. An Early Modern Irish Translation of a Section of the Mediaeval Medical Text-Book of John of Gaddesden* edited with introduction, glossary and English version by Winifred Wulff M.A., London [1923] 1929 [= Irish Texts Society (Cumann Na Sgríbheann Gaedhilge) Volume XXV (1923): 1929].

Rosenthal, F. (1978): "The Physician in Medieval Muslim Society" – The Fielding H. Garrison Lecture, in: *BHM* 52, 475-491. [Reprint in: F. Rosenthal, *Science and Medicine in Islam. A Collection of Essays* [Variorum Reprints CS 330], Aldershot 1990 under No. X].

Rosenthal, F. (1975): *The Classical Heritage in Islam*, London. [= (E) tr. of (G): *Das Fortleben der Antike im Islam*, Zürich/Stuttgart 1965].

Rosenthal, F. (1970): *Knowledge Triumphant. The Concept of Knowledge in Medieval Islam*, Leiden.

Rosenthal, F. (1969): "The Defense of Medicine in the Medieval Muslim World", in: *BHM* 43, 519-532. [Reprint in: F. Rosenthal, *Science and Medicine in Islam. A Collection of Essays* [Variorum Reprints CS 330], Aldershot 1990 under No. VIII].

Rosenthal, F. (1966): "Life is short, The Art is Long": Arabic Commentaries on the First Hippocratic Aphorism", in: *BHM* 40, 226-245. [Info on ALB on 230 and 237-40].

Rosenthal, F. (1950-51): "Sedaka, Charity", in: *Hebrew Union College Annual*, Cincinnati (Ohio), vol. XXIII, Part I, 411-430.

Rosenthal, F. (1937): "Die arabische Autobiographie", in: *Studia Arabica* I (*Analecta Orientalia* 14), Rome, 1-40. [Reprint in: F. Rosenthal, *Muslim*

Intellectual and Social History [Variorum Reprints CS 309], Aldershot 1990 under No. B V].

Rousseau, G.S., see: Porter, R. and G.S. Rousseau (1998).

Rutten, A.M.G. (2005, in [D]): *Heksen, Heiligen en Hallucinogenen. Medische toverkunsten*, Rotterdam.

Sabra, A. (2000): *Poverty and Charity in Medieval Islam. Mamluk Egypt, 1250-1517*, Cambridge. [= Cambridge Studies in Islamic Civilization].

Sanagustin, F. (1997): "Princes et médecins dans l'orient musulman classique", in: *Annales Islamologiques* XXXI, 169-180.

Sanders, P. (1994): *Ritual, Politics, and the City in Fatimid Cairo*, Albany.

Sanders, P. (1993), see: Goitein, S.D. and Paula Sanders (1993). [= *A Mediterranean Society. The Jewish Communities of the Arab World as portrayed in the Documents of the Cairo Geniza*, Volume VI: *Cumulative Indices*].

Saunders, R.H. (1924, editor): *The First Successful Attempt to Broadcast Spirit Voices, at the Hall of the Art Worker's Guild...July 24th, 1924* (copy of shorthand notes, 20 pp. [edited by R.H. Saunders]), London.

Savage-Smith, E. (2006): "New Evidence for the Frankish Study of Arabic Medical Texts in the Crusader Period", in: *Crusades* 5 (2006), 99-112.

Savage-Smith, E. (2005): "Between Reader & Text: Some Medieval Arabic *Marginalia*", in: Danielle Jacquart et Charles Burnett (editors): *Scientia in Margine. Études sur les marginalia dans les manuscrits scientifiques du moyen âge à la renaissance* [= École Pratique des Hautes Études: Sciences historiques et philologiques V – Hautes Études Médiévales et Modernes 88], Genève, 75-101.

Savage-Smith, E. (2000): art. "Ṭibb" in: *EI²*, vol. X, 452a-460a.

Savage-Smith, E. (1997): "Europe and Islam", in: Irvine Loudon (editor): *Western Medicine: an illustrated history*, Oxford/New York, 40-53.

Savage-Smith, E. (1983): "Islamic science and medicine", in: Pietro Corsi and Paul Weindling (editors): *Information Sources in the History of Science and Medicine*, [= Butterworths Guides to Information Sources], London/Boston/ Durban/Singapore/Sydney/Toronto/Wellington, 437-455.

Savage-Smith, E., see also: Pormann, P.E. and E. Savage-Smith (2007).

Sayili, A. (1981): "Certain aspects of medical instruction in medieval Islam and its influences on Europe", in: *Belleten* (Türk Tarih Kurumu) 45, 9-21.

Scarfe Beckett, K. (2003): *Anglo-Saxon Perceptions of the Islamic World*, Cambridge. [Cambridge Studies in Anglo-Saxon England 33].

Schacht, J., see: Meyerhof, M. and J. Schacht (1931 & 1937).

Schipperges, H. (1976): "Arabische Medizin im lateinischen Mittelalter", in: *Sitzungsberichte der Heidelberger Akademie der Wissenschaften, Mathematisch-naturwissenschaftliche Klasse*; Jahrgang 1976, 2. Abhandlung, Berlin/Heidelberg/New York, 91-274.

Schipperges, H. (1971): "Zum Bildungsweg eines arabischen Arztes", in: *Orvostörténeti Közlemények* (Budapest). Communicationes de Historia Artis Medicinae 60-61, 13-31.

Schipperges, H. (1964): *Die Assimilation der arabischen Medizin durch das lateinische Mittelalter* (Sudhoffs Archiv Beiheft 3), Wiesbaden.

Schipperges, H. (1960a): "Der Scharlatan im arabischen und lateinischen Mittelalter", in: *Zur Geschichte der Pharmazie. Geschichtsbeilage der Deutschen Apotheker-Zeitung*, 12. Jahrgang, Nr. 2, 9-13.

Schipperges, H. (1960b): "Der ärztliche Stand im arabischen und lateinischen Mittelalter", in: *Materia Medica Nordmark* 12, 109-118.

Schipperges, H. (1959): "Die arabische Medizin als Praxis und als Theorie", in: *Sudhoffs Archiv* 43, 317-328.

Schipperges, H. (1957): "Aus dem Alltag arabischer Ärzte", in: *Deutsche medizinische Wochenschrift* 45, Jahrgang 82, 1929-1932.

Schippers, A. (1995): "Autobiography in Medieval Arabic Literature", in: Concepción Vázquez de Benito and Miguel Ángel Manzano Rodríguez (editors): *Actas XVI Congreso UEAI* [Union Européenne d'Arabisants et d'Islamisants, celebrado en Salamanca durante los días 27 de agosto a 2 de septiembre de 1992], Salamanca, 481-487.

Schramm, M. (1959): "Zur Entwicklung der physiologischen Optik in der arabischen Literatur", in: *Sudhoffs Archiv* 43, 289-316.

Schregle, G. (1961): *Die Sultanin von Ägypten. Šağarat ad-Durr in der arabischen Geschichtsschreibung und Literatur*, Wiesbaden.

Scully, T. (1995): *The Art of Cookery in the Middle Ages*, Woodbridge.

Scully, T. (1992): "The Sickdish in Early French Recipe Collections", in: Sheila Campbell, Bert Hall, David Klausner (editors) [Centre for Medieval Studies, University of Toronto]: *Health, Disease and Healing in Medieval Culture*, Basingstoke and London, 132-140.

Segal, D.S. (2001, tr. [E]): *Judah al-Ḥarizi: The Book of Taḥkemoni.* Jewish Tales from Medieval Spain translated, explicated, and annotated by David Simha Segal, Oxford/Portland (Oregon). [The Littman Library of Jewish Civilization].

Serri, Yaron, see: Amar, Zohar and Yaron Serri (2003).

Sezgin, F. (1967-84; 1995; 2000, editor): GAS = *Geschichte des arabischen Schrifttums*, vols. 1-9: Leiden 1967-84; Indices: Frankfurt am Main 1995; vols. 10-12: Frankfurt am Main 2000.

Shaham, R. (2010): *The Expert Witness in Islamic Courts: Medicine and Crafts in the Service of Law*, Chicago & London.

Shaḥḥādah, 'Abd al-Karīm (1977): "Al-Baghdādī al-atharī al-'arabī al-rā'id", in: *Majallat 'Ādiyāt Ḥalab*, al-kitāb ath-thālith, 177-200.

Shatzmiller, J. (1984): "Doctors' Fees and Their Medical Responsibility. Evidence from Notarial and Court Records", in: Paolo Brezzi and Egmont Lee (editors): *Sources of Social History: Private Acts of the Late Middle Ages*. Papers of the Colloquium sponsored by the Istituto di Studi Romani,

the University of Calgary and the Canadian Academic Centre in Italy, Rome, 16-18 june 1980, Toronto/Rome, 201-208. [= Papers in Mediaeval Studies 5].
Shefer-Mossensohn, M. (2009): *Ottoman Medicine: Healing and Medical Institutions 1500-1700*, Albany (NY).
Shiloah, A. (1972): "Ibn Hindū, le médecin et la musique", in: *Israel Oriental Studies*, II, 447-462.
Siegel, R.E. (1970): *Galen on sense perception*, Basel.
Siegel, R.E. (1968): *Galen's System of Physiology and Medicine: an Analysis of his Doctrines and Observations on Bloodflow, Respiration, Humors and Internal Diseases*, Basel/New York.
Siggel, A. (1953, tr. [G]): "Die propädeutischen Kapitel aus dem Paradies der Weisheit über die Medizin des 'Alī b. Sahl Rabban aṭ-Ṭabarī", in: *Akademie der Wissenschaften und der Literatur in Mainz: Abhandlungen der Geistes- und sozialwissenschaftlichen Klasse*; Jahrgang 1953 – Nr. 8, 1-109.
Siggel, A. (1951): *Decknamen in der arabischen alchemistischen Literatur*, Berlin [= Deutsche Akademie der Wissenschaften zu Berlin. Institut für Orientforschung. Veröffentlichung Nr. 5].
Siggel, A. (1950): *Arabisch-Deutsches Wörterbuch der Stoffe* [aus den drei Naturreichen, die in arabischen alchemistischen Handschriften vorkommen, nebst Anhang: Verzeichnis chemischer Geräte], Berlin.
Siraisi, N.G. (1997): *The Clock and the Mirror. Girolamo Cardano and Renaissance Medicine*, Princeton.
Siraisi, N.G. (1990): *Medieval & Early Renaissance Medicine. An Introduction to Knowledge and Practice*, Chicago and London.
Siraisi, N.G. (1987): *Avicenna in Renaissance Italy*. The *Canon* and Medical Teaching in Italian Universities after 1500, Princeton.
Siraisi, N.G. (1981): *Taddeo Alderotti and His Pupils. Two Generations of Italian Medical Learning*, Princeton (NJ).
Skinner, P. (1997): *Health and Medicine in Early Medieval Southern Italy*, Leiden/New York/Köln.
Slomp, J. (1997, in [D]): "Geneeskunde in de islamitische traditie. Suggesties voor verdere studie", in: Dik Pranger (editor): *Islam en gezondheidszorg* [= Annalen van het Thijmgenootschap jaargang 84 (1996), aflevering 3], Baarn, 177-185.
Sobhy Bey, G.P., see: Meyerhof, M. and G.P. Sobhy Bey (1932-1940).
Sommer, J.H. (2001, in [D]): *Spiritisme*, Kampen.
Somogyi, J. (1957): "Medicine in ad-Damīrī's *Ḥayāt al-ḥayawān*", in: *JSS* 2, 62-91.
Spencer, J. (1984, tr. [E] from [It]): *The Four Seasons of the House of Cerrutí*, New York/Bicester. [= a facs. ed. and tr. of a 14th century Latin manuscript, known as the *Tacuinum Sanitatis in Medicina*, based on the *Taqwīm al-ṣiḥḥa* (*Regimen of Health*) by Ellbochasim de Baldach or: Ibn Buṭlān of Baghdād].
Speziale, F. (2010): *Soufisme, religion et médecine en Islam indien*, Paris.

Spies, O. and H. Müller-Bütow (1964): "Drei urologische Kapitel aus der arabischen Medizin", in: *Sudhoffs Archiv* 48, 248-259.

Stathakopoulos, D. Ch. (2004): *Famine and Pestilence in the Late Roman and Early Byzantine Empire: A Systematic Survey of Subsistence Crises and Epidemics*, Aldershot/Burlington. [= Birmingham Byzantine and Ottoman Monographs volume 9].

Stearns, J.K. (2011): *Infectious Ideas. Contagion in Premodern Islamic and Christian Thought in the Western Mediterranean*, Baltimore.

Steinschneider, M. (1869): *Al-Farabi (Alpharabius), des arabischen Philosophen Leben und Schriften, mit besonderer Rücksicht auf die Geschichte der griechischen Wissenschaft unter den Arabern. Nebst Anhängen etc.*, Mémoires de l'Académie Impériale de St. Pétersbourg. VIIIe Série. Tome XIII. No. 4, St. Petersburg. [Reprint: Amsterdam 1966].

Steinschneider, M. (1866): "Wissenschaft und Charlatanerie unter den Arabern im neunten Jahrhundert. Nach der hebräischen Uebersetzung eines Schriftchens von Rhases", in: *Archiv für pathologische Anatomie und Psychologie und für klinische Medicin* (Herausgegeben von Rudolf Virchow), Berlin, 36, 570-586.

Stillman, N.A. (1975): "Charity and social service in medieval Islam", in: *Societas. A Review of Social History* V (2), 105-115.

Street, T. (1997): "Concerning the Life and Works of Fakhr al-Dīn al-Rāzī", in: Peter G. Riddell and Tony Street (editors): *Islam: Essays on Scripture, Thought and Society. A Festschrift in Honour of Anthony Hearle Johns* [= Islamic philosophy, theology, and science; Vol. 28], Leiden/New York/Köln, 135-146.

Strohmaier, G. (1999): *Avicenna*, München.

Strohmaier, G. (1998): "Reception and Tradition: Medicine in the Byzantine and Arab World", in: Mirko Drazen Grmek (editor)/ Bernardino Fantini (coordinator)/Antony Shugaar (translator): *Western Medical Thought from Antiquity to the Middle Ages*, Cambridge (Mass.)/London, 139-169 & 372-377.

Strohmaier, G. (1987): "«Von Alexandrien nach Baghdad» - eine fiktive Schultradition", in: J. Wiesner (editor): *Aristoteles, Werk und Wirkung (Paul Moraux gewidmet)*, vol. 2, Berlin and New York, 380-89.

Strohmaier, G. (1980): "Der arabische Hippokrates. Bemerkungen zu einem Aufsatz von Dieter Irmer", in: *Sudhoffs Archiv* 64 (3), 234-249.

Strohmaier, G. (1979): "Ärztliche Ausbildung im islamischen Mittelalter", in: *Klio* 61, 519-24.

Stroumsa, S. (2009): *Maimonides in His World. Portrait of a Mediterranean Thinker*, Princeton and London.

Sudhoff, K. (1914-18): *Beiträge zur Geschichte der Chirurgie im Mittelalter*, 2 Vols., Studien zur Geschichte der Medizin, Heft x-xii, Leipzig.

Sugg, R. (2011): *Mummies, Cannnibals and Vampires: The History of Corpse Medicine from the Renaissance to the Victorians*, Abingdon (Ox)/New York.

Tabbaa, Y. (1997): *Constructions of Power and Piety in Medieval Aleppo*, University Park, (Penn.).
Talmon-Heller, D. (2007): *Islamic Piety in Medieval Syria. Mosques, Cemeteries and Sermons under the Zangids and Ayyūbids (1146-1260)*, Leiden/Boston.
Taschkandi, Schah Ekram (1969, tr. [G]): *Übersetzung und Bearbeitung* des *Kitāb at-Tashwīq aṭ-ṭibbī des Ṣā'id b. al-Ḥasan. Ein medizinisches Adabwerk aus dem 11. Jahrhundert*, (Diss.) Bonn.
Taylor, C.S. (1999): *In the Vicinity of the Righteous. Ziyāra and the Veneration of Muslim Saints in Late Medieval Egypt*, Leiden/Boston/Köln.
Temkin, O. (1979): "Medical Ethics and Honoraria in Late Antiquity", in: Charles E. Rosenberg (editor): *Healing and History. Essays for George Rosen*, New York, 6-26.
Temkin, O. (1977): *The Double Face of Janus and other essays in the history of medicine*, Baltimore.
Temkin, O. (1973): *Galenism: Rise and Decline of a Medical Philosophy*, Ithaca and London.
Temkin, O. (1955): "Medicine and Graeco-Arabic Alchemy", in: *BHM* 29, 134-153.
Temkin, O. (1945, [2]1971): *The Falling Sickness. A History of Epilepsy from the Greeks to the Beginnings of Modern Neurology*, Baltimore and London.
Teule, H. (2003): "Gregory Barhebraeus and his Time: The Syrian Renaissance", in: *Journal of the Canadian Society for Syriac Studies* 3, 21-43.
Thierry de Crussol des Epesse, B. (2010): *La psychiatrie médiévale persane: La maladie mentale dans la tradition médicale persane*, Berlin/ Heidelberg/New York.
Tobyn, G. (1997): *Culpeper's Medicine. A Practice of Western Holistic Medicine*, Shaftesbury (Dorset)/Rockport (Mass.)/Brisbane (Queensland).
Toonder, M. (1972, in [D]): "De loodhervormer", in: *Een groot denkraam*, Amsterdam, 185-245. [separate edition (in [D]): Amsterdam 2005].
Truong, N., see: Le Goff, J. and N. Truong (2004).
Ullmann, M. (1978): *Islamic Medicine* (Islamic Surveys, 11), Edinburgh. [Info on ALB on 48, 71, 79-80, 104].
Ullmann, M. (1972): *Die Natur- und Geheimwissenschaften im Islam* (Handbuch der Orientalistik, I. Abt., Erg.-Bd. VI, 2), Leiden/Köln. [Info on ALB esp. on 5, 9, 31, 56, 69, 81, 254].
Ullmann, M. (1970): *Die Medizin im Islam* (Handbuch der Orientalistik, I. Abt., Erg.-Bd. VI, 1), Leiden/Köln. [Info on ALB esp. on 29, 68, 94, 170-72, 226].
Unschuld, P.U. (2003): *Was ist Medizin? Westliche und östliche Wege der Heilkunst*, München.
Urvoy, D. (1998): *Averroès. Les ambitions d'un intellectuel musulman*, Paris.
Vallance, J. (2000): "Doctors in the Library: The Strange Tale of Appolonius the Bookworm and Other Stories", in: Roy MacLeod (editor): *The Library of Alexandria: Centre of Learning in the Ancient World*, London/New York, 95-113.

Van Bladel, K. (2009): *The Arabic Hermes From Pagan Sage to Prophet of Science*, Oxford/New York.

Van Gelder, G.J. (2005): *Close Relationships. Incest and Inbreeding in Classical Arabic Literature*, London/New York.

Van Gelder, G.J. (2000): *God's Banquet. Food in Classical Arabic Literature*, New York/Chichester (West Sussex).

Van Gelder, G.J. (1995): "The joking doctor: Abū l-Ḥakam 'Ubayd Allāh Ibn al-Muẓaffar (d. 549/1155)", in: Concepción Vázquez de Benito and Miguel Ángel Manzano Rodríguez (editors): *Actas XVI Congreso UEAI* [Union Européenne d'Arabisants et d'Islamisants, celebrado en Salamanca durante los días 27 de agosto a 2 de septiembre de 1992], Salamanca, 217-228.

Van Ginkel, J.J. (1998): "Making History: Michael the Syrian and his Sixth-Century Sources", in: René Lavenant (editor): *Symposium Syriacum VII* (Uppsala University, Department of Asian and African Languages, 11-14 August 1996), [OCA 256], Roma, 351-358.

Von Staden, H. (1982): "Hairesis and Heresy: The Case of the *haireseis iatrikai*", in: Ben F. Meyer and E.P. Sanders (editors): *Jewish and Christian Self-Definition, III: Self-Definition in the Graeco-Roman World*, London, 76-100.

Waddington, K. (2011): *An Introduction to the Social History of Medicine: Europe Since 1500*, Basingstoke.

Waines, D. (1995): "Medicinal nutriments as home remedies: a case of convergence between the medieval islamic culinary and medical traditions", in: Concepción Vázquez de Benito and Miguel Ángel Manzano Rodríguez (editors): *Actas XVI Congreso UEAI* [Union Européenne d'Arabisants et d'Islamisants, celebrado en Salamanca durante los días 27 de agosto a 2 de septiembre de 1992], Salamanca, 551-558.

Wallis, F. [ed.] (2010): *Medieval Medicine: A Reader*, Toronto.

Wear, A. (2000): *Knowledge and Practice in English Medicine, 1550-1680*, Cambridge.

Webster, C. (2008): *Paracelsus: Medicine, Magic and Mission at the End of Time*, New Haven and London.

Wedeen, R.P. (1984): *Poison in the Pot: The Legacy of Lead*, Carbondale and Edwardsville (Illinois).

Wehr, H. (1976, 1979): *A Dictionary of Modern Written Arabic (Arabic-English)*, ed. J. Milton Cowan, 3rd ed.: Münster/Ithaca/New York 1976; 4th ed.: Wiesbaden 1979.

Weisser, U. (1991): "Unter den Künsten die nützlichste: Aspekte des ärztlichen Berufs im arabisch-islamischen Mittelalter" – Charles Lichtenthaeler zum 75. Geburtstag gewidmet, in: *Medizinhistorisches Journal* 26, 3-25.

Weisser, U. (1985): "Zwischen Antike und europäischem Mittelalter. Die arabisch-islamische Medizin in ihrer klassischen Epoche", in: *Medizinhistorisches Journal* 20, 319-341.

Weisser, U. (1983): "Ibn Sīnā und die Medizin des arabisch-islamischen Mittelalters – Alte und neue Urteile und Vorurteile", in: *Medizinhistorisches Journal* 18, 283-305.

Weltecke, D. (2003): *Die «Beschreibung der Zeiten» von Mōr Michael dem Grossen (1126-1199). Eine Studie zu ihrem historischen und historiographie geschichtlichen Kontext*, Louvain-la-Neuve. [= CSCO: Vol. 594, Subsidia Tomus 110].

Westendorf, W. (1999): *Handbuch der altägyptischen Medizin*, Bd. 1-2, Leiden/Boston/Köln. [= Handbuch der Orientalistik, Abteilung 1: Der Nahe und Mittlere Osten; Bd. 36].

Westerink, L.G. (1964): "Philosophy and Medicine in Late Antiquity", in: *Janus* 51, 169-177.

Wharton Epstein, A., see: Kazhdan, A.P. and A. Wharton Epstein (1985).

Wiedemann, E. (1911): "Über Charlatane bei den Muslimen nach al-Gaubarī", in: *Sitzungsberichte der Physikalisch-medizinischen Sozietät zu Erlangen* Bd. 43, 206-232. [Reprint in: E. Wiedemann, *Aufsätze zur arabischen Wissenschaftsgeschichte* I (Collectanea VI/1) mit einem Vorwort und Indices herausgegeben von Wolfdietrich Fischer, Hildesheim/New York 1970, 749-775].

Wiedemann, E. (1909): "Kleinere Arbeiten von Ibn al-Haiṯam – 1. Eine philosophische Studie von Ibn al-Haiṯam über den Ort", in: *Sitzungsberichte der Physikalisch-medizinischen Sozietät zu Erlangen* Bd. 41, 1-11. [Reprint in: E. Wiedemann, *Aufsätze zur arabischen Wissenschaftsgeschichte* I (Collectanea VI/1) mit einem Vorwort und Indices herausgegeben von Wolfdietrich Fischer, Hildesheim/New York 1970, 519-29].

Wiet, G. (1962, tr. [F]): "Le Traité des famines de Maqrīzī", in: *Journal of the Economic and Social History of the Orient* 5, 1-90. [= A French translation of al-Maqrīzī's *K. Ighāthat al-umma bi-kashf al-ghumma*].

Wild, S. (1975): "Jugglers and fraudulent sufis", in: Frithiof Rundgren (editor): *Proceedings of the VIth Congress of Arabic and Islamic Studies, Visby 13-16 August, Stockholm 17-19 August 1972* [= Filologisk-filosofiska serien 15 Kungl. Vitterhets Historie och Antikvitets Akademien], Uppsala, 58-63.

Williams, S.J. (1997): "Roger Bacon and the *Secret of Secrets*", in: Jeremiah Hackett (editor): *Roger Bacon and the Sciences. Commemorative Essays*, Leiden/New York/Köln, 365-393. [= Jan A. Aertsen *et alii* (editors): Studien und Texte zur Geistesgeschichte des Mittelalters, Bd. LVII].

Woolgar, C.M. (2006): *The Senses in Late Medieval England*, New Haven and London.

Wootton, D. (2006): *Bad Medicine. Doctors Doing Harm Since Hippocrates*, Oxford.

Wright, R. (1988): *Hafed & Hermes*, London.

ZDMG = *Zeitschrift der Deutschen Morgenländischen Gesellschaft.*

ZGAIW = *Zeitschrift für Geschichte der Arabisch – Islamischen Wissenschaften.*

Ziai, H. (1997): art. "al-Suhrawardī, Shihāb al-Dīn Yaḥyā b. Ḥabash b. Amīrak, Abu 'l-Futūḥ", in: *EI²*, vol. IX, 782a-784b.

Al-Ziriklī, Khayr al-Dīn (1373-1378/1954-1959): art. "Ibn al-Raḥbī", in: *Al-A'lām, qāmūs tarājim li-ashhar ar-rijāl wa-n-nisā' min al-'arab wa-l-musta'ribīn wa-l-mustashriqīn*, vol. 5 (1374/1955), 187-88. [vols. 1-4: 1373/1954; vols. 5-6: 1374/1955; vols. 7-8: 1375/1956; vol. 9: 1376/1957; vol. 10: 1378/1959: al-Qāhira].

Index of Terms Relating to the English Translation of the Medical Section of the *Kitāb al-Naṣīḥatayn*

The numbers refer to the folios of the Bursa manuscript, not to the page numbers in this volume. The English translation of the *Kitāb al-Naṣīḥatayn* can be found on the pages 63-93 of this volume.

General Index

A

Aleppo: 69r, 77r
Alexandria: 75v
Antidote (or: Theriac): 65r, 72r, 76r
Abridgment(s): 74r
Abyssinians: 75r
Agriculture: 63r
'Ain Zarbā [*Anazarbus* in Asia Minor]: 75v
Alcohol: 66v
-alcoholics: 67r
Apoplexy: 75r
Apothecary: 77v
aqrabādhīnāt: 75v
Arabic language: 70v, 71r
Archery: 64v
Arithmetic(ians): 63r, 64v
Asafetida resin: 76r
Asclepiades: 73r
Astringents: 70r
Astronomy: 63r
Authority: 62v, 63r

B

Baghdād: 69r, 74r, 75r, 75v, 77r
Barley-water: 70v, 72v
basfā'ij: 65r
Bat: 66r
Bile (black): 76r
Blood: 67v, 68r, 73r
Blood-letting (or: Bleeding): 67v, 69v, 70r, 72r, 73r, 75r, 76r
Byzantine(s): 69r

C

Cairo: 69r, 77r
Carnal (desire): 77v
Cassia senna: 65r
Chicken broth: 70r
Christian: 63v
Cleanse(d): 63v, 70r
Colic: 75r
Conditions: 64r, 64v, 65v, 68r
- (pre)conditions: 65r, 75v, 76r
Conjecture: 64v
Colocynth leaves: 71v
Convonvulus scammonia L.: 65r
Constantinople: 68v, 69r

D

Damascus: 69r
Dancing (girls): 67r
Delay: 73r
- delay of diagnosis: 76v, 77r
Diagnosis: 68r, 76r, 76v, 77r
Diagnostics: 65v
dinar: 66v

D

Dioscorides: 75v
dirham: 65v, 66r, 66v, 67r, 68v, 69v
Disease(s): 64v, 65r, 65v, 66v, 67r, 69r, 70r, 70v, 71r, 71v, 72r, 72v, 74v, 75r, 76r, 76v, 77r
-phlegmatic [mucous]: 70v, 74v, 75r
-choleric [bilious]: 70v, 75r
-sanguinary: 70v, 75r, 76r
Dropsy: 75r
Drugs: 65r, 67r, 70r, 71r, 71v, 72r, 72v, 73r, 74r, 74v, 75r, 75v, 77v
dūlāb: 76r

E

Egypt(ian): 75v
Electuary: 76r
Empiricist (sect): 67r, 67v
Enema: 70r
Engineering: 63r
Epilepsy (Epileptic): 75r, 76r
Error: 62v, 64v, 65r, 75r, 76v

F

Fanaticism: 62v
Fever: 67v, 72v, 73r, 73v, 74v, 76r
- tertian: 74
- quartan: 74v, 75r
- double quartan: 75r
- quotidian: 74v, 75r
- nocturnal: 75r
fiqh: 68v
Franks: 69r

G

Galen: 64r, 65v, 66r, 67r, 71r, 72r, 72v, 73r, 73v, 74r, 74v, 75r, 75v, 77r, 77v, 78r
Generalities: 73v
Genus: 67v
Geometry: 63r
God: 62v, 63r, 64r, 68v, 70v, 73r, 75v, 77v, 78r
Greece (Greeks, Greek): 74r, 74v, 75r, 75v

H

Hemiplegia: 74v, 75r
Hippocrates: 65r, 67r, 72r, 73r, 73v, 74r, 74v, 77v
Hippocratic Oath: 69r

I

Ibn abī l-Ash‘ath, Abū Ja‘far Aḥmad ibn Muḥammad: 73r
Ibn Hibat Allāh (ibn) Ṣā‘id, (Raḍī al-Dawla Abū Naṣr): 77r
Ibn Sarābiyūn: 74r
Ibn at-Tilmīdh 77r
Ibn Waḥshīya: 74v
India(n): 75v
Insomnia: 69v
Intellect: 64v, 66r, 66v, 67r, 68v
Ipomoea turpethum L.: 65r
Iraq: 74r, 75r
Islam: 69v
Islamic: 73r

J

Jew(ish): 63v, 69v
jins: 67v

J

Jumādā I: 69v
Jurisprudence: 68v

K

Kill(ing): 65r, 68v, 69v, 70v
Knowledge: 62v, 63r, 63v, 64r, 66r, 66v, 67r, 68r, 68v, 69r, 71v, 74r, 74v, 76r, 77v
kullīyāt: 73v

L

Legal (questions): 68v
Lubricants: 72v, 73r

M

maghribī: 69v, 77r
Malaṭya [Malatya]: 75v
al-Malik al-Ẓāhir Ghāzī ibn Yūsuf: 69v
Mazdean: 63v
Medicament(s): 71r, 72r, 75v, 76r
Methodist (sect): 67r, 67v
al-Mubarrad, Abū al-'Abbās: 70v
Mucilaginous (decoctions): 72v
Muḥammad (prophet): 62v, 78r

N

Nabataean(s): 74v
Navigation: 63r
North African: 69v, 77r
Nourishment: 73r

O

Old women (medicine of): 71r
Organs: 72v, 73r
Overweight: 69v

P

Paralysis (facial): 75r
Peasants: 72r
Phthisis: 70v, 76r
Plato: 63v, 66r
Pleurisy: 76r
Poets: 67r
Poison(ous): 65r, 65v, 72r, 72v, 73r
Polypodium vulgare L.: 65r
Potion(s): 65r, 70r, 71r, 71v
Pulpa colocynthidis: 65r
Purgation/Purgative (drugs): 65r, 69r, 70r, 70v, 71r, 72r, 72v, 73r
Pus: 76r

Q

Quack: 65r, 65v, 68v
Qūnyah, [Konya, the ancient *Iconium* in Asia Minor]: 75v

R

Rationalist (sect): 67v, 68r
ar-Rāzī, Abū Bakr: 71r
Recipe: 77v
Recompense: 64r
Remedy: 71r, 71v, 72v, 76r, 77r, 77v
Retentive faculty/power: 70r, 72v
Reward: 63r, 63v
rizq: 64r, 71r
Rose syrup: 70v

S

sanā: 65r
saqmūnīyā: 65r
Sense-perception: 64v

S

shaḥm al-ḥanẓal: 65r
sharīʿah: 69v
shurūṭ: 64r
Slavs: 75r
Species: 67v, 71v
Spongers: 71v, 77r (cf. likewise 64r, 67v, 71r, 77v)
Spurges: 71v
Stricture: 67v
Substance: 72r, 74v, 75r, 76r
Suppositories: 70r
Syria(n): 74r, 75v

T

Target: 64v, 67r, 67v, 70r
Temperament (bodily mixtures): 71v, 72r, 72v, 73r, 73v

T

Ten Commandments: 69v
Tolerance: 64v, 75r
Torah: 69v
Treatment: 66v, 70r, 70v, 72r, 72v, 74r, 75r, 77v
turbid: 65r

V

Venom: 65r
Veterinarians: 68v

W

Wine: 67r

Index of Authors and Works Cited in the Medical Section of the *Kitāb al-Naṣīḥatayn*

'Abd al-Laṭīf ibn Yūsuf al-Baghdādī:
Treatise on the man who started the medical art [*Maqāla fī al-bādi' bi-ṣinā'at al-ṭibb*]: 73r

Abū 'Alī al-Ḥusayn ibn Sīnā [Avicenna]:
Canon of Medicine [*K. al-Qānūn (fī al-ṭibb)*]: 73v, 74r

Abū Sahl al-Masīḥī:
The Hundred Books on the Medical Art [*al-Kutub al-Mi'ah fī al-ṣinā'a al-ṭibbīya*]: 74r

'Alī ibn al-'Abbās al-Majūsī [Haly Abbas]:
The Royal Book [*K. al-Malakī*]: 74r

Galen:
Book on the Examination of the Physician [*K. fī Imtiḥān aṭ-ṭabīb*]: 65v, 66r
Book on Compound Drugs according to Places [*K. al-Mayāmir*]: 67r
Book on Compound Drugs according to Types [*K. al-Qaṭājānis*]: 67r
Book on the Sects (for Beginners) [*K. al-Firaq*]: 67r
Book on the Stratagem of Healing [*K. Ḥīlat al-bur'*]: 72v
The Compendium of the Book on the Stratagem of Healing [*Ikhtiṣār Ḥīlat al-bur'*]: 73v
Book on Mixtures/On Temperaments [*K. al-Mizāj*]: 73v
The Small Book on the Pulse [*K. an-Nabḍ aṣ-ṣaghīr*]: 73v
The Large Book on the Pulse [*K. an-Nabḍ al-kabīr*]: 73v [?], cf. footnote 249
The Book on the Pulse [*K. an-Nabḍ*]: 76r
The Small Book on the Art of Medicine [*K. aṣ-Ṣinā'a aṣ-ṣaghīra*]: 73v
The Book to Glauco [*K. (ilā) Ighlūqun*]: 73v
The Two Treatises on the Restoration of Health [*al-Maqālatān al-Shāfiyatān*]: 73v

Hippocrates:
Book on Regimen in Acute Diseases [*K. al-Amrāḍ al-ḥādda*]: 65r, 67r
Book on the Rules of Conduct and Manners of Doctors [*K. fī Adab aṭ-ṭabīb*]: 65r
How it is appropriate (for a doctor) to act and (be)have [*Kayfa yanbaghī an yakūna*]: 65v
Book on Aphorisms [*K. al-Fuṣūl*]: 72r, 76r

Book on Urinary Science [*K. ʿIlm al-baul*]: 76r
Book of the Forecasting of Knowledge [*K. Taqdimat al-maʿrifa*] or *Prognosticon*: 76r
Book of Airs and Places [*K. al-Ahwiya wa-l-buldān*]: 76r

Ibn Sarābiyūn:
The Small Compendium [*al-Kunnāsh aṣ-ṣaghīr*]: 74r

Ibn Waḥshīya:
Book of (Nabataean) Agriculture [*K. al-Filāḥa an-nabaṭīya*]: 74v

Plato:
Book on Politics [= *Politeia, The Republic*]: 63v

Appendix: The Arabic Originals of the Medical Section of the *Kitāb al-Naṣīḥatayn* - Ms. Bursa (Turkey): Hüseyin Çelebi 823 (fol. 62r-78r)

62

وَقَد رَأيتُ أن أقتصرَ علي هذا القدر إذ هُوَ كافٍ في بُلوغ ما أردتُ

هذه المقالة له وهي مع صغر حجمها تقدح زناد الفهم وتورثُ نار المعرفة

وتوطئ الذهن على فهم كتابِ الكون والفساد وفهم كتابِ المزاج وتقف الذهن على كثير من الشكوك

ومن الله استمد المعونة بمنه وجوده ∴ ه ه ه

والحمدُ لله رب العالمين وصلى الله على سيدنا نبيه محمد وآله

الطيبين الطاهرين ∴

كتاب النصيحتين

من عبد اللطيف بن يوسف

إلي الناس كافة ∴

بسم الله الرحمن الرحيم

هذا كتاب من المتقرب الى خالقه سبحانه وتقدس سند بن جهد منجويا
في المناصحة والارشاد ؛ الى اخلصائه واودائه على تفرقهم في
البلاد وتنقلهم في القرى وفي الامصار ؛ ثم الى ملوك الاطراف
والولاة والامراء ؛ ثم الى السواد كافة ممن يؤثر الخير لنفسه والسعادة
لها بترك الهوى والعصبية والانفة من التقليد على الحمية وباستعمال
النظر والتامل والروية ؛ فاول ما ابتدي به حمد الله
سبحانه الذي هو مفتاح كل خير واستيفاقه الذي هو قايد الى
كل مكرمة والثنا عليه بما هو اهله ؛ ثم الصلوة على نبي الرحمة
ومرشد الامة والمنقذ من كل ضلالة وعمة ؛ والدال على سبل النجاة والسعادة
محمد النبي الامي وعلى اله الطاهرين وعلى الاوليا والشهداء
والصديقين ؛ ثم الشكر للحكما العظما الذين اقتدوا بالانبياء على غاية
الامكان بان اصلحوا انفسهم اولا ثم نحلوا العامة النصيحة بما وضعوا لهم
من العلوم الفاضلة والصنايع النافعة ؛ فجعلوا الحكمة غايتهم
من حياتهم الداثرة وزادهم الى الدار الآخرة وصرفوا وقتهم وقوتهم في
اقتنايها وغنوا بها عن المقتنيات الفانية والاعراض البالية واقتصروا
من ضرورة البدن على ما يوصلهم الى الاجل ولا يصدهم عن المبتغى وعزفت نفوسهم

عن كل ما سوى الحكمة وراوا ان اقتنايها افضل القرب الى الحكيم
الازلي الواحد الفرد القديم الابدي وصرفوا افضل حكمتهم الى ما يعود على
العامة بالمنفعة في نفوسهم وابدانهم وبثوا فيهم من اصناف العلوم والصنايع
النافعة في دنياهم واخراهم ما اثاره مشكورة وافعاله ظاهرة محمودة
كالطب والنجوم والفلاحة والملاحة والحساب والهندسة والمساحة
وكل من جا بعدهم وامر حذوهم واخذ اخذهم وامتثل سمتهم كان
معدودا منهم ومحسوبا في زمرتهم وله اجر مثل اجورهم واستحق الحمد والشكر
بقدر عنايته وصدق قصده ∴ ومن اعان على ذلك من الملوك واولي
الامر كان له الاجر اضعافا والفضيلة اصلا وضعفا لان الملك تبعه
الناس ويتشبهون به وما يامرون له ويقبلونه وهذا لهم في اصل
فطرهم ومعجون بجبلتهم كما ترى الصبي يحاكي شيم والديه ومؤدبه ثم
لهم منه الرغبة والرهبة ومن خذل عن ذلك كان عليه من الوبال كفاء
ما للاول من الثواب اذ الحسنات اضداد السيئات ∴

وقصدي في هذا الكتاب الى خاصاي ان شدهم الله واحسن توفيقهم
ان اخلص لهم النصيحة او اوقظهم من رقدة الغفلة وسنة الالف والعادة
وانبههم على بلية انتشرت يعم ضررها النفوس والابدان واحذرهم من
الوقوع فيها فمن كان عارفا بصحة ما اقول ازداد تمسكا به وثقة ومن لم

يكن عارفا رجوت له ان يعرف ولو اهتدى بما اقول واحد من العالم
لحسبني اجره وكفاني فخره ونكاية هذه البلية في الملوك والعظما
اضعاف نكايتها في الرعاع والغثا وافتها اعظم من افة عدم الحكمة
فان سالت وقلت اي افة هي اعظم من عدم الحكمة فاقول اسمع
مني وافهم عني واعلم ان اقتنا الحكمة المموهة اشد افة واعظم مضرة من
عدم الحكمة الحقة فان من عدم الحكمة راسا شعر بالخلو عنها والفراغ
منها والحاجة اليها فكان يتشوقها ويطلبها ويحرص مجتهدا في
اقتنايها فاما من عنده حكمة مموهة فانه يظن انه غني وهو افقر
الفقرا ويوهل نفسه للتعليم والاصلاح وهو احوج الى التعلم والصلاح
فمن لا دين له اسرع اجابة ممن له دين فاسد ومن ينطوي على اعتقاد
خطا اعسر اجابة ممن لا اعتقاد له ولذلك كانت العوام اسرع
تعلما واسلس قيادا ممن تمكنت فيه اعتقادات فاسدة كمن
صحيفة بيضا واخرى مشغولة بخطوط فاسدة وقد اشارت النبوة
المقدسة الى هذا المعنى بهذا القول كل مولود يولد على الفطرة حتى يكون
ابواه هما اللذان يهودانه وينصرانه ويمجسانه ∴ وقال افلاطن في
كتاب السياسة ان الشر اشد مضادة للخير من سلب الخير ∴ وقال العلم
صبغ النفس وليس يشرق صبغ الشي حتى ينظف ادناسه ∴ وهذه البلية

64 العظمى والفادحة الكبرى التي قصدت الاجر في التنبيه عليها وقعت
في الطب الموضوع لخلاص الابدان من الاسقام وفي الحكمة الموضوعة
لخلاص النفوس من الام الجهل الى سلامة المعرفة وصحة ادراك الحق
ونحن نشرح اولا البلية الواقعة من جهة الطب اذ كان شرها عاما
للجمهور ولكل احد فيها نصيب اذ كل احد يهمه خلاص بدنه من
الالام وليس كل احد يهمه خلاص نفسه من الجهل فنقول ان صناعة
الطب خطيرة شريفة قد اقر بفضلها الجمهور واصفقت الامم مع
تباينهم على جلالتها وعظم الحاجة اليها وفيها ما هو وحي والهام ورؤيا في المنام
صادقة وهي منسوبة الى الانبيا عليهم السلم والى الحكما الربانيين وجعلت
من اعظم القرب الى الله سبحانه وتقدس ولمن يعانيها مرتبة من الشرف
لا تدفع ومدح من جميع الطوايف لا تجحد وذلك لما يظهر من
فضلها ونفعها وافعالها التي تشبه السحر لكن هولا المسترقة
بها اطفوا نورها واخمدوا ذكرها ومحوا محاسنها واساوا سمعتها
واذالوا اقدارها والحقوا بها العجز والقصور وصناعة الطب
اذا استوفيت شرايطها لا تخطي ابدا وانما يخطي الطبيب الحاذق
فيها مرة ويصيب مايه مرة كما قال جالينوس ولا يكون خطوه
قطعا ولا كبيرا ولا بعيدا من الصواب ومثاله الحاذق في الرماية فانه

يصيب الغرض الباً وان اخطا فلا يبعد عنه بعداً كثيراً وانما يقع سهمه
قريباً من الغرض سدداً واما ان يقع في ضد الجهة وكلا فهكذا
يكون خطأ الطبيب وانما قلنا ان الطب لا يخطي بل الطبيب الحاذق
يخطي على الاقل ويصيب على الاكثر من قبل ان الصنايع التي شانها ان يعمل
في المادة لها شروط كثيرة من جهة الصورة وشروط كثيرة من جهة المادة
وكل ذلك من جهة الامر الكلي ومن جهة الامر الجزي فاما الكلي فعليه يقع التعليم
والتعلم واما الجزي اعني الاشخاص فلا ياتي عليه القول وانما الملكة
الحاصلة بالمزاولة هي التي تحدس عليه وتقارب فيه والمسامحة
اليسيرة من شان الطبيعة لا تعبا بها وتستدركها ولا سيما في
الامراض التي ليست في غاية الحدة والخطر وانا اضرب لك مثلاً من
مساحة الدايرة وجذر الاصم كالعشرة مثلاً فان الحاذق في الصناعة
يستخرج ذلك على اقرب ما يمكن ويسامح باقل جزء مما لا يظهر له تفاوت
في الحس ولا كبير اختلاف عند العقل فهذا الحكم يعد صواباً وان كان فيه
تسامح حيث اخل بجزء لا يكاد يعتد به وكلما قل ذلك الجزء المتسامح
به كان الحكم اصح وصاحبه احذق فالحدس الصناعي في الطب بهذه المنزلة
وما خالف ذلك وبعد عنه فهو ظاهر الخطا وصاحبه لا يعد من اهل
الصناعة كما ان من قال ان جذر العشرة مثلاً ثلثة لم يعد حاسباً ولم يوخذ

بقوله وكذلك من كان بهذه المثابة ممن يدعي صناعة الطب لم يكن 65
طبيبا وينبغي ان يردع عنها ويخرج من اهلها ويحذر اشد من حذر السباع
الضارية والسموم للموجية وجميع الآفات التي تاتي على النفوس
لانها اعلا مكاشرة قد استعد لها وحذر منها ∴ واما الطبيب الجاهل
فانه عدو مبين في ثياب صديق وسم في صورة ترياق وهو
يعطي ادوية مشهورة بالنفع فيقتل بها اذا لم يصادف موقعها فيكون لذلك
سما قاتلا وان شربه ما في غير وقتها او بغير شرطها قد يقتل فدع ادوية مسهلة
سمية كالسنا والسباح والتربد وشحم الحنظل والسقمونيا وامثال ذلك
مما هو سم او سمي وكلما كان المرض احد واخطر كان الضرر في خطا الطبيب
اعظم حتى ان بعض المرضى يكون شفاؤه في شربه ما اذا منعها
هلك واخر شفاؤه المنع منها اذا اعطيها هلك ولا يحقرن احد
خطا الطبيب فقليله كثير ويسيره له وقع عظيم ∴
وقد قال بقراط انه لما كان الطبيب يستعمل الاسما
التي يستعملها المتطبب لم يفرق العامة بين الطبيب والمتطبب وذلك
ان الطبيب يصادف بها الوقت والمتطبب يخطيه وهذا المعنى لا
تدركه العامة ∴ وقد قال في مبتدا كتاب الامراض الحادة
نحو هذا القول وله كتاب في ادب الطبيب وكتاب اخر في صفة الطبيب

كيف ينبغي ان يكون وجالينوس كتاب في امتحان الطبيب
وهو كتاب فاضل حقيق من يحتاج ان يستطب ان يقف عليه
ويتادب بما فيه فمما قال فيه انه لما كان كثير من الروسا وارباب
الثرا لا يتسع وقتهم للاشتغال بصناعة الطب وكانوا يحتاجون
الى الاطبا عندما يقعون في الامراض وكان الطبيب الحاذق ينجيهم من
الالام والجاهل يوقعهم فيما هو اشد منها وهو الهلاك وجب ان يكون
عندهم علامات يفرقون بها بين الطبيب والمتطبب
ويسبرون بها احوالهما حتى يتوقوا هذا ويسلموا مهجهم الى الاخر كما
يجب على الانسان ان يكون عنده معرفة بالفرق بين السم والغذا فلا يلتبس
عليه احدهما بالاخر ثم قال فيجب ان يتامل ويسبر من يدعي الطب
فيما ذا صرف صدر عمره وفيما ذا يصرفه في حالته الراهنه بعد ان
يعلم جودة فطرته وحسن استعداده وصحة عقله وفطنته التي
وهبت له من اصل مولده ثم يسبر دينه وامانته ومروته وكتمانه
للسر ويتفقد ذلك كله في افعاله لا من اقواله فان كل احد يحسن في قوله
ويتجمل فيما يظهر من فعله للناس وانما يجب ان يتتبع حاله في خلواته وما
يبدو منه عند من ينبسط اليه ثم يمتحن عفته في بطنه وفرجه ومقدار حرصه
في تحصيل الدرهم فان كان عنده ذلك فلا خير عنده فانه لا يومن ان يبيع

66 ذبياه واخوته بدرهم واحد وبفستقة واحدة فان كان غبيا
بالفطرة ردي الطباع بالجبله فلا ترج منه خيرا ولا توقع منه فضيله
وايس من فلاحه ولا تطمع في صلاحه ولا تتربص به ان تصلحه الرياضة
بالعلوم بل توقع ان تزيده شرا وفسادا كما قال بعض الشعراء

العلم للرجل اللبيب زيادة ونقيصة للاحمق الطياش
مثل النهار يزيد ابصار الورى نورا ويعشي اعين الخفاش

وكان هذا ماخوذ من قول افلاطون العلم يزيد الشرير شرا لانه يقوم له مقام
الانياب والمخالب للسباع ∴ فان كان فيه مع ذلك
حسد وملق وجشع فقد اجتمعت فيه الات الشر كلها ودواعيه فان
اضاف الى ذلك الكذب وقلة التدين فاحذر منه كل الحذر ∴
فان كان مطبوعا جيد الفهم والفطنة لكنه اذهب صدر عمره في
البطاله والتجارة فلا ترج منه الحذق في الصناعة (البراعه) ولا تيئس
منه كل الياس فان صرف وقته الزاهر في اللذات فذلك
بعيد من الفضيلة بقدر استغراقه في الرذيلة ∴ وقد قال في هذا الكلام
يجب ان تنظر فيما اذا يصرف الطبيب وقته ووكده فان صرفهما
بالليل في نيل اللذات وبالنهار في لقا الروساء في الاهنيه والاعزيه
فلا خير عنده ولا فضل لديه وان كان يصرف ليله وساعات فراغه

في القراءة والتعلم والتفكر والتزيد وتصرف ساير وقته في مصالح
الناس ومعالجة المرضى وبذل الجهد في نفعهم والحرص على تخليصهم
من الالام والاسقام على سبيل الفرح بذلك والابتهاج والتقرب به
الى خالق الكل والمطلع على خفيات القلوب فمثل ذلك طبيب
فاضل يجب ان يوثق بعلمه ويستنام الى تدبيره ورايه ومن صفاته
ان يكون مع ذلك فيه رافة ورحمة وشفقة بعيدا عن القساوة والغلظة
ويكون فرحه بما اصابته في حدسه اضعاف فرحه بتحصيل الدرهم والدينار
وكيف يحسن بعاقل ان يسلم مهجته الى من يبيت سكران
ويصبح مخمورا فمثل هذا مريض النفس والجسم فكيف يداوي صاحب
مرضين صاحب مرض واحد وحال المعاقر للشراب مضاد لحال العالم
الحاذق فان المعاقر مريض بتواتر الابخرة المتصاعدة الرطبة الضبابية
المتراكمة في بطون الدماغ فانها تسد منافس البدن وتكدر الارواح
وتظلم قوى الحواس وتطفي نور الحياة وبهجة النفس وتعطل موضع الفكر
وتخرب بيت الراي فهل يستوي هذا ومن بات ليلته مكبا على
التعلم والتفكر والبحث والتحري يصقل مراة عقله ويشحذ غرار فهمه ويرهف
قواه ويستثير خواطره وسوانحه ويصبح وهمه افادة الناس بعلمه وعمله
وتجربه ما علمه وحدسه هل يستوي هذا ومن يصبح والدنيا غاية

همه يسعى لغايته ودرهم يقتنيه احب اليه ∴ ولبعض الشعراء 67

في ذم المعاقر للشراب ش

ذر الخمر تسلم من عيوب كثيرة واياك ان تزداد ما يورث الجهلا

فما عاقل يرضى باتلاف عقله على الخمر ان الخمر تستلب العقلا

وما زال بقراط وجالينوس ومن سلك سبيلهما يشكون
من جهل اطبا ازمنتهم وقلة معرفتهم وكثرة تهجمهم ولقد تكلم بهم بقراط
كثيرا في كتابه في الامراض الحادة ∴ واما جالينوس فانه
يشتغل جل كتبه بمناقضتهم والتحذير منهم والاعلان بنقصهم ومع
هذا فانه لم يشاهد زماننا ولم ير ما راينا ولم يبل بما ابلينا
به فان شكواه كانت من فرقة اصحاب الحيل وفرقة
اصحاب التجربة وكل هولاء لهم مع تقصيرهم ضوابط ومع نقصهم فضايل
يصلح ان تقتني وتعلم ولسيما اصحاب التجربة فان جالينوس ينقل
عنهم كثيرا من اعمالهم في الميامر وفي قاطاجانس واما اهل
زماننا فليسوا من الفرق الثلث الذين حددهم في كتاب الفرق
وانما هم من باب البخت والاتفاق مثل الاعمى يرمي
ولا يدري في اي جهة هو الغرض فان فرقتي الحيل والتجربة تعلمان
جهة الغرض ولكن برمانه مع عدم تحصيل موضعه الخاص واما

واما ارباب القياس فيعلمون الجهة ويحصلون موضع الغرض
ويسددون نحوه السهم اكمل تسديد وافضل تصويب واهل التجربة
يحصلون عرضا من اعراض الغرض كظله مثلا فهم جديرا بالاصابة
فاما اهل نباتنا فلا يحصلون الغرض ولا جهته فلذلك صار العجب
من صوابهم لا من خطئهم ∴ واما ارباب القياس فالعجب من خطئهم
لا من صوابهم لانهم يصيبون على الاكثر وبالذات ويخطئون على الاقل وبالعرض
واما هولا المسترزقة فصوابهم على الاقل وبالعرض وخطوهم على الاكثر
وبالذات ∴ ونحن نريد ذلك بيانا بمثال نصفه فاترك
رجلا حم فاتاه من كل فرقة طبيب اما صاحب الحيل فانه يقصد
للحمى لحتقانا ∴ واما صاحب التجربة فيقول اني رصدت مرات كثيرة
مرية مثل هذه الحمى ففصدته واخرجت له من الدم مقدار كذا وكذا
بالان غشي عليه فافرق دفعة واحدة ∴ ولما صاحب القياس
فانه يجعل الحمى جنسا ويقسمها بفصول ذاتيه الى انواعها الثلث
ويطرح حمى هذا الرجل من اى هذه الثلث هي فيجدها من الحمى ذات المادة ثم
يقسم هذه الحمى الى انواعها بحسب المواد فيجدها دموية ويقسم الدموية
الى الخالصة والمشوبة فيجدها خالصة ويقسم هذه الخالصة الى ما عفن
والى ما اخذ في الغليان فيجدها مما اخذ في الغليان ثم يعتبر الملة والسن

والوقت الحاضر والعادة وسالف التدبير وساير ما شانه ان يغير 68
الحكم ثم يستخرج من مجموع ذلك كله صورة التدبير الواجب ثم يقصد حسم
عرض الغشي فمن ترى ليت شعري اقمن بالصواب وابعد من الخطا من هولا الثلثة
الاطبا فلا عاقل الا وهو يختار صاحب القياس ويحكم له بالحذق ويرجوا
له الظفر والفلح. فاما الواحد من اطبا زماننا فانه يتقدم فيفصد
او يمنع من فصده كيف جا واتفق لا عن معرفة بشي من هذه
القوانين المذكورة بل بحسب ما يظن ظنا غير صناعي ويحدس حدسا
بحسب ما يقع في خياله لا عن قياس وحجة او تجربة ورصد هذا هو
الغالب فيهم ولا احد من يعتبر بعض الشروط المذكورة الا الواحد بعد
الواحد. واظن ان هذا الفساد كله راجع الى اهمال الملوك
والروسا امتحان الاطبا وربما قدموا الناقص ورفعوه على الكامل فانكسر
همته وهمه الشادي وراوا ان الدنيا انما تنال بالبخوت لا بالفضيلة
فقصروا في طلبها. والعجب ان الملك ينظر من يتولى طعامه
وشرابه ويتفقد احواله وينظر مثل ذلك لرعيته وخاصته ويهمل
جانب الطب وهو اشرف واهم واعلى وانفس واخطر وهو احق
بالنظر والرعاية والحياطة من جميع ما عددناه لان التفريط في ذلك
يخل بالالذ والانفع والتفريط في حال الطب يخل بالمهج فيجب ان يكون للملك

عناية بشي اكثر من عنايته بامر الطب والاطبا والعجب من انسان يختار
لحماره و فرسه اجود البياطرة واحذقهم ثم يسلم مهجته الى من لا يثق
بحذقه ولا معرفته والعجب ممن يحتسب على السوقة في
الطبخ والشوا والخبز ويهمل جانب الاطبا ويتركهم يتلاعبون بالمهج
والعجب من اهمال الفقها هذا الباب واحتياطهم على باب الاموال
فلا يثقون عليها الا الامين ولا يقبلون على الدرهم الا شهادة العدل ويقبلون
قول الواحد من هولا في المهج من غير اختبار دينه وامانته وعلمه وفهمه
والعجب من فقيه قد بلغ درجة الاجتهاد او كاد ويسلم مهجته الى عامي
كراسة واحدة والعجب منهم كيف اهملوا ذلك ولم يعملوا بقول
النبي صلى الله عليه وسلم من تطبب ولم يعلم منه طب فقتل فهو ضامن
والعجب انه قد سبق في لسان الجمهور لمن اخطا عليه الاطبا ان يقولوا
مات باجله وان الله قضى عليه مع انهم يعتقدون ان جميع افعال
العباد خلق الله سبحانه وتعالى ومع هذا فيقتلون القاتل ويقتصون
من الجاني كان الله سبحانه انما تولى قتل من يخطي عليه الاطبا دون
من يذبح وتضرب عنقه ولم اسمع بقوم يحتاطون على صناعة الطب
ويعتبرون الاطبا وياخذون على ايديهم كاهل قسطنطينيه فانهم
لا يمكنون احدا من مزاولة الطب دون ان يكون قد تدرج في اجزايه

69 R

ويمرن في اشغاله ومضى عليه سنون كثيرة وشهد له بذلك الشيوخ

الافاضل ثم يعقد مجلس ويمتحن في محفل منهم بان يحضر له عدة مرضى مختلفي

الامراض وقد يدبرهم بحضرة جميع الافاضل فاذا رضوا افعاله بعدما رضوا

قوله اخذوا عليه عهد ابقراط الذي كان عهده الى الغربا حتى دخلوا

به في زمرة الاولاد والاقربا. وهذه كانت حالهم لما كان ملكهم

الروم وفي هذه السنين انتقل الملك الى الافرنج وغيروا كثيرا من

الاوضاع الحسنة ومحوا معظم الرسوم القديمة فلا ادري كيف حالهم

اليوم. ورايت لاهل بغداد للاطبا بعض العناية

وكذلك لاهل مصر لا يطلق المباشرة الا من معه محضر فيه خطوط

شيوخ الصناعة وعلى نحو هذا يجري حال الاطبا بدمشق

ولم ار اشد اهمالا من هذه الصناعة بمدينة حلب فلذلك كانت سيرهم

في غاية الرداه وطرق اطبايها على حال من الفساد لا يكون احط منها

فلا سلطان يزعهم ولا دين يردعهم ولا علم يرشدهم ولا رئيس عليهم يرشدهم

ويرهبهم ولهم اسلوب متشابه قلما يخالفونه وهو ان

كل من شكا اليهم مرضا عاجلوه بشربة مسهل ليتعجلوا ثمنها

وليغتنموا فضلتها ولا يعتبرون نجحا ويهملون ساير الشرايط وطلقون

ذلك لمن سمعوا خبره من غير معاينة وليس همهم سوى اختلاس ثمن المسهل

والتحيل عليه بكل وجه

كيف قتلوا ابها ويبيعون مهجة انسان بربع درهم ∴ واظن
ان الذي جراهم على هذه الافعال القبيحة والشيم الرذلة شيخ فيهم مغربي
كان مسلما وارتد وعاد يهوديا في الظاهر وهم يعتقدون انه مهمل
لجانب دينهم متهاونون بوظايف عباداتهم منحل في الشريعة اكذب
ما يكون اذا حلف بالتوراة والعشر الكلمات وكان
فقيرا انتركض في البلاد بخدمة التجار وعانى صناعة الطب على
الكبر وفيه من الحرص على الدنيا وشدة الكلب والجشع
ما يحمله على الفتك بالمهج والاقدام على النفوس اقدام الضرغام على
الفريسة واجمعوا على انه لا يخاف خالقا ولا مخلوقا واهون شي عليه
قتل الف نفس في ساعة واحدة قالوا وانه يلتذ بذلك ويسره ∴
وقتل في سنة ثلث عشرة واربع عشرة وستماية جماعة من الملوك والاكابر
شهدت بعضهم والباقي اتصل بي خبرهم وممن قتل في سنة ثلث عشرة
سلطان المدينة للملك الظاهر غازي بن يوسف فانه حم يوم
السبت السادس والعشرين من جمدى الاولى من السنة المذكورة وكان
قد ناهز الاربعين سنة وتقدم له فكر وهموم في تعبيه عساكر
وملابسه حروب ونفقات فهو لاجل ذلك الشراب واقل الطعام
واكثر السهر واعمال الفكر فاشار طبيب مسلم بفصده ووافقه على ذلك

الاطباء فمنعهم هذا الملعون من الفصد وقال لهم في السر ان فصده 70
هذا الخطي عنده ونقدم عليكم فصد فوه عن الفصد فسقاه شربته
المجربة في اليوم السادس من مرضه قبل النضج فمشاه اربعة وعشرين والعشرين
مجلسا سقطت قوته في المجلس الرابع وبرد جسمه وبطلت حركته
نحو ثلثين ساعة ويئسوا منه وفعل الملعون يضحك ويعمل رايه
فيمن يكون بعده فقام منهم رجل ذو حمية ومعرفة لينظر قوته فطتروا
به وقالوا انت تريد ان تحيي الموتى قال فطمعت في حياته اذ كان
سقوط قوته من قبل التدبير لا من قبل خبث المرض فسقاه
شيئا من امراق الفراريج بعد ان فتح فاه بجهد فتراجع نبضه وقوته وفتح
عينه وتكلم ثم طلب الماء والغذاء ونهض على نفسه فعادوا
اليه وكان هذا الملعون الى ان سهمه لم ينفذ فاعطاه حقنة بعد اخرى
وفي اثنائهما قتلا كثيرة ورفقاؤه من الاطباء ينهونه ويردعونه وهو
يكبهم في وجوههم ويسبهم ويستحمقهم ويقول انما قصدي ان اغسل
بدنه وبهذا وامثاله كان يقنع خدمه واهله الى ان وثقه واسلمه
الى المنون فانحلت القوى الماسكة وانشق فاخذوا حينئذ في المقبضات
المفرطة يظنون ان الادوية تعمل بانفسها من غير ان يكون في البدن قوة
تدبرها وتفعل بها وانا اقول ان الادوية لا تفعل بانفسها انما هي آلات

لقوي البدن فاذا افسد ذو الاله وبطلت الآلة ولم تفعل ولذلك لا
يحدي ولم يزل رحمه الله سبيل حتى مات في الرابع والعشرين
من مرضه .:. واجتمع في كل واحد من الاطبا الذين كانوا معه
وصرحوا بانه قتله ووصف كل واحد منهم صنفا من التدبير
الردي الذي ارتكبه غير ما وصفه الاخر ومن دقيق مكره في هذه المرضة
انه اوهم من تولى امره من الخدم ان كثرة الاطبا تضجره فاقتصروا على اثنين
يشير الى نفسه والى مشيخ فهو صالح العلاج متلطف ولو قدر على العاده
لفعل فاحتال بالسلطان والشيخ مغلوب معه فحكم فيه كيف شا حتى
افاق السلطان وطلب احرمهم كان بانسرته وهو رجل كهل
حسن التدبير سديد الراي فتسلمه ولكن بعد ان تقدم ذلك الملعون فاسلمه
وكثيرا ما رايت هذا الملعون يروم ان يحفظ الصحة بالضد ويزيل
المرض بالشبيه فيسقي في الامراض البلغمية بزر القثا وما الشعير وشراب
الورد وفي الامراض الصفراوية والدموية والمسلولين المعالي الملفتحه
المسخنة والمسهلات الحارة وقد ظن بعض العقلا ان فعله هذا عن قصد
منه لاهلاك النفوس والتلذذ بافساد الصور .:. وحكي عن المبرد انه مر
بطريق يلحن في هاذورة لحنا مفرطا فقال لصاحبه اظن هذا يعرف
طرفا من العربية فقال له ممّاذا عرفت فقال رايته يتوقى الصواب يوقي

من يعرفه فوقف حتى يفرق الناس عنه وسأله هل يعرف من 71
العربية شيئا فقال نعم وانما اعدل عنها لئلا يلحقني حرفة الادب ∴
ونعود فنقول ما قال بقراط ترك الطبيعة مع المرض
خير من تسليمها الى طبيب سوء ∴ وقال الرازي من جمع اطبا اوشك
ان يجمع خطاهم ∴ واما جالينوس فقد شحن كتبه بالتحذير منهم
والتنبيه على اصناف خطيهم فمن ذلك قوله ان حال الفقرا في امراضهم خير
من احوال الروسا والمياسير لان الفقير لا يقدر على طبيب فيبقى
مع طبيعته والغني يجتمع اليه الاطباء ويصبون عليه اصناف الادوية
والاشربة وفنون العلاج لخطا فيصدون الطبيعة عن جهتها ويقهرونها
ويحيرونها ثم قال فمقدار ما يخرج جنازة الغني يكون الفقير
قد ابل وربما شيع جنازته وانا اقول ان طب العجاير افضل من طب هولاء
لان العجوز يعمل ما رات نجحه وجربت نفعه فهي قريبة من فرقة التجارب
واما هولا فيقدمون بقياس فاسد وظن مختل ثم ان العجوز فلما تقدم
على دوا قوي ومسهل خطر وان اقدمت على شي منه لم تلح فيه ولم تبالغ لكن
ان رات امارات النجح ثبتت والا اقلعت وهولا المسترقه يتقدمون
بتهور ويصفون ادوية لا يعرفون صورها ولا جربوا قواها ولا شاهدوا
اثارها وكثيرا ما اسال الواحد منهم بعد الواحد عن مفردات ادويتهم فلا

احدهم يعرفون صورها فضلاً عن قواها وغاية الفاضل منهم ان يسند
ذلك الى كتاب ويحيله على نقل فلا يعرفون قوى الادوية المفردة معرفة
امتحان وتجربة ولا القوة الحاصلة للمركب عنها وليتهم اقتصروا على
التركيب المذكور في الكتب وتركوا عنهم ان يركبوا من قبل
انفسهم ويتصرفون في الكيفيات والكميات مع جهل بهما
وبالامراض التي يقصدون مقابلتها وهم يقصدون ازديادها والضد
بالضد مع جهل بهما وبمقدار البعد بينهما وبما بينهما من التضاد النوعي
فضلاً عن جهلهم بالتضاد الشخصي فان الطبيب لا يكتفي في صواب العلاج
بمعرفة التضاد النوعي دون الشخصي فانه انما يداوي الاشخاص لا الانواع
وكذلك الحال في حفظ الصحة بالشبيه يجب عليه ان يعرف الشبيه
الشخصي فانه اياه يحفظ ولا يقتصر في شيء من ذلك على معرفة
النوع فان هذا غير كاف فان هذه المعرفة ليست مقصودة لذاتها
بل لاجل الشخص وليتوصل بها الى معرفة الشخص واقول ان الغربا
الذين يسقون الشرابات على قوارع الطرقات امثل من هولا اما اولا
فلان اكثر الناس وخواصهم يحذرونهم ولا يسلمون نفوسهم اليهم
واما ثانيا فانهم يسقون المنوعات والسنبوس الذي هو ورق الحنظل
للاصحا وامزجتهم يحتمل الخطا اكثر مما يحتمله المرضى واكثر ما يسقون

72 ادويتهم الفلاحين وارباب الكد وامزجتهم تحتمل الادوية القوية
ثم ان الغربا عندهم ادوية مجربة ممتحنة واعشاب مجربة ثم يحتنونها
ويمتحنونها ويتناقلون العلم بها ∴ ويجب على الطبيب الحاذق العاقل
الشفوق ان يحذر من شرب الدوا المسهل اشد الحذر ولا يقدم عليه
الا عند تحقق الضرورة وتوفر الدواعي والموجبات ويكون حذره منه
في المرضى اشد من حذره في الاصحا ويكون من الاسهال اشد حذرا من
الفصد وانما حذرنا من المسهلات لانها انما تسهل بسمية فيها
والطبيعة تستعين بما فيها من السمية على دفع سمية مادة المرض
فاذا وافق غرضها سهل احتمالها سمية الدوا اذ تدفع به سمية اعظم
منه كما تدفع الشر بشر والعدو بعدو فلذلك اذا صادف الدوا
وقته ومحله خف على الطبيعة وسهل احتماله وحصلت الراحة
والخف عقيبه واذا لم يصادف محله تمحضت مضرته وتضاعفت
بليته وقد قالت الحكما ان الادوية الترياقية اذا شربت
وفي البدن سم ظهر نفعها واذا شربت والبدن نقي عادت سما وقالوا
ان الترياق طبيعة متوسطة بين طبيعة السم المحض والدوا المحض وقال
بقراط في كتاب الفصول من كان بدنه صحيحا فاسهل او قيّ بدوا
اسرع اليه الغشي وكذلك من كان يغتذي باغذية ردية وجالينوس

من سقي المسهل المزمن به كثير الامتلا وقد شرح ذلك في كتاب حيلة
البرء وذكر خطا الاطبا على من هذه حاله ثم ذكر الحيلة في استفراغه
بالدلك الدايم المتناسب والمرخ والدهن وتكرير ذلك حتى يستفرغ
بعض المادة وتنضج الباقي فحينئذ يمكنه اسهاله ان احتاج الى ذلك او
فصده ∴ وانما قلنا ان الحذر من المسهل في المرضى اشد منه
في الاصحا من قبل ان الاصحا موفورو القوة صحيحو الاعضا فمع هذا فهو
يضعفهم وينكي فيهم اذا صادف محلة فضلا عن ان لا يصادف فما
ظنك بالمرضى الذين قد ضعفت قواهم ونكى المرض اعضاهم الرييسة وانما
كان الدوا يضعف القوى وينكي الاعضا من قبل ان المسهلات سموم وانما
تسهل ما ان ينكي القوى الماسكة لامشاج البدن فتخلى عنها ولذا
لا تعطى الا مصلحة ومكسورة السورة ومقدرا افضل ويستدرك [illegible]
التي تخلفها في البدن في عدة ايام حتى ان التي تسهل بالترليق وهي قريبة من طبيعة
الغذا مثل الاجاص وتمر الهندي والاعبة فمن شانها ان ترخي وتحل القوة
الماسكة وانما يقاوم اليبس الحادث عن الحمى في المعدة والامعا وما يلي هذه
الاعضا فاذا اتفق ان لم يكن يابسة نكت فيها وقد حذروا من الشعير مع
فضله ومدحه وانه غذا فاضل صالح ومع هذا فاذا لم يصادف موضعه
اضر وقد عددوا اضراره في الامراض المزمنة وفي الحادة اذا تجاوزت

[illegible]

73 وإذا كنا نحذر مضار المسهل في الصحيح الموفور القوى فما أجدرنا
بالحذر منه في المريض المنهوك القوى فينبغي أن نحذره فيهم غاية الحذر
ولا سيما في أصحاب الحميات الحادة مع أن المسهلات حارة
ولهذا قد احتال لهم الأطباء بما يسهل بالتزليق وفيه تبريد وترطيب ∴
ومن هذا تبين أن الخطر في الفصد أقل منه في شرب الدواء لأن الفصد
ينقص الامشاج والقوى موفورة والأعضاء الرئيسة على حالها فيمكنها
أن تعوض عن الدم الصالح في أمد قريب وأما الإسهال فلا ينفع الأبدان
يضعف الأعضاء الباطنة فيعجز عن العوض إلا في زمان طويل وبقدر إضعاف
الدواء لها ونكايته فيها يتأخر العوض لأن هذه الأعضاء هي التي تفعل العوض
فإذا حلت بها آفة نقص فعلها عنه إن الآفة هذا في الأصحاء فلا يمكنهم الاغتذاء
والعوض وإن تناولوا الغذاء فبمقدار ما لا يفي بسد الفايت ∴ وقد كنا
بينا في مقالة لنا مفردة في البادي بصناعة الطب وأنها ماشية معه [مع الانسان]
حيث كانت حاجته إليها معه وأنها كلما اخلقت على طول الزمان
قيض الله سبحانه وتعالى لها من يحيي آثارها ويجدد ما انمحى من رسومها
وتهدم من أركانها كما جرى ذلك على عهد أبقراط فإنه أحيا طب جده
الأكبر اسقليبيادس ثم على عهد جالينوس فإنه أحيا طب أبقراط
وآخر من أعرفه في ملة الإسلام أبو جعفر أحمد بن محمد بن أبي الأشعث

واما المشتغلون في هذا الزمان بالطب فشانهم ان يقروا اشيا من كليات
كتاب القانون فيحفظون حد الطب وحد الاسطقس وحد المزاج
وامثال ذلك ويتجادلون فيه ويرفعون بذلك اصواتهم في المجالس
والاسواق ثم يتقدمون على العلاج ظنا منهم ان ذلك يجدي عليهم وانه
كافيهم وان من حقق حد الطب قدر ان يبري من الحميات وغيرها
ويعرف اصنافها .. وانا اشير على من يقبل نصيحتي ان شا ان يكون طبيبا
الا يعدو كتب جالينوس وبقراط وان استغشني في نصيحتي
فليفعل ذلك في جزء من اجزا الطب واوضحه كتاب المزاج مثلا فيقروه
ثم يقرا ما في هذا المعنى من كلام القانون وغيره فان وجد في شي مما عدا كلام
جالينوس مغني عنه فلا يقبل مني سائر اقوالي ان وجد في نفسه عند قراة
كلام جالينوس قوة على عمل تصنيف مثل تصانيفهم فليثق بقولي وليمض قدما
ويفعل ذلك في كتاب النبض الصغير لجالينوس والنبض من كتاب القانون
ويمتثل في جميع كتب جالينوس ما امتثله في كتاب المزاج الذي جعله
كالانموذج والتجربة والامتحان ثم في كتاب النبض الصغير وهكذا جميع كتبه
العلميه والعملية وان استطالها فليقتصر على ما احب من مختصراتها مثل
كتاب الصناعة الصغير التي هي مدخل ومثل النبض الصغير واغلوقن لاختصاره
حيلة البرء والمقالتين الشافيتين له وان يشا ان يقرا كلام المتاخرين على جهة

التنزم على مقادير العلما في علمهم وتفاوتهم في فهمهم وبعض اختصارهم 74.
وبسطهم فذلك لينه ومن زعم ان في الملكي او في كتاب المايه او في القانون
كفاية عن كتب جالينوس فقد زعم بطلا ولم يقل ذلك عن اختبار ولا
عن اطلاع على كلام جالينوس بل عن تقليد اقرا وما استخرج من
كلام جالينوس شيء الا وكلامه افضل منه ولا دخل كلامه قلب
احد فوسع كلام سواه ولا ارا قوله غيره ولا اطناه ما عدا الا على ان كتاب
المايه كتاب فاضل واما كناش ابن سرابيون فهو مادة تصانيف اكثرهم ولا
اعرف كناشا افضل منه ∴ وقد رايت جماعة ممن اعرض
عن كلام جالينوس وحدث نفسه انه ممن قد اطلع على اسرار الوجود ووقف
على غوامض العالم يقول ان طب اوليك قد بطل اليوم واختلف الزمان
بحركة الكواكب الثابته واستقلت الطبايع ويورخ ان اهل بغداد كانوا يعالجون
بالادوية الحارة ∴ واما اليوم فلا يقدرون عليها اصلا وانما يكبون
على المبردات ∴ وقد يقول من هولا ان طب بقراط وجالينوس كان
بحسب بلاد اليونان واما بلاد الشام والعراق فلا يحتمل ذلك وهذا حال من
لم يقرا كتب القدما ولا جرب شيئا مما فيها الا ترى الكواكب حيث دارت
غيرت طبايع الناس فقط دون النبات وسائر الحيوان ان كان هكذا
فان ذلك لعجيب وان غيرت الجميع فانه سيصير الافيون حارا او الفلفل باردا

ولحم السمك حارا ولحم الاسد باردا ونصف الاسد جبانا والارنب شجاعا
ومنذ لحكمهم على طبائع الادوية والاغذية من النبات والحيوان والمعادن
ثم انا نجد ابقراط يوافق من قبله بالاحقاب الطويلة على طبايع الاشيا
وامتحن ما قالوه قديما فوجده في زمانه على ما حكموا عليه لم يتبدل وكذلك
امتحن جالينوس على ابقراط جميع ما حكم به فوجده موافقا وبينهما من
الزمان ستماية سنه ومازال الناس يمتحنون ما قال جالينوس الى زماننا
هذا فوجدوه موافقا ولجالينوس نحو الف سنه ومايتي سنه ∴
وهذا كتاب الفلاحة الذي نقله ابن وحشيه من لغه النبط له مدد متكاثره
والطبايع فيه ثابته على حال واحدة وهذا القول يستخف جدا لولا انه
قد سطر في الكتب المحسن في منا قصته وحكايته ورايت من
يعتقده ويغرب بذكره ويتبجح بمعرفته ومثله في السخافه قولهم ان طب
ابقراط وجالينوس كان بحسب بلاد اليونان وما علم ان اقوالهم امور
كلية لا تقبل التبدل ولا التغير فان قولهم ان الضد شفا الضد وان الصحة
تحفظ بالشبيه وان الحمى تقاوم بالتبريد والترطيب وان الغب الخالصه
تحتاج من التبريد والترطيب الى مقدار كثير وليس كذلك البلغمية
والربع وان النائبه لا يستعمل في اولها ما يسخن بافراط بل برفق فاذا نضجت
المادة اعطي ما يسخن بقوة وقد حذر من استعمال ما يسخن بقوة في اول الفالج

75 وانما يستدرج فيه وقد حكى جالينوس ان فلانا كان به ربع فاشار عليه
الاطبا بادوية حارة فنهيته عنها وقلت ان فعلت عادت داءين فلما قبل
منهم عادت ربعين فلما سلم الي علاجه رفقت به حتى نضجت المادة ثم
اعطيته تلك الادوية الحارة بعينها فاقلعتا جميعا عنه وهكذا
جميع ما في كتب القوم ليس فيه ما يقبل التبدل والتغير وانما هي قوانين
كلية ثابتة على حالة واحدة ثم ان القوم قد ملوا كتبهم بالوصية
بان تعتبر السن والبلد والعادة والهوا واوقات السنة والوقت
وغير ذلك وعابوا من اغفل النظر في ذلك ونسبوه الى الغلط والخطا
فطبهم منطبق على الصقالبة وعلى الحبشان جميعا وما بين هذين الطرفين
واهل بغداد لا يخرجون عن الوسط فضلا عن الاطراف ∴ ثم انا ل
نقول ان اهل بغداد لا يعرض لهم امراض البلغم كالفالج واللقوة والسكتة
والصرع والاستسقا ونحو ذلك افترى نعالج هولا بالاشيا البارده
لاجل حركة الكواكب الثابتة اتراهم لا يعرض لهم حميات نايبة وليلية
وربع اترانا نعالجها بما نعالج به الدموية من الفصد والتبريد والتخفيف
والصفراوية من التبريد والترطيب اتراهم امنوا القولنج البلغمي فليت
من الطبايع تغيرت بحركة الكواكب الثابتة ام اي علاج خاص ببلاد اليونان
لا يستعمل في العراق ان هذا السخف بين وعقل ما نورق هذا طب الهند

قد نقل الينا وشحنت به كتبنا ومعاجينهم الكبار مشوثه في
الاقراباذينات هذا مع انهم من الاقليم الاول وبلاد يونان
من الاقليم الرابع والخامس والعراق من الثالث والرابع فهو اقرب الى بلاد
اليونان من الهند ثم ان مصر والشام قد كانت داخلة في كثير من
الاوقات في ولاية القوم متصلة بهم وجالينوس قد سلك مصر والشام
وحكم على طبايعها وشاهد عادات اهل الاسكندريه وحكاها
في كتبه وعرضها لب وعرض بغداذ لج واما
دسقوريدس فمن عين زربي وكثير من حكما اليونان من مصر والشام
وقونيه قد كانت من بلاد الحكما وكذلك ملطيه وقد كان بها خزانه
كتب عظيمه وكان بها دار تعليم للحكمه وملطيه مختلطة بالشام
وهذا دسقوريدس تفسير اسمه عشاب الله لانه اقام ثلثين
سنه يسيح في اقطار الارض ليعرف اعيان النبات ومنافعه وياخذ
ذلك عمن وقع اليه فيه تجربة وقيل انه كان يحكم عليه ثم يجربه فيصدق
حكمه :. وانا اقول قولا اختم به هذا الفصل هل
جربتم ادوية القدما بشرايطها فلم تنجح وحقا اقول ان الواحد منكم ليبلغ
من العمر تسعين سنه يعالج المرضى ولم يستعمل شيا مما في كتب القدما
ولا يعلم اصحيح هو ام باطل ولعمر الله ان طب القدما منزول

76 عندكم لعجزكم عن استعماله وجهلكم بشروطه فمن فيكم يقدر ان يفصد المحموم
حتى يعرض له الغشي ويبريه في الحال او من فيكم يجسر ان يسقي الما المبرد
بالثلج حتى يخصر المحموم وينطفي حماه على المكان ام من فيكم من يسقي في ذات
الجنب الحريق ويستفرغه السودا او من يعلم العلة في الحاجة الى استفراغ
السودا من المجنوب وكيف تتولد في بدنه مع ان مادة مرضه دموية
ومن ذا الذي يقدر ان يلحم وجه الرية في مسلميها بالترياق الفاروق ويمنع
من تولد المدة فيها والوقوع في السل ومن يقدر منكم ان يداوي صاحب
الصرع بالدولاب —— والحكما القدما انما يفخرون بحسم الامراض
قبل تمكنها فانها اذا تمكنت قلت فيها الحيلة ومن فيكم من يقدم فيسقي
الخل في قرحة الرية فاذا كنتم لا تجربون طب القدما فمن اين لكم انه
صواب او خطا او انه يوافق بلد كذا ويضر ببلد كذا ∴ اترى
كتاب النبض وعلم البول وما في كتاب الفصول وتقدمة المعرفة
وكتاب الاهوية والبلدان بتغيير علم ما فيها حركات الكواكب الثابتة
اترى دوا الحلتيت والمعجون لغلاء يبطل فعله ولا يوجد مرض لا يحتاج
اليه ∴ وقد بذلت لك نصيحتي وبحتك حمي دخلتي فان قبلت فلك
وان ابيت فعليك ∴ وانا اوصيك بما اوصي به نفسي اذا استفتيت
في امر مريض تصل الا تعجل بالحكم بل تميز وتتثبت وتكشف وتسال

وتجبل فكرك وتتوهم انك انت صاحب المرض فتحكم له بما تحكم
به على نفسك لو حلّ بك وتخاف من الغلط عليه كما تخاف من الغلط
على نفسك ولو كان عدوك وانا اطرفك بعجيبة كثيرا ما يقع لي وهو
ان الواحد من الاطبا اذا حلّ به مرض او بولده وعزيز عليه شاور
فيه وتوقف وتحيّر فاذا عرض عليه مريض غريب بادر وحكم
وسارع واستبدّ ولم يشاور كانه احكم طب الاجانب دون الاقارب
فيجب عليك ان تتفكّر ثم تتكلم فان الصواب مع تأخر الجواب لا يخرج
الانسان عن مرتبة العلما واما المخطي فلا حظّ له من الفضيلة اسرع
او ابطأ واذا عوّد نفسه اعمال فكرته صارت تجيبه باهون سعي
فيصير يسرع ويصيب واذا عوّدها الاهمال والتسرع من غير حقيقة وروية
صارت لنفسه ملكة ردية لو اراد ان يزول عنها عند الحاجة
الى غيرها لم يقدر على ذلك ولم ينقد له مثل من يعوّد لسانه اللحن
واذا اخذت نفسك بالسداد والصواب هان عليك وصار ذلك
ملكة لك يعمل عنها بسهولة واكثر ما يحملهم على المسارعة في الجواب
ايثارهم الا يظهر للناس نقصهم كان التوقف في الجواب يحط قدرهم
فلا يزالون يسرعون في الخطا حتى يصير ذلك ملكة وعادة سو لو
ارادوا الانتقال عنه لما قدروا ولو توقفوا وتفكروا وظهر عليهم بشر الظفر

وهشاشة المعرفة لكانت الثقة بهم من العامة اكثر واعتقدوا فيهم 77
الفضيلة والحرص والاجتهاد والعجب ان جالينوس ونظراه يتوقفون
في كثير من الامراض عن الحكم الى اليوم الثاني والثالث واكثر من ذلك
ولا تجد الواحد من هولا المسترزقة يشكل عليه مرض اصلا بل يعلم كل
شي ويحكم في كل شي فانت ايها الناصح لنفسه المحب لها اقتنا الفضيلة
اياك ثم اياك والعجلة فانها من الشيطان وعليك بالتاني والرفق وتحبب
الحق والالتذاذ بالاصابة فانك اذا كنت كذلك انكشف لك المستور
وانقادت لك الامور وعاجلك الحق عن امم ولبالك الصواب من كثب
فالحق يتبعك عند حصوله ثم ينفعك في جميع المستقبل كالاساس
الصحيح واما الباطل فيريحك في الاول ويتعبك دايما كالبيت المبني
على اساس واه لا يزال ينهدم ∴ وقد رايت من اطبا مصر وبغداد وما
بين ذلك ومن ورد الي ممن قرات —— عليه او قرا علي فلم ار اسوا حالا
من هذا الملعون المغربي الذي بحلب ولا احسن حالا من ابن هبة الله صاعد
المعروف بابن التلميذ لا الشيخ المصنف فان ذلك لم ادركه بل ولده وكان
قد تجاوز سبعين سنة فشاهدت له ملكة عجيبة كان يحكم على الامراض
كانه يعاينها وكان البدن زجاج شفاف يصف ما وراه وكان كما
يقال لا يسطو ولا يخطي ولا يبطيل الصفات ولا ينكر التركيبات وشاكله ما كان

يعالج به المفردات فإن ركب فتركيبًا يسيرًا ولا ينتقل من علاج إلى
علاج لقوة ثقته بل كان يثبت عليه حتى يظهر له ما كان يتوقعه كما قال بقراط
إذا أنت فعلت جميع ما ينبغي ولم تر ما ينبغي فلا تنتقل عما ينبغي ما دام ما رأيته
منذ أول الأمر ثابتًا ∴ ومن مخرقتهم وتمويههم تطويل النسخ وتكثير
المفردات عن غير موازنة بين قواها ولا تجربة لما يكون عنها ويفعلون ذلك
إما ليتعجب العامة منهم ومن سعة علمهم وإما ليحصل لهم ربح إذا اشتريت الحوائج
منهم أو من عطار هو شريكهم وقد يدخل الواحد منهم على المريض في اليوم مرات
يصف في كل دخلة علاجًا جديدًا وقصده في ذلك أن يكون لدخوله أثر ويظهر
له في كل مرة عمل والفاضل منهم يجعل التغييرات متشابهة وربما
عرضت عليه نسخة طبيب آخر فيزيد وينقص ما لا ينفع ولا يضر وقصده
بذلك أن يري لنفسه فضيلة على غيره وينبه على مكانه وهذا ونحوه
فلا أكرهه كما أكره الأول لأن هذا ينفعه ولا يضر به أحدًا وأما الذي
أكرهه جدًا فما يضر به الناس أعاذنا الله وإياك أن نكون ممن يبيع آخرته بدنياه
ويؤثر على دينه هواه ∴ هذا آخر ما أريد أن أقوله في هذه النصيحة
للناس كافة وفي صناعة الطب خاصة وليس بك عندك حاجة
سوى أن تقرأ كتب جالينوس وليس في هذا مشقة عليك ولا كلفة
بالحق ولا تحتاج أن أشير عليك بترك كتب المتأخرين فإنك إذا

قرات كتب جالينوس تركت ما عداها وحدثتك نفسك بعمل مثلها وان قراتها 78

مع قراة كتب جالينوس فلا ضير عليك والسلم عليك ∴

والحمد لله رب العالمين وصلى الله على سيدنا محمد نبيه وعلى اهل بيته

الطيبين الطاهرين ∴